HIPAA Plain & Simple

AFTER the FINAL RULE

Third Edition

Carolyn P. Hartley, MLA
Edward D. Jones III

Foreword by Louis W. Sullivan, MD

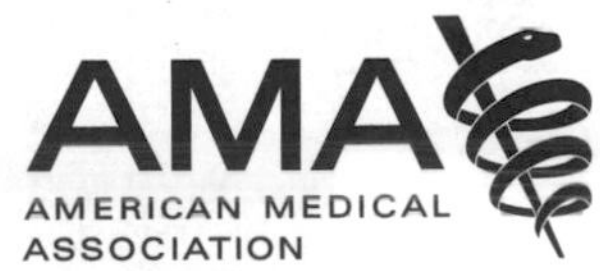

Printed in the United States of America

13 14 15 16 17 18 19 20/TB-PH/ 9 8 7 6 5 4 3 2 1

Internet address: www.ama-assn.org

The American Medical Association (AMA) and its authors and editors have consulted sources believed to be knowledgeable in their fields. However, neither the AMA nor its authors or editors warrant that the information is in every respect accurate and/or complete. The AMA, its authors, and editors assume no responsibility for use of the information contained in this publication. Neither the AMA, its authors or editors shall be responsible for, and expressly disclaims liability for, damages of any kind arising out of the use of, reference to, or reliance on, the content of this publication. This publication is for informational purposes only. The AMA does not provide medical, legal, financial, or other professional advice and readers are encouraged to consult a professional advisor for such advice.

The contents of this publication represent the views of the authors and should not be construed to be the views or policy of the AMA, or of the institution with which the authors may be affiliated, unless this is clearly specified.

Additional copies of this book may be ordered by calling 800 621-8335 or from the secure AMA Web site at www.amastore.com. Refer to product number OP 320712.

AMA publication and product updates, errata and addendum can be found at ama-assn.org/go/ProductUpdates.

Library of Congress Cataloging-in-Publication Data
Hartley, Carolyn P., author.
HIPAA plain and simple : after the final rule / Carolyn P. Hartley, Edward D. Jones III. -- Third edition.
p. ; cm.
Includes bibliographical references and index.
ISBN 978-1-60359-657-2
I. Jones, Ed, III, author. II. American Medical Association, issuing body. III. Title.
[DNLM: 1. United States. Health Insurance Portability and Accountability Act of 1996. 2. Medical Records Systems, Computerized--United States. 3. Confidentiality--legislation & jurisprudence--United States. 4. Practice Management, Medical--organization & administration--United States. WX 173]
R728
610.68--dc23

2013028158

BP02:13-P-033:07/13

Dedications

To Michyla, Logan, Jackson, Brooks, Emily, and Easton, and their parents, already HIPAA-aware, wise health care consumers.

To Eliza Gayle . . . and in loving memory of my wife and your paternal grandmother, Ann Maynard Jones.

Ancillary Content

HIPAA Plain and Simple: After the Final Rule, third edition, provides forms and checklists from the text of this book in Microsoft Word format. Ancillary content can be downloaded from this URL: www.ama-assn.org/go/OP320712aae.

Use the tools listed below as advised in the book, and modify them to suit your office environment. Retain these and other documents as evidence of your compliance activities.

- Business Associate Agreements Tracking Form
- Privacy Official Job Responsibilities
- Workforce Training Session Attendee List
- Notice of Privacy Practices Receipt
- Sample Authorization Form
- Sample Verification Form/Patient Certification
- Sample Consent to Disclose PHI for Treatment, Payment, and Health Care Operations
- Sample Marketing Authorization Form
- Request to Access Records
- Response to Request to Access Records
- Access Denial Log
- Request to Amend Records
- Response to Request to Amend Records
- Request for Accounting of Disclosures
- Response to Request for Accounting of Disclosures
- Request to Restrict Disclosure
- Request to Terminate Restrictions
- Disclosure Log
- Request for Alternative Communications
- Sample Complaint Form
- Sample Privacy Complaint Log
- Minimum Necessary Checklist
- De-identification Checklist

- Security-related Repair Form
- Emergency Access Log
- Electronic Media and Hardware Movement Log
- Acknowledgement of Responsibilities Regarding Access to Practice's Electronic Systems Containing Electronic Protected Health Information
- Consequences of Unauthorized Access to the Practice's Electronic Protected Health Information
- Workforce Member Exit Interview Checklist
- Workforce Member Acknowledgement of Awareness and Understanding of Practice's Exit Interview
- Otherwise Permitted Uses and Disclosures (45 CFR164.512)
- Communicating with a Patient's Family, Friends, or Others Involved in the Patient's Care
- Common Questions About HIPAA
- HIPAA Privacy Rule Disclosures to a Patient's Family, Friends, or Others Involved in the Patient's Care or Payment for Care
- Emergency and Disaster Disclosure
- Decision Tree

Table of Contents

Reviewer

Carol Scheele, JD

Foreword

Louis W. Sullivan, MD

I am pleased to write the Foreword for the third edition of *HIPAA Plain and Simple: After the Final Rule*.

During my tenure as Secretary of the US Department of Health and Human Services (HHS) from 1989 to 1993, I recognized that the federal government had to address the problem of rapidly rising health care costs. In 1991, I asked leaders in the health care industry, from both business and government, to come together in a collaborative effort to examine ways to lower administrative costs, particularly those associated with paper transactions, and to ascertain how electronic technology could help. This collaborative effort was the genesis of the Workgroup for Electronic Data Interchange (WEDI) and the *1993 WEDI Report*, a road map for a more efficient health care information system.

The work of WEDI in the early 1990s provided the framework for the administrative simplification provisions that were enacted as part of the Health Insurance Portability and Accountability Act of 1996 (HIPAA). WEDI was one of four organizations designated in the HIPAA statute to advise the Secretary of HHS and the National Committee on Vital and Health Statistics (NCVHS) on the adoption of HIPAA administrative simplification standards. To facilitate its advisory role, WEDI created the Strategic National Implementation Process (SNIP) initiative in 2000 as a forum for health care industry participants to collaborate on addressing and resolving business and technical issues associated with implementing standards for the electronic exchange of health care information. Many of those standards were adopted by regulation and required compliance in the 2003-2006 period.

In response to recommendations from WEDI and other organizations, in February 2009, Congress enacted privacy and security modifications to HIPAA administrative simplification standards and provided for breach notification standards in the Health Information Technology for Economic and Clinical Health (HITECH) Act, which was included in the American Recovery and Reinvestment Act. Then, in March 2010, Congress addressed transaction, code set, and identifier standard issues in the Patient Protection and Affordable Care Act (ACA).

Administrative simplification statutory and regulatory provisions of HIPAA, the HITECH Act, and the ACA are the subject of *HIPAA Plain and Simple: After the Final Rule*, which also includes provisions of the January 25, 2013, HITECH

Act final rule modifications that require compliance on September 23, 2013. Fortunately, the authors of *HIPAA Plain and Simple* have taken the details and complexities of these provisions and turned them into understandable explanations of actions that health care providers, particularly physician practices, must take to become HIPAA compliant. As you read through the chapters on HIPAA administrative simplification transactions, the Privacy Rule, and the Security Rule, you will find the following sections (with examples) particularly useful:

- What to Do
- How to Do It
- Critical Point

As you move toward HIPAA compliance, I would like you to keep in mind the original objectives of the administrative simplification provisions, which were to:

- Attain more efficient and effective exchange of administrative and financial health care system information using electronic transaction standards
- Realize increased protection of such information and patients' medical records
- Reduce costs of health care transactions

I am as confident today as I was in 1991 that in the years ahead the health care system in the United States will realize these objectives. Further, with a more efficient and less costly administrative structure, the health care system can devote more of its resources to improving the quality of health care delivered.

Access to health care and improving the quality of health care are significant focal points of my career as a physician, as the Secretary of HHS, and as founding dean and president of Morehouse School of Medicine (MSM) in Atlanta, Georgia. The mission of MSM, a historically black institution, is to recruit and train minority and other students as physicians, biomedical scientists, and public health professionals committed to meeting the health care needs of the underserved in our society. Enhancing that mission is MSM's new National Center for Primary Care. The center's focus is on "improving health care and health care access for low-income, minority, and other underserved populations using a number of strategies—research, health policy alternatives, cost-effective programs, professional training, and supporting collaborative efforts."

For clinical staff, like those at MSM, *HIPAA Plain and Simple: After the Final Rule* presents a set of understandable explanations, tools, examples, and references that will help health care providers become compliant with HIPAA administrative simplification standards. Many underserved provider communities will gain by having access to the information presented in the book, including references to additional sources of information that can be accessed through the Internet.

HIPAA compliance opens up new possibilities for improving access to and delivery of quality health care in all medical practices. The electronic standards and accompanying privacy and security mandates discussed herein are just the beginning of the electronic revolution in health care. Electronic methods of communicating data, including e-mail, text messaging, and increasingly popular smart phone and tablet technologies, facilitate collaboration. Electronic data interchange opens new ways for patients to communicate with medical staff and physicians. It also supports an easier way for physicians, specialty organizations, and academic medical centers to communicate with one another and with remote health care facilities. The development of electronic medical records will provide greater access to health care resources and enable the delivery of quality health care to all of our citizens.

Today, WEDI is a vibrant organization of more than 400 participants engaged in furthering efficient use of electronic tools and standards in the health care system to improve health care delivery and quality of care at a lower cost. I was asked by WEDI in March 2013 to serve as honorary chair of a steering committee of business and government leaders preparing a 20th anniversary WEDI report. This report will serve as a road map for the future, identifying priorities for avoiding or overcoming barriers and accelerating innovations that will help the nation realize the benefits of electronic exchange of health care information. Identifying these priorities will help make the road ahead less bumpy as we continue to embrace electronic processes and technologies in health care. Those are the goals that we all strive for as we advance into the future.

I recommend *HIPAA Plain and Simple: After the Final Rule* and wish you successful compliance with HIPAA administrative simplification standards.

Louis W. Sullivan, MD
President Emeritus, Morehouse School of Medicine
Former Secretary, US Department of Health and Human Services

About the Authors

Carolyn P. Hartley, MLA

Carolyn is President and CEO, Physicians EHR, Inc., a North-Carolina-based company that serves as coaches and EHR project managers for customized EHR selection through detailed implementation and preparedness for quality incentives. Most recently, she and her team have been called upon to diagnose and stabilize (rescue) implementations for oncologists, nephrologists, neurologists and community health centers in 23 states. She and her health IT leadership team also serve as contracted EHR technical advisors to national and state medical societies, including the American Medical Association, American Society of Clinical Oncology, American Dental Association, and Texas Association of Community Health Centers.

As sub-contractor to two GSA contractors, Carolyn serves as subject matter expert for multiple DHHS agencies and health information management companies striving to make sense of data, current and future. Carolyn's future health information technology focus is on the 29+ million family caregivers and how technology can help improve their lives and the lives of the loved ones for whom they provide care. Central to her mission is protecting the confidentiality and security of individuals relying on health care professionals for accurate and secure information.

She is lead author of multiple books focused on meaningful use, health IT, HIPAA, and risk mitigation. Two of her 2011 AMA bestselling books include *EHR Implementation: A Step by Step Guide for the Medical Practice, 2nd Edition*, and *HIPAA Plain & Simple*, 2nd Edition. *A Guide to Achieving Meaningful Use* is scheduled for release in 2013. She also is co-host with Jim Tate of the Tate & Hartley internet radio show sponsored by HITECH Answers, and broadcast on HealthcareRadioNow.

She holds a Master of Liberal Arts degree with an emphasis in medical anthropology and philosophy from Baker University. Carolyn can be reached at Carolyn@physiciansehr.com, #CarolynPHartley, or #PhysiciansEHR.

Edward D. Jones III

Ed Jones is a full-time resident of Seabrook Island, SC, author, managing member and CEO of three Cornichon Healthcare companies, and president of HIPAA, LLC, Beaufort, South Carolina.

Ed and his colleagues at HIPAA, LLC offer federal health care legislative and regulatory information source material and commentary at HIPAA, LLC's Web site, www.hipaa.com, and offer online HIPAA and HITECH Act privacy and security training for covered entities and business associates at www.HIPAASchool.com. In partnership with the American Medical Association, HIPAA, LLC has tailored these CME-accredited courses for AMA members at http://AMA.HIPAASchool.com.

Ed and his colleagues at Cornichon consult with health care stakeholders on enabling regulations and electronic business strategies related to the Health Insurance Portability and Accountability Act (HIPAA), the Health Information Technology for Economic and Clinical Health Act (HITECH Act), and the Patient Protection and Affordable Care Act. In addition, they consult with electronic health record (EHR) systems vendors on certification requirements and with hospitals and physician groups on implementation of EHR and practice management systems, management of the revenue cycle, and evaluation of gaps in HIPAA privacy and security compliance. For business associates, they consult on risk assessment, sample policy and procedure, and documentation management solutions for achieving HIPAA privacy and security compliance and in support of cyber-security insurance underwriting.

Ed brings considerable health care industry and business leadership to these companies. His peers elected him for two terms as the 2003-2004 chair of the board of directors of WEDI—the Workgroup for Electronic Data Interchange, an association of more than 400 corporate and government members. WEDI was founded by former secretary of Health and Human Services (HHS) Louis W. Sullivan, MD, and is an advisor to the secretary of HHS and National Committee on Vital and Health Statistics (NCVHS) on design and implementation of HIPAA and HITECH Act administrative simplification standards and on electronic business and clinical tools in health care. Ed also was a founding commissioner of the Electronic Healthcare Network Accreditation Commission (EHNAC) and an architect of its accreditation criteria for security, serving from 1994 to 2003. He currently serves on EHNAC's Policy Advisory Board.

In March 2013, after a national Request For Quotation competition, WEDI selected Ed to manage the 2013 WEDI Report project and write the *2013 WEDI Report*. This project's mission, under the auspices of former HHS Secretary Sullivan and a consortium of major health care stakeholder CEOs, association leaders, and HHS agency heads, is to identify priorities for overcoming barriers to efficient electronic health care information exchange and accelerating business-driven incentives for such exchange beginning in 2014.

Until it was acquired in December 1999, Ed served as senior vice president and member of the CEO's Executive Operations Committee of the NYSE-company, The Centris Group, Inc., which comprised seven subsidiary companies with a core focus on underwriting, insuring, and reinsuring self-funded health plans for US employers. Before joining Centris in 1993, Ed served as executive vice president and as a member of the board of directors of Medical Review Systems, a firm that he co-founded in 1990 and that was acquired in 1995 by Equifax. Before that, he served as a consultant to the

National Research Council of the National Academy of Sciences, the US Sentencing Commission, and firms in insurance and other industries; and held senior positions in the US Department of Justice and Central Intelligence Agency.

Ed is the co-author with Carolyn Hartley of several books for AMA and the American Dental Association (ADA), including:

HIPAA Transactions: A Nontechnical Business Guide for Health Care (AMA, 2004)

HIPAA Security Kit for Dentists (ADA, 2004)

Technical and Financial Guide to EHR Implementation (AMA, 2007)

Policies and Procedures for the Electronic Medical Practice (AMA, January 2010); *Addendum*, July 2010

ADA Practical Guide to HIPAA Compliance: Privacy and Security Kit (ADA, 2010)

HIPAA Plain & Simple: A Health Care Professional's Guide to Achieve HIPAA and HITECH Compliance, 2nd Edition (AMA, 2010)

EHR Implementation: A Step-by-Step Guide for the Medical Practice, 2nd Edition (AMA, 2012)

Ed is the solo author of *HITECH Act Final Rule Sample Policies and Procedures: Privacy, Security, Breach Notification, and Meaningful Use Security for the Busy Healthcare Practitioner,* an updatable eBook and App to be published in Summer 2013 through Cornichon Healthcare's Web site, www.HIPAASafeguardPoliciesandProcedures.com.

Ed holds degrees in economics from the University of Chicago and Washington University in St. Louis. He can be reached at edj3@me.com.

Introduction

Last year AMA published the second edition of *EHR Implementation: A Step-by-Step Guide for the Medical Practice,* our guide to help health care providers understand how to adopt and meaningfully use certified electronic health record (EHR) technology. While health care providers were busily adapting to new clinical workflows and requirements as part of the meaningful use program, the federal government was readying new administrative requirements for transactions and code sets, privacy, security, and identifiers. We anticipated these in the second edition of *HIPAA Plain & Simple*, published in 2011, but much has transpired in the administrative arena since then, so it is now time for a third edition to discuss new and modified requirements and compliance dates. As examples, a new standard transaction version, 5010, required compliance on January 1, 2012, and standard transaction operating rules for eligibility and claim status began a rollout on January 1, 2013; compliance with a new code set, ICD-10, was delayed a year until October 1, 2014; and a unique health plan identifier requires compliance on November 5, 2014 and use in standard transactions by November 7, 2016.

With regard to privacy and security, the federal government published in the *Federal Register,* on January 25, 2013, its long-awaited *Modifications to the HIPAA Privacy, Security, Enforcement, and Breach Notification Rules Under the Health Information Technology for Economic and Clinical Health Act (HITECH Act) and the Genetic Information Nondiscrimination act; Other Modifications to the HIPAA Rules: Final Rule*, which requires compliance by covered entities and business associates by September 23, 2013. When you add Stage 2 Meaningful Use adaptation of workflows and reporting into the mix, with accompanying risk management and security measures to implement and attest, you know that your organization will be busy writing new and revising existing safeguard policies and procedures to achieve compliance. We trust that this third edition will help make your efforts on the administrative front easier.

The HITECH Act modifications to HIPAA make good business sense. The provisions tighten control over patients' protected health information by extending federal regulation to business associates and their subcontractors—now deemed business associates, too—and require business associates to implement the HIPAA Security Rule. In addition, the provisions change the definition of breach, now presuming a breach has occurred unless the breaching party can demonstrate a "low probability" of "impermissible use or disclosure" based on specific factors of consideration, but they leave the notification substantially as under the earlier interim final rule. The provisions also streamline the process of providing student immunization records to schools. We discuss these and other provisions of the January 25, 2013, Final Rule in detail in this book.

The American health care system is at a critical juncture. Since passage of HIPAA in August 1996, and the beginning of promulgation of enabling regulations in the last decade (see Table 1.1 in Chapter 1), the federal government in collaboration with business has developed a number of electronic tools for the health care industry. The health care industry has tried to follow the path of other industries by automating many redundant and costly processes and eliminating wasteful workflows, with mixed success, while at the same time safeguarding patients' protected health information. Technology is changing rapidly as new portable and mobile devices such as smartphones and tablets proliferate, and new options for maintaining data, such as the cloud, emerge. Health care providers are under pressure to keep up not only with the regulatory environment, but also with the rapid change in technology that challenges return on investment in their business venues. The challenge has been, and will continue to be, to realize the benefits of electronic processes enjoyed by other industry sectors, such as greater efficiency and reduced costs of operations, while enhancing the quality of health care delivered.

This is not news to those of us who have been in health care for decades. Now, under the HITECH Act, the federal government is investing tens of billions of dollars to help health care providers make the transition to an electronic environment. This is the carrot. At the same time, again under the HITECH Act, the federal government has strengthened federal enforcement of privacy and security rules, required breach notification rules, established compliance audits, and substantially increased the financial penalties for noncompliance. This is the stick, and represents the accountability factor of using taxpayer dollars to build consumer confidence in the electronic health care information exchange system.

These are the themes we discuss in the third edition of *HIPAA Plain & Simple*. In Chapter 1, we provide a timeline and overview of HIPAA and the HITECH Act regulations, with significant explanatory detail of January 25, 2013, Final Rule modifications from the preamble of the Final Rule. In Chapter 2, we discuss transactions and code sets, including information on operating rules and the tools available to assist the transition from ICD-9 to ICD-10. In Chapters 3 and 4, we discuss the January 25, 2013, modifications to the HIPAA Privacy Rule and HIPAA Security Rule, respectively. Chapter 4 also presents the Department of Health and Human Services' *Guidance Specifying Technologies and Methodologies that Render Protected Health Information Unusable, Unreadable, or Indecipherable to Unauthorized Individuals,* which was included in the August 24, 2009 Breach Notification Interim Final Rule and is applicable today and reinforced in the January 25, 2013, Final Rule. Finally, in Chapter 5, we pull the story together, giving you tools that you can use to implement HIPAA and HITECH Act regulatory safeguards in your organization, facilitate communication about them with workforce members and patients, and build a culture that sustains your organization as a health care provider and ongoing business.

Like our previous editions, this third edition of *HIPAA Plain & Simple* is designed to uncomplicate "HIPAA heavy." It is not "HIPAA light" but rather "HIPAA easy to understand." It is your reference tool when the legal dossier seems a little over the top. HIPAA and the HITECH Act require certain levels of legal and documentation accuracy, so we didn't substitute a simplified approach for the language of the regulation. Your management team responsible for implementing HIPAA and HITECH Act regulations should consult a health-law attorney when you are dealing with contracts, such as the business associate agreement that must clearly state the covered entity's protected health information use and disclosure permissions for all business associates downstream (contractors and subcontractors), and when responding to a compliance audit or complaint or breach investigation.

This book is also for nurses who spend the majority of their time in clinical and personal patient interaction, and are likely to field privacy and security questions for the physician. It's also for the vulnerable receptionist and scheduler, workforce members frequently confronted by patients with near-impossible questions even as they keep the office running smoothly. It also is for the billing and insurance specialists required to stay current with the 5010 version and operating rules transaction standards and the resultant code set changes with Version 5010, to say nothing of the challenges of the transition from ICD-9 to ICD-10. These are your guides through the detailed workflow redesigns and data capture changes in your organization.

The third edition of *HIPAA Plain and Simple* also is designed for persons taking on new responsibilities within the health care community; not only those in the medical practice but also in health plans and health care clearinghouses; business associates; and, especially, new workforce members with responsibilities for protected health information outlined in their job descriptions.

Use this book as a resource to explore the practical integration of complex HIPAA and HITECH Act strategies and to identify and specify required policies and procedures. You need not hunt through copies of the *Federal Register* or the *Code of Federal Regulations.* We tell you where in those documents you can find additional information if you are of a mind to do so.

Our readers have been on our minds throughout the entire process of revising this book. We spoke with many friends and business colleagues who, like you, are in the trenches making HIPAA and HITECH Act modifications happen. We've guided health care providers through the risk analysis and security implementation process, designed safeguard policies and procedures, assisted in the transition to Version 5010 and electronic health record software, and supported users when problems or issues arose.

Each chapter contains What to Do and How to Do It directions, along with Critical Points, in which we highlight key learning objectives. The book is loaded with checklists, charts, quick reference guides, timelines, training strategies, and communication plans to make HIPAA and HITECH Act modifications easier to understand.

With the help of a dynamic team of publisher, editors, reviewers, and marketers, we fully deconstructed the original "HIPAA heavy" products so that we could confidently bring you this plain and simple version. We are better authors for knowing the professionals at AMA, and we're sure you'll find that they had you in mind when publishing this valuable addition to your compliance library.

Warmest wishes as you continue your HIPAA/HITECH Act journey. We hope you'll let us know how you're doing.

Carolyn P. Hartley
Edward D. Jones III

chapter 1

HIPAA, HITECH Act, and Breach Notification Overview

In the early 1990s, health care leaders came to then Secretary of Health and Human Services (HHS), Louis W. Sullivan, MD, and asked for help to simplify the health care industry's complex and costly administrative mess. The biggest problem at the time was that the administrative process to manage health information, including billing and claims processes, had become out-of-sync with the clinical process and burdensome to health care practitioners. For example, let's say a Blue Cross/Blue Shield (BCBS) health plan indicated that it would pay for a physician to conduct chest percussion therapy on a 60-year-old male patient, but to get paid for the treatment, the physician would need to use a special procedure number that only BCBS recognized. Those numbers were called *local codes*. But if the physician ordered the same procedure for a Cigna patient, the physician would need to search for the Cigna number because the BCBS local code would not apply. If you multiply this example by the number of payers, then by the number of diagnoses and procedures, and again by the number of physicians, you definitely have a complex administrative mess.

Physicians wanted to provide care to patients and get paid for the service, but they faced a barrier in that few payers spoke the language of conducting business. Language barriers in an industry where the national health expenditure in 1990 was $724.3 billion, or 12.5% of gross domestic product (GDP), and today is $2.7 trillion (2011 data), or 17.9% of GDP,[1] can create significant inefficiencies, processing errors, and large administrative costs. The result was wasted time and effort; repeated filings; denied claims; payment collection debates between payers, providers, and patients; distrust and anxiety; confusion over the status of claims; excessive postage costs; and overall headache.

At that meeting with Dr Sullivan, health care leaders expressed their exasperation with the clumsy, fragmented system, and nearly everyone agreed that the administrative management process needed a major overhaul. Leaders also agreed that the health care industry couldn't come to an agreement on standard language formats by itself; rather, it needed a regulatory body to unravel proprietary, state, and federal codes. As we shall see, this is very much a work in progress two decades later, in 2013.

Dr Sullivan assigned the following four agencies and organizations to work together and come to an agreement on how to simplify the administrative process:

- National Committee on Vital and Health Statistics (NCVHS)
- Centers for Disease Control and Prevention (CDC)
- National Institutes of Health (NIH)
- Workgroup for Electronic Data Interchange (WEDI)[2]

The specific challenge to WEDI, a collaboration of government and private industry, was to find a way to decrease administrative costs of health care, eliminate software adaptations for multiple formats, agree on one standard for sending and receiving electronic data, and still allow room for electronic commerce to flourish in the health care industry—a huge undertaking!

To begin, WEDI examined the effect of electronic technology in minimizing administrative costs of health care transactions. WEDI's findings, published in a 1993 report,[3] indicated that the savings from using electronic technology to process health care transactions would be substantial. This report provided the foundation for the administrative simplification provisions in the Health Insurance Portability and Accountability Act of 1996 (HIPAA), which President Clinton signed on August 21, 1996.[4]

The word *portability* in the title of the law guaranteed that an employee could obtain health insurance if he or she changed jobs. The word *accountability* in the title of the law began to identify *who*, *what*, *when*, and *how* for specific health care activities and assigned specific job roles for accountability for compliance. One part of accountability is administrative simplification, which was designed to address the messy administrative systems in health care. Figure 1.1 gives you a quick overview of the structure of administrative simplification and how it fits into the HIPAA statute. Our focus in this book is on the transactions and code sets (Chapter 2), the Privacy Rule (Chapter 3), and the Security Rule (Chapter 4). We will briefly outline national identifiers later in this chapter.

FIGURE 1.1

Overview of the Structure of Administrative Simplification

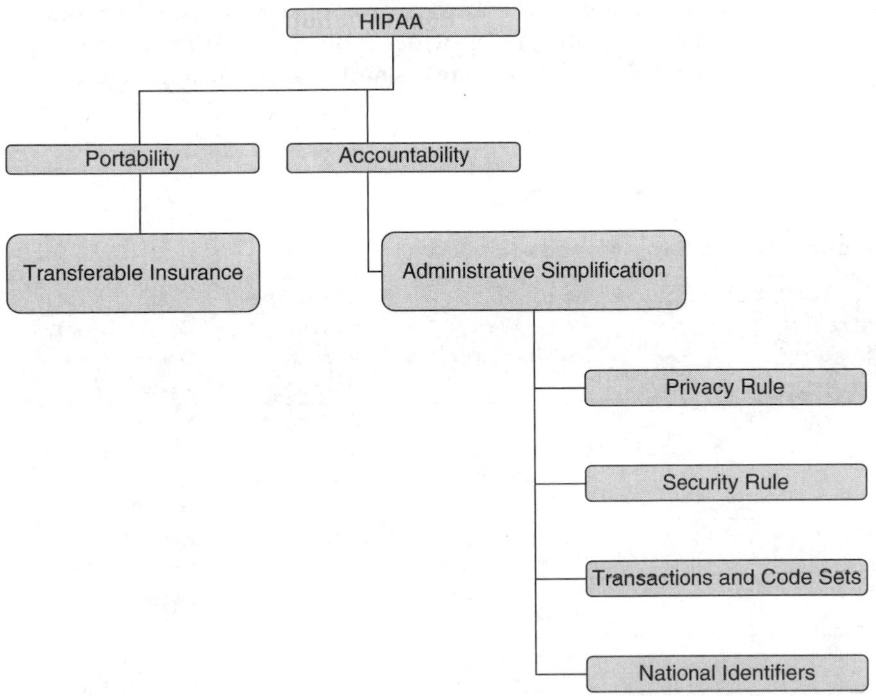

The overall objectives of HIPAA administrative simplification are to:

- Improve efficiency and effectiveness of the health care system via electronic exchange of administrative and financial information
- Protect the security and privacy of transmitted and stored administrative and financial information
- Reduce high transaction costs in health care, which include, but are not limited to:
  - Paper-based transaction systems
  - Multiple, nonstandard health care data formats
  - Misuse of, errors related to, and loss of health care records

Reduced to these objectives, HIPAA administrative simplification appears manageable; that is, simplify transactions so that all entities filing electronic transactions use the same set of codes, and keep patient information safe and secure while doing it. As the 17 years that have passed since the enactment of HIPAA administrative simplification have shown, it has been easier to specify those objectives in writing than to accomplish them in practice.[5]

BUILDING THE INFRASTRUCTURE

The procedural mechanisms for building the HIPAA administrative simplification infrastructure are the enabling regulations promulgated under the federal Administrative Procedure Act. Table 1.1 provides a timeline of the status of enabling regulations for HIPAA administrative simplification through early June 2013.

TABLE 1.1

HIPAA Administrative Simplification Timeline

HIPAA Administrative Simplification Rule	Status	Federal Register Publication Date	Compliance Date for Covered Entities	Other Compliance Date, If Applicable
Transactions and Code Sets	Final	August 17, 2000[i]; modifications: February 20, 2003[ii]	October 16, 2003	N/A
Privacy	Final	December 28, 2000[iii]; modifications: August 14, 2002[iv]	April 14, 2003	April 14, 2004 (small health plans)
National Employer Identifier	Final	May 31, 2002[v]	July 30, 2004	August 1, 2005 (small health plans)
Security	Final	February 20, 2003[vi]	April 20, 2005	April 20, 2006 (small health plans)
National Provider Identifier	Final	January 23, 2004[vii]	May 23, 2007	May 23, 2008 (small health plans)
Claim Attachment	Notice of Proposed Rulemaking	September 23, 2005[viii]		Withdrawn, January 25, 2010[ix]
Enforcement	Final	February 16, 2006[x]	March 16, 2006	N/A
Modification to Transactions and Code Sets: Version 5010	Final	January 16, 2009[xi]	January 1, 2012	Compliance date changed to October 1, 2014 (see table note xxi)
Modification to Transactions and Code Sets: ICD-10	Final	January 16, 2009[xii]	October 1, 2013	N/A

Continued

TABLE 1.1 (continued)

HIPAA Administrative Simplification Timeline

HIPAA Administrative Simplification Rule	Status	Federal Register Publication Date	Compliance Date for Covered Entities	Other Compliance Date, If Applicable
HHS Secretary's Delegation of Authority to HHS's Office for Civil Rights (OCR) to Enforce HIPAA Security Rule	Notice	August 4, 2009[xiii]	July 27, 2009	N/A
Breach Notification for Unsecured Protected Health Information	Interim Final Rule	August 24, 2009[xiv]	September 23, 2009 (effective date for breaches of protected health information occurring on or after this date, with enforcement commencing for breaches occurring on or after February 22, 2010)	N/A
Enforcement	Interim Final Rule	October 30, 2009[xv]	November 30, 2009 (effective date for violations occurring on or after February 18, 2009)	N/A
Modifications to the HIPAA Privacy, Security, and Enforcement Rules Under the [HITECH Act] National Plan Identifier	Notice of Proposed Rulemaking	July 14, 2010[xvi]		Comments to HHS on or before September 13, 2010
Privacy Rule Accounting of Disclosures Under the HITECH Act	Notice of Proposed Rule Making	May 31, 2011[xvii]		
Adoption of Operating Rules for Eligibility and Claim Status Transactions	Interim Final Rule	July 8, 2011[xviii]	January 1, 2013	CMS Notice to Industry changed to final rule, effective December 7, 2011

Continued

TABLE 1.1 (continued)

HIPAA Administrative Simplification Timeline

HIPAA Administrative Simplification Rule	Status	Federal Register Publication Date	Compliance Date for Covered Entities	Other Compliance Date, If Applicable
Adoption of Standards for Electronic Funds Transfers (EFTs) and Remittance Advice	Interim Final Rule	January 10, 2012[xix]	January 1, 2014	
Adoption of Operating Rules for Electronic Funds Transfers (EFTs) and Remittance Advice	Interim Final Rule	August 10, 2012[xx]	January 1, 2014	CMS Notice to Industry changed to final rule, effective April 19, 2013
Adoption of Standard for Unique Health Plan Identifier; Additional National Provider Identifier (NPI) Requirements; Change in Compliance Date for ICD-10	Final Rule	September 5, 2012[xxi]	Health Plan ID: November 5, 2014 (small health plans have until November 5, 2015); NPI: May 6, 2013; ICD-10: October 1, 2014	
Modifications to HIPAA Privacy, Security, Enforcement, and Breach Notification Rules Under the HITECH Act and Genetic Information Nondiscrimination Act (GINA)	Final Rule	January 25, 2013[xxii]	September 23, 2013	Effective date: March 26, 2013; date to conform business associate contracts: September 22, 2014
Technical Corrections to the HIPAA Privacy, Security, and Enforcement Rules	Final Rule	June 7, 2013[xxiii]		Effective date: June 7, 2013

[i] HHS, Office of the Secretary, 45 CFR Parts 160 and 162: Health Insurance Reform: Standards for Electronic Transactions; Final Rule, *Federal Register*, v. 65, n. 160, August 17, 2000, pp. 50312-50372. Available at http://www.cms.gov/Regulations-and-Guidance/HIPAA-Administrative-Simplification/TransactionCodeSetsStands/Downloads/txfinal.pdf; and 45 CFR Parts 160 and 162: Health Insurance Reform: Standards for Electronic Transactions; Corrections, *Federal Register*, v. 65, n. 227, November 24, 2000, p. 70507. Available at http://www.cms.gov/Regulations-and-Guidance/HIPAA-Administrative-Simplification/TransactionCodeSetsStands/Downloads/StandardsForElectronicTransactions-Corrections.pdf.

[ii] HHS, Office of the Secretary, 45 CFR Part 162: Health Insurance Reform: Modifications to Electronic Data Transaction Standards and Code Sets; Final Rule, *Federal Register*, v. 68, n. 34, February 20, 2003, pp. 8381-8399. Available at http://www.gpo.gov/fdsys/pkg/FR-2003-02-20/pdf/03-3876.pdf.

[iii] HHS, Office of the Secretary, 45 CFR Parts 160 and 164: Standards for Privacy of Individually Identifiable Health Information; Final Rule, *Federal Register*, v. 65, n. 250, December 28, 2000, pp. 82462-82829. Available at http://www.hhs.gov/ocr/privacy/hipaa/administrative/privacyrule/prdecember2000all8parts.pdf.

[iv] HHS, Office of the Secretary, 45 CFR Parts 160 and 164: Standards for Privacy of Individually Identifiable Health Information; Final Rule, *Federal Register*, v. 67, n. 157, August 14, 2002, pp. 53182-53273. Available at http://www.hhs.gov/ocr/privacy/hipaa/administrative/privacyrule/privrulepd.pdf.

[v] HHS, Office of the Secretary, 45 CFR Parts 160 and 162: Health Insurance Reform: Standard Unique Employer Identifier; Final Rule, *Federal Register*, v. 67, n. 105, May 31, 2002, pp. 38009-38020. Available at http://www.cms.gov/Regulations-and-Guidance/HIPAA-Administrative-Simplification/EmployerIdentifierStand/Downloads/emplDfinal.pdf.

[vi] HHS, Office of the Secretary, 45 CFR Parts 160, 162, and 164: Health Insurance Reform: Security Standards; Final Rule, *Federal Register*, v. 68, n. 34, February 20, 2003, pp. 8334-8381. Available at http://www.hhs.gov/ocr/privacy/hipaa/administrative/securityrule/securityrulepdf.pdf.

[vii] HHS, Office of the Secretary, 45 CFR Part 162: HIPAA Administrative Simplification: Standard Unique Health Identifier for Health Care Providers; Final Rule, *Federal Register*, v. 69, n. 15, January 23, 2004, pp. 3434-3469. Available at http://www.gpo.gov/fdsys/pkg/FR-2004-01-23/pdf/04-1149.pdf.

[viii] HHS, Office of the Secretary, 45 CFR Part 162: HIPAA Administrative Simplification: Standards for Electronic Health Care Claims Attachments; Proposed Rule, *Federal Register*, v. 70, n. 184, September 23, 2005, pp. 55990-56025. Available at http://www.gpo.gov/fdsys/pkg/FR-2005-09-23/pdf/05-18927.pdf.

[ix] HHS, Office of the Secretary, Semiannual Regulatory Agenda, *Federal Register*, v. 75, n. 79, April 26, 2010, p. 21804. Available at http://www.gpo.gov/fdsys/pkg/FR-2010-04-26/pdf/2010-8934.pdf. Please see the discussion in Chapter 2 about the administrative simplification provisions of the Patient Protection and Affordable Care Act, which was enacted on March 23, 2010, for the new statutory adoption date deadline of January 1, 2014, and effective date deadline of January 1, 2016, for the health claims attachment standard.

[x] HHS, Office of the Secretary, 45 CFR Parts 160 and 164: HIPAA Administrative Simplification: Enforcement; Final Rule, *Federal Register*, v. 71, n. 32, February 16, 2006, pp. 8390-8433. Available at http://www.gpo.gov/fdsys/pkg/FR-2006-02-16/pdf/06-1376.pdf.

[xi] HHS, Office of the Secretary, 45 CFR Part 162: Health Insurance Reform; Modifications to the Health Insurance Portability and Accountability Act (HIPAA); Final Rule, *Federal Register*, v. 74, n. 11, January 16, 2009, pp. 3296-3328. Available at http://www.gpo.gov/fdsys/pkg/FR-2009-01-16/pdf/E9-740.pdf.

[xii] HHS, Office of the Secretary, 45 CFR Part 162: HIPAA Administrative Simplification: Modifications to Medical Data Code Set Standards to Adopt ICD-10-CM and ICD-10-PCS; Final Rule, *Federal Register*, v. 74, n. 11, January 16, 2009, pp. 3328-3362. Available at http://www.gpo.gov/fdsys/pkg/FR-2009-01-16/pdf/E9-743.pdf.

[xiii] HHS, Office of the Secretary, Office for Civil Rights; Delegation of Authority: Notice, *Federal Register*, v. 74, n. 148, August 4, 2009, p. 38630. Available at http://www.hhs.gov/ocr/privacy/hipaa/administrative/securityrule/srdelegation.pdf.

[xiv] HHS, Office of the Secretary, 45 CFR Parts 160 and 164: Breach Notification for Unsecured Protected Health Information; Interim Final Rule, *Federal Register*, v. 74, n. 162, pp. 42740-42770. Available at http://www.gpo.gov/fdsys/pkg/FR-2009-08-24/pdf/E9-20169.pdf.

[xv] HHS, Office of the Secretary, 45 CFR Part 160: HIPAA Administrative Simplification: Enforcement; Interim Final Rule, *Federal Register*, v. 74, n. 209, October 30, 2009, pp. 56123-56131. Available at http://www.gpo.gov/fdsys/pkg/FR-2009-10-30/pdf/E9-26203.pdf.

[xvi] HHS, Office of the Secretary, 45 CFR Parts 160 and 164: Modifications to the HIPAA Privacy, Security, and Enforcement Rules Under the Health Information Technology for Economic and Clinical Health Act; Proposed Rule, *Federal Register*, v. 75, n. 134, July 14, 2010, pp. 40868-40924. Available at http://www.gpo.gov/fdsys/pkg/FR-2010-07-14/pdf/2010-16718.pdf.

[xvii] HHS, Office of the Secretary, 45 CFR Part 164: HIPAA Privacy Rule Accounting of Disclosures Under the Health Information Technology for Economic and Clinical Health Act; Proposed Rule, *Federal Register*, v. 76, n. 104, May 31, 2011, pp. 31426-31449. Available at http://www.gpo.gov/fdsys/pkg/FR-2011-05-31/pdf/2011-13297.pdf.

[xviii] HHS, Office of the Secretary, 45 CFR Parts 160 and 162: Administrative Simplification: Adoption of Operating Rules for Eligibility for a Health Plan and Health Care Claim Status Transactions; Interim Final Rule, *Federal Register*, v .76, n. 131, July 8, 2011, pp. 40458-40496. Available at http://www.gpo.gov/fdsys/pkg/FR-2011-07-08/pdf/2011-16834.pdf. By Notice to Industry, CMS converted the interim final rule to a final rule on December 7, 2011. Available at http://www.cms.gov/Regulations-and-Guidance/HIPAA-Administrative-Simplification/Affordable-Care-Act/CMS-0032-IFC.pdf. CMS announced on January 1, 2013, the compliance date for operating rules for the eligibility for a health plan and health care claim status transactions, that it was implementing a 90-day period, until March 31, 2013, of "enforcement discretion" to give the health care industry more time to implement these operating rule transactions. Available at http://www.cms.gov/Outreach-and-Education/Outreach/OpenDoorForums/Downloads/010213Sec1104ofACAAnnouncement.pdf.

[xix] HHS, Office of the Secretary, 45 CFR Parts 160 and 162: Administrative Simplification: Adoption of Standards for Health Care Electronic Funds Transfers (EFTs) and Remittance Advice; Interim Final Rule, *Federal Register*, v. 77, n. 6, January 10, 2012, pp. 1556-1590. Available at http://www.gpo.gov/fdsys/pkg/FR-2012-01-10/pdf/2012-132.pdf.

[xx] HHS, Office of the Secretary, 45 CFR Part 162: Administrative Simplification: Adoption of Operating Rules for Health Care Electronic Funds Transfers (EFT) and Remittance Advice Transactions; Interim Final Rule, *Federal Register*, v. 77, n. 155, August 10, 2012, pp. 48008-48044. Available at http://www.gpo.gov/fdsys/pkg/FR-2012-08-10/pdf/2012-19557.pdf. By Notice to Industry, CMS converted the interim final rule to a final rule on April 19, 2013. Available at http://www.caqh.org/pdf/CMSEFTERAFinalRuleAnnouncement.pdf.

[xxi] HHS, Centers for Medicare & Medicaid Services, 45 CFR Part 162: Administrative Simplification: Adoption of a Standard for a Unique Health Plan Identifier; Addition to the National Provider Identifier Requirements; and a Change to the Compliance Date for the International Classifications of Diseases, 10th Edition (ICD-10-CM and ICD-10-PCS) Medical Data Code Sets; Final Rule, *Federal Register*, v. 77, n. 172, September 5, 2012, pp. 54664-54720. Available at http://www.gpo.gov/fdsys/pkg/FR-2012-09-05/pdf/2012-21238.pdf.

[xxii] HHS, Office of the Secretary, 45 CFR Parts 160 and 164: Modifications to the HIPAA Privacy, Security, Enforcement, and Breach Notification Rules Under the Health Information Technology for Economic and Clinical Health Act and the Genetic Information Nondiscrimination Act; Other Modifications to the HIPAA Rules; Final Rule, *Federal Register*, v. 78, n. 17, January 25, 2013, pp. 5566-5702. Available at http://www.gpo.gov/fdsys/pkg/FR-2013-01-25/pdf/2013-01073.pdf.

[xxiii] HHS, Office for Civil Rights, 45 CFR Parts 160 and 164: Technical Corrections to the HIPAA Privacy, Security, and Enforcement Rules, *Federal Register*, v. 78, n. 110, June 7, 2013, pp. 34264-34266. Available at http://www.gpo.gov/fdsys/pkg/FR-2013-06-07/pdf/2013-13472.pdf.

The chapters of this book will explore the content of the administrative simplification enabling regulations. Note in Table 1.1 that it was almost seven years after enactment of HIPAA administrative simplification, in April 2003, that the first standard requiring health care industry compliance—privacy—was in place. The Administrative Procedure Act provides for a relatively slow process, and the health care industry is complex. Yet, as we pass the 17th anniversary of the enactment of HIPAA administrative simplification, we are still wrestling with proposals for and implementation of HIPAA administrative simplification standards, well beyond the timeframes for implementation that Congress envisioned. Given the rapid change in electronic technologies—the growth of the Internet as a source of information and as a vehicle for transactions, and the increasing switch of financial transactions from cash and check to debit and credit cards and online and mobile payments—since the enactment of HIPAA administrative simplification, can the relatively slow federal initiative processes keep up with market developments, or do they impede progress?[6] You be the judge as we explore HIPAA administrative simplification standards and their implementation specifications in this book.

FOUR SETS OF STANDARDS

In this section, we outline the characteristics of each of the four sets of standards:[7] transactions and code sets, privacy, security, and identifiers.

Transactions and Code Sets

In past decades, a very complicated network of billing and software companies was retained by physician practices to facilitate payment of claims. Prior to the promulgation of the HIPAA administrative simplification transaction rules, most of the companies used different formats, which sometimes made it difficult for payers to understand the connection between treatment and payment. Also, each payer required different information about the treatment or the individual. The result was a proliferation of nonstandard transaction formats and data-content requirements that complicated and slowed the claim-payment process. Each side blamed the other for these complications, but one thing was certain: everyone was unhappy with the process, including the patient. So HHS, through HIPAA, said that health plan payers, health care providers, and health care clearinghouses—HIPAA's covered entities—must send or receive transactions using standard formats and data content.

The Transaction and Code Sets rule required compliance on October 16, 2003, by covered entities: health plans, health care clearinghouses, and health care providers. Compliance with a modification of the Accredited Standards Committee (ASC) X12[8] transaction standards—from Version 4010 to Version 5010—was required on January 1, 2012. Covered entities have begun implementing operating rules. Compliance with the first set of transactions—eligibility and claim status—was required by January 1, 2013, and compliance with the second set of transactions—electronic funds transfers (EFTs) and remittance advice—is required by January 1, 2014. Operating rules are discussed further in Chapter 2 in the context of the Patient Protection and Affordable Care Act. See Appendix C for additional AMA resources and information on transactions and code sets.

A *transaction* refers to the electronic transmission of information between two parties to carry out financial or administrative activities. *Code sets* are data sets that identify diagnoses, treatment procedures, drug codes, equipment codes, financial codes, location codes, and other codes necessary to effect a transaction by identifying a value that will populate a specified data element in a transaction. The required diagnosis code set will change from the *International Classification of Diseases, Ninth Revision, Clinical Modification* (ICD-9-CM) to the *International Classification of Diseases, Tenth Revision, Clinical Modification* (ICD-10-CM) on October 1, 2014.

We identify and discuss transaction standards and code sets in detail in Chapter 2.

The importance of codes to the physician practice is as follows: when the diagnostics match a complicated set of health plan payer-approved procedure codes, then the payers understand how the provider intends to treat the patient, and payers pay the provider for services rendered. If the codes are accurate and properly inserted as data element values in a transaction, then appropriate claim information moves from the provider to the payer, and payment moves from the payer to the provider, with few interruptions or disruptions.

As you will see in Chapter 2, use of situational variables and companion guides continued to frustrate the transaction process, but ASC X12 Version 5010 of the transaction standards, with which compliance has been required since January 1, 2012, addresses those uses and, along with operating rules, expedites the transaction process.

Achieving agreement on standard formats for electronic transactions is a challenge, but the standards development process allows all parties—vendors, payers, providers, clearinghouses, and government—to come together to make their business cases for what should be reflected in the standards. Each of the parties has an opportunity to identify information that it needs to complete a transaction. Then, the parties as a group negotiate a common set of requirements that they would use to transact business. That process is ongoing because the parties continue to meet to discuss new or revised data requirements in response to innovations in technology that may further improve business processing or removal of barriers that impede electronic health care information exchange in the health care industry.

CRITICAL POINT

Your practice must ensure that your software vendor, as a business associate, can send and receive electronic health care information using required transaction standard data formats and data content. The financial penalty for not doing so has increased from $100 per violation to up to $50,000 per violation.

HIPAA provides for a Designated Standard Maintenance Organization (DSMO)[9] process to handle industry-recommended modifications to the standards. Health care stakeholders have expended considerable time and money not only in the development of standards, but also in the implementation process, including the testing of transactions among trading partners. Although health plan payers and health care providers use the electronic transactions process as a business tool, ultimately it is the responsibility of their system vendors and health care clearinghouses to make the process work as seamlessly as possible. You also will see in Chapter 2, in the discussion of the background relating to ASC X12 Version 5010 and in the new administrative simplification provisions of the Patient Protection and Affordable Care Act, that the *adoption and implementation* of the transaction standards is still very much a work in progress.

Privacy Standards

HHS recognized that if it required covered entities to use a standard set of formats and data content to transmit files electronically, consumers would expect their medical files to be kept confidential. That is why HHS also developed standards that protect patients' rights, including unauthorized use and disclosure of their protected health information (PHI). The Privacy Rule requires that you change some of your day-to-day tasks so that information used to identify a patient is protected and that this protected health information is safeguarded to prevent unauthorized use or disclosure. Protected health information is individually identifiable health information that is transmitted or maintained in electronic media or in any other form or medium.

The HIPAA Privacy Rule has garnered considerable attention because it is nontechnical—mainly addressing policies and procedures—and is an important issue to patients. Compliance with the Privacy Rule was required on April 14, 2003, with small health plans having an additional year to comply.

Table 1.2 outlines the HIPAA Privacy Rule standards, which cover requirements related to PHI: use and disclosure, notice of privacy practices, access, restrictions, amendment, accounting, and administrative safeguards. These requirements are covered in detail in Chapter 3, along with new restrictions on use or disclosure of PHI in marketing and fundraising communications with which compliance is required by September 23, 2013. Later in this chapter, we examine the HITECH Act provisions related to breach notification for impermissible use or disclosure of unsecured PHI.

TABLE 1.2

HIPAA Privacy Rule Standards

Subpart E: Privacy of Individually Identifiable Health Information
164.502 Uses and disclosures of protected health information: General rules
Standard: A covered entity or business associate may not use or disclose PHI, except as permitted or required.
Covered entities: Permitted uses and disclosures
Covered entities: Required disclosures
Business associates: Permitted uses and disclosures
Business associates: Required uses and disclosures
Prohibited uses and disclosures
Use and disclosure of genetic information for underwriting purposes
Sale of protected health information
Standard: Minimum necessary
Standard: Uses and disclosures of protected health information subject to an agreed upon restriction
Standard: Uses and disclosures of de-identified protected health information
Standard: Disclosures to business associates

Continued

TABLE 1.2 (continued)

HIPAA Privacy Rule Standards

Standard: Deceased individuals

Standard: Personal representatives

Standard: Confidential communications

Standard: Uses and disclosures consistent with notice

Standard: Disclosures by whistleblowers and workforce member crime victims

164.504 Uses and disclosures: Organizational requirements

Standard: Business associate contracts

Standard: Requirements for group health plans

Standard: Requirements for a covered entity with multiple covered functions

164.506 Uses and disclosures to carry out treatment, payment, or health care operations

Standard: Permitted uses and disclosures

Standard: Consent for uses and disclosures permitted

164.508 Uses and disclosures for which an authorization is required

Standard: Authorizations for uses and disclosures

164.510 Uses and disclosures requiring an opportunity for the individual to agree or to object

Standard: Use and disclosure for facility directories

Standard: Uses and disclosures for involvement in the individual's care and notification purposes

164.512 Uses and disclosures for which an authorization or opportunity to agree or object is not required

Standard: Uses and disclosures required by law

Standard: Uses and disclosures for public health activities

Standard: Disclosures about victims of abuse, neglect, or domestic violence

Standard: Uses and disclosures for health oversight activities

Standard: Disclosures for judicial and administrative proceedings

Standard: Disclosures for law enforcement purposes

Standard: Uses and disclosures about decedents

Standard: Uses and disclosures for cadaveric organ, eye, or tissue donation purposes

Standard: Uses and disclosures for research purposes

Standard: Uses and disclosures to avert a serious threat to health or safety

Standard: Uses and disclosures for specialized government functions

Standard: Disclosures for workers' compensation

164.514 Other requirements relating to uses and disclosures of protected health information

Standard: De-identification of protected health information

Requirements for de-identification

Re-identification

Standard: Minimum necessary requirements

Standard: Limited data set

Standard: Uses and disclosures for fundraising

Standard: Limited data set

Standard: Uses and disclosures for fundraising

TABLE 1.2 (continued)

HIPAA Privacy Rule Standards
Fundraising requirements
Standard: Uses and disclosures for underwriting and related purposes
Standard: Verification requirements
164.520 Notice of privacy practices for protected health information
Standard: Notice of privacy practices
164.522 Rights to request privacy protection for protected health information
Standard: Right of an individual to request restriction of uses and disclosures
Standard: Confidential communications requirements
164.524 Access of individuals to protected health information
Standard: Access to protected health information
164.526 Amendment of protected health information
Standard: Right to amend
164.528 Accounting of disclosures of protected health information
Standard: Right to an accounting of disclosures of protected health information
164.530 Administrative requirements
Standard: Personnel designations
Standard: Training
Standard: Safeguards
Standard: Complaints to the covered entity
Standard: Sanctions
Standard: Mitigation
Standard: Refraining from intimidating or retaliatory acts
Standard: Waiver of rights
Standard: Policies and procedures
Standard: Changes to policies and procedures
Standard: Documentation
Standard: Group health plans

Security Standards

Security standards go hand in hand with privacy standards. The Security Rule is about controlling access to electronic protected health information (ePHI) only, while the Privacy Rule, as indicated above, covers oral, hard copy, and electronic PHI.

CRITICAL POINT

Security is about controlling access to ePHI. Privacy is about controlling how oral, hard copy, and electronic PHI is used and disclosed.

Compliance with the Security Rule by covered entities was required on April 20, 2005 (with small health plans having an additional year to comply). Under the HITECH Act, and the enabling regulation of January 25, 2013, discussed later in this chapter, business associates of covered entities are required to comply with the Security Rule by September 23, 2013, and business associate agreements between a covered entity and its business associates have to be updated or amended to incorporate specific compliance responsibilities, in addition to the other satisfactory assurances regarding safeguarding the covered entity's ePHI.[10]

In Chapter 4, we examine each of the security standards and implementation specifications in detail. It is important to note the following key attributes of the Security Rule. Each workforce member in your practice should have a working knowledge of these attributes because they are the key components of your policies, procedures, actions, and assessments that will underpin your practice's security strategy and successful compliance efforts.

1. The Security Rule is a set of standards and implementation specifications that your practice, as a covered entity, must comply with by federal law. Your business associates, as of September 23, 2013, must comply with them, too.
2. The Security Rule standards are always required for compliance by your practice, while implementation specifications are either *required* or *addressable*.
3. The Security Rule is scalable, taking into consideration the size of your practice, and flexible, taking into consideration the structure of the practice, costs of security measures, and probability and criticality of potential risks (threats and vulnerabilities).
4. The Security Rule is reasonable and permits your practice to implement security safeguards that are appropriate.
5. The Security Rule is built on the key principles of availability, confidentiality, and integrity of patients' health information.
6. The Security Rule, with one exception,[11] is technology neutral: the choice of protection measures (inputs) is up to your practice, as long as the safeguard performance measures (outputs) are achieved.
7. The Security Rule is based on risk analysis and mitigation of risk: identifying potential vulnerabilities in and threats to the practice, and taking risk avoidance measures.
8. The Security Rule is built on a foundation of safeguarding ePHI, so maintaining the availability of electricity is a key factor.
9. The Security Rule formalizes many of the policies, procedures, actions, assessments, and documentation requirements that you likely use in your practice today.
10. Complying with the Security Rule is an investment in the future of your practice as a successful business.

Identifiers

Four identifiers are specified in the HIPAA administrative simplification standards:

- The National Employer Identifier,[12] with compliance required on July 30, 2004[13]
- The National Provider Identifier,[14] with compliance required on May 23, 2007[15]
- The National Health Plan Identifier (HPID),[16] with compliance required by November 5, 2014.[17] Covered entities must use the HPID in standard transactions by November 7, 2016.
- The National Individual Identifier (Congressional hold on development)[18]

Identifiers are numeric electronic addresses for participants in health care electronic exchange. To learn more about identifiers, visit the Centers for Medicare & Medicaid Services (CMS) Web site HIPAA—General Information at http://www.cms.gov/Regulations-and-Guidance/HIPAA-Administrative-Simplification/HIPAAGenInfo/index.html?redirect=/hipaageninfo/.

CHANGE IN FOCUS: ADMINISTRATIVE TO CLINICAL PROCESSES

In the early part of the first decade of the 21st century, the federal government initiated a fundamental shift in how it implemented health care policy, especially as it related to adoption of electronic processes. Previously, the federal government's focus was on administrative processes, using the authority of HIPAA administrative simplification. Although the federal government continued with its efforts to implement administrative simplification standards under the Administrative Procedure Act, the process was slow. The federal government also began implementing electronic *clinical* standards using a different approach.

In December 2002, the Bush administration began implementing the E-Government (E-Gov) initiatives, following the enactment of HR 2458, the E-Government Act of 2002.[19] In July 2003, then HHS Secretary Tommy Thompson announced two initiatives designed for "building a national electronic healthcare system that will allow patients and their doctors to assess their complete medical records anytime and anywhere they are needed."[20]

> First, the Secretary announced that the Department has signed an agreement with the College of American Pathologists (CAP) to license the College's standardized medical vocabulary system and make it available without charge throughout the U.S. This action opens the door to establishing a common medical language as a key element in building a unified electronic medical records system in the U.S.
>
> Secondly, the Secretary announced that HHS has commissioned the Institute of Medicine to design a standardized model of an electronic health record. The health care standards development organization known as HL7 has been asked to evaluate the model once it has been designed. HHS will share the standardized model

> record at no cost with all components of the U.S. health care system. The Department expects to have a model record ready in 2004.
>
> Today's announcements are part of the ongoing HHS effort to develop the National Health Information Infrastructure by encouraging and facilitating the widespread use of modern information technology to improve the nation's health care system.

Then, in May 2004, Thompson announced the appointment of David Brailer, MD, PhD,* as the first National Health Information Technology Coordinator to coordinate and accelerate US "health information technology efforts."[21]

In July 2004, Thompson initiated "a 10-year plan [known as the Decade of Health Information Technology (HIT), 2004–2014] to build a national electronic health information infrastructure in the United States" and outlined "four major collaborative goals" and "12 strategies for advancing and focusing future efforts."[22] We discuss these efforts in detail in our book *EHR Implementation: A Step-by-Step Guide for the Medical Practice,* 2nd Ed.[23]

In August 2006, the federal government marked the 10th anniversary of the enactment of HIPAA administrative simplification. The question then was, if the goals of HIPAA administrative simplification could not be accomplished within 10 years, how likely would it be that the nation could achieve the objectives relating to the Decade of HIT, ending in 2014?

While the federal government was emphasizing clinical initiatives, the standards groups and health care stakeholders were busy trying to solve a number of problems and barriers that impeded the smooth working of electronic transactions from a business perspective. We discuss these issues in the next chapter.

On August 22, 2008, HHS published two Notices of Proposed Rulemaking (NPRMs): one related to a change in version of the transaction standards, and the other related to a change in code set from ICD-9 to ICD-10. Four days before the end of George W. Bush's presidency, the Bush administration published in the *Federal Register* the final rules related to these changes. We discuss both the NPRMs and the final rules in the next chapter.

THE HITECH ACT

President Obama signed into law the American Recovery and Reinvestment Act of 2009 (ARRA), known as the "stimulus bill," on February 17, 2009. Included in this legislation was the Health Information Technology for Economic and Clinical Health (HITECH) Act. The HITECH Act comprises Title XIII (Health Information Technology) of Division A of ARRA (123 STAT. 226-279) and Title IV (Medicare and Medicaid Health Information Technology; Miscellaneous Medicare Provisions) of Division B of ARRA (123 STAT. 467-496).[24]

The HITECH Act provisions of ARRA in Title XIII include important changes in Subtitle D (Privacy), Section 13401 at 123 STAT. 260, that provide for federal regulation of business associates for the first time [emphasis added]:

* David Brailer wrote a Foreword to the second edition of *HIPAA Plain & Simple.*

(a) Application of Security Provisions.—Sections 164.308, 164.310, 164.312, and 164.316 of title 45, Code of Federal Regulations, **shall apply to a business associate of a covered entity in the same manner that such sections apply to the covered entity**. The additional requirements of this title that relate to security and that are made applicable with respect to covered entities shall also be applicable to such a business associate and shall be incorporated into the business associate agreement between the business associate and the covered entity.

(b) Application of Civil and Criminal Penalties.—In the case of a business associate that violates any security provision specified in subsection (a), sections 1176 and 1177 of the Social Security Act (42 U.S.C. 1320d–5, 1320d–6) **shall apply to the business associate with respect to such violation in the same manner such sections apply to a covered entity that violates such security provision**.

(c) Annual Guidance.—For the first year beginning after the date of enactment of this Act and annually thereafter, the Secretary of Health and Human Services shall, after consultation with stakeholders, annually issue guidance on the most effective and appropriate technical safeguards for use in carrying out the sections referred to in subsection (a) and the security standards in subpart C of part 164 of title 45, Code of Federal Regulations, including the use of standards 3002(b)(2)(B)(vi) of the Public Health Service Act, as added by section 13101 of this Act, as such provisions are in effect as of the date before the enactment of this Act.

Note that in subsection (a), business associates must apply the Security Rule in the same way that the rule applies to covered entities,[25] which we discuss later in this chapter. Also, note in subsection (b) that business associates are subject to penalties for noncompliance with the Security Rule in the same way that covered entities are, which we discuss later in this chapter. Finally, we also discuss guidance, mentioned in (c), later in this chapter.

Next, we discuss how the definition of business associate was modified in the January 25, 2013, final rule.

Final Rule Modification of Business Associate Definition

The January 25, 2013, final rule, often called the HIPAA Omnibus Rule,[26] modified the HIPAA definition of business associate in several ways. We start with the modified definition of business associate:[27]

(1) Except as provided in paragraph (4) of this definition, business associate means, with respect to a covered entity, a person who:

(i) On behalf of such covered entity or of an organized health care arrangement (as defined in this section) in which the covered entity participates, but other than in the capacity of a member of the workforce of such covered entity or arrangement, creates, receives, maintains, or transmits protected health information for a function or activity regulated by this subchapter, including claims processing or administration, data analysis, processing or administration, utilization review, quality assurance, patient safety activities listed at 42 CFR 3.20, billing, benefit management, practice management, and repricing; or

(ii) Provides, other than in the capacity of a member of the workforce of such covered entity, legal, actuarial, accounting, consulting, data aggregation (as defined in §164.501 of this subchapter), management, administrative, accreditation, or financial services to or for such covered entity, or to or for an organized health care arrangement in which the covered entity participates, where the provision of the service involves the disclosure of protected health information from such covered entity or arrangement, or from another business associate of such covered entity or arrangement, to the person.

(2) A covered entity may be a business associate of another covered entity.

(3) *Business associate* includes:

(i) A Health Information Organization, E-prescribing Gateway, or other person that provides data transmission services with respect to protected health information to a covered entity and that requires access on a routine basis to such protected health information.

(ii) A person that offers a personal health record to one or more individuals on behalf of a covered entity.

(iii) A subcontractor that creates, receives, maintains, or transmits protected health information on behalf of the business associate.

(4) *Business associate* does not include:

(i) A health care provider, with respect to disclosures by a covered entity to the health care provider concerning the treatment of the individual.

(ii) A plan sponsor, with respect to disclosures by a group health plan (or by a health insurance issuer or HMO with respect to a group health plan) to the plan sponsor, to the extent that the requirements of §164.504(f) of this subchapter apply and are met.

(iii) A government agency, with respect to determining eligibility for, or enrollment in, a government health plan that provides public benefits and is administered by another government agency, or collecting protected health information for such purposes, to the extent such activities are authorized by law.

(iv) A covered entity participating in an organized health care arrangement that performs a function or activity as described by paragraph (1)(i) of this definition for or on behalf of such organized health care arrangement, or that provides a service as described in paragraph (1)(ii) of this definition to or for such organized health care arrangement by virtue of such activities or services.

By no later than February 17, 2010, business associates were required statutorily to implement HIPAA Administrative Simplification Security Rule administrative, physical, and technical safeguards, based on having conducted a risk analysis; develop and implemented related policies, procedures, actions, and assessment; and comply with written documentation and workforce training requirements. Compliance, as stated in the portion of ARRA quoted above, "shall apply to a business associate of a covered entity in the same manner that such sections apply to the covered entity. The additional requirements of this title that relate to security and that are made applicable with respect to covered entities shall also be applicable to such a business associate and shall be incorporated into the business associate agreement between the business associate and the covered entity."[28]

Here are three key modifications in section 1 of the definition:

- "Individually identifiable health information" in the predecessor version—discussed in the second edition of *HIPAA Plain & Simple*—is modified to "protected health information" here. The reason for the modification, as stated by HHS, is that: "a business associate has no obligation under the HIPAA Rules with respect to individually identifiable health information that is not protected health information." 78 *Federal Register* 5574
- "Performs, or assists in the performance of an activity involving the use or disclosure of protected health information" in the predecessor version is modified to "creates, receives, maintains, or transmits protected health information." The reason for the modification, according to HHS, is "to clarify that a business associate includes an entity that 'creates, receives, maintains, or transmits' protected health information on behalf of a covered entity. The change is to make the definition more consistent with language at §164.308(b) of the Security Rule [the *Business associate contracts and other arrangements* standard] and §164.502(e) of the Privacy Rule [the *Disclosures to business associates* standard], as well as to clarify that entities that maintain or store protected health information on behalf of a covered entity are business associates, even if they do not actually view the protected health information." 78 *Federal Register* 5574
- The modified version includes a new type of activity, *patient safety activities,* performed by a Patient Safety Organization (PSO) as a business associate. The Patient Safety and Quality Improvement Act of 2005 (PSQIA) "provides that Patient Safety Organizations (PSOs) must be treated as business associates when applying the Privacy Rule. . . . A reporting provider may be a HIPAA covered entity and, thus, information reported to a PSO may include protected health information that the PSO may analyze on behalf of the covered provider. The analysis of such information is a patient safety activity for purpose of PSQIA and the Patient Safety Rule, 42 CFR 3.10, et seq. While the HIPAA Rules as written would treat a PSO as a business associate when the PSO was performing quality analyses and other activities on behalf of a covered health care provider, . . . this change to the definition of 'business associate' [is] to more clearly align the HIPAA and Patient Safety Rules." 78 *Federal Register* 5570

Section (2) in the modified version of the business associate definition is identical to (3) in the predecessor definition. An example is a health care clearinghouse in a business associate role with a health care provider.

We now turn our focus to the role of the "subcontractor" in section (3) (iii).[29] The January 25, 2013, final rule defines a subcontractor as a business associate, and as modified, §164.314(a)(2)(iii) of the Security Rule provides for the following (emphasis in bold added):

> (a) *Standard: Business associate contracts or other arrangements*. . . .
>
> (2) *Implementation specifications (Required)*. . . .
>
> (iii) *Business associate contracts with subcontractors.* **The requirements of paragraph (a)(2)(i) [Business associate contracts] and (a)(2)(ii) [Other arrangements] of this section apply to the contract or other**

arrangement between a business associate and subcontractor required by §164.308(b)(3) in the same manner as such requirements apply to contracts or other arrangements between a covered entity and business associate.

Under this final rule, the definition of subcontractor was added to 45 CFR 160.103 (Definitions), as follows: "*Subcontractor* means a person to whom a business associate has delegated a function, activity, or service, other than in the capacity of a member of the workforce of such business associate." [78 Federal Register 5689] Again, as a reminder, as also defined at 45 CFR 160.103, *person* means "a natural person, trust or estate, partnership, corporation, professional association or corporation, or other entity, public or private."

The final rule goes on to clarify further: "A subcontractor is then a business associate where that function, activity, or service involves the creation, receipt, maintenance, or transmission of protected health information," . . . and it "**makes clear that a covered entity is not required to enter into a contract or other arrangement with a business associate that is a subcontractor**" [78 Federal Register 5573] [emphasis added].

As for "satisfactory assurances" that a subcontractor will appropriately safeguard PHI, the final rule states:

> [C]overed entities must ensure that they obtain satisfactory assurances required by the Rules from their business associates, and business associates must do the same with regard to subcontractors, and so on, no matter how far "down the chain" the information flows. This ensures that individuals' health information remains protected by all parties that create, receive, maintain, or transmit the information in order for a covered entity to perform its health care functions. For example, a covered entity may contract with a business associate (contractor), the contractor may delegate to a subcontractor (subcontractor 1) one or more functions, services, or activities the business associate has agreed to perform for the covered entity that require access to protected health information, and the subcontractor may in turn delegate to another subcontractor (subcontractor 2) one or more functions, services, or activities it has agreed to perform for the contractor that require access to protected health information, and so on. Both the contractor and all of the subcontractors are business associates under the final rule to the extent they create, receive, maintain, or transmit protected health information. [78 Federal Register 5574]

Here are several things to remember about subcontractors:

- Subcontractors are business associates to the extent they create, receive, maintain, or transmit protected health information.
- Subcontractors are not business associates of covered entities, but rather of another business associate.
- If a subcontractor discovers a breach, the subcontractor reports it up the line through the hierarchy of subcontractors, if applicable, to the business associate that is the contractor to the covered entity, and it is the business associate contractor that reports the discovered breach to the covered entity.

Finally, with regard to business associate exclusions in the definition, in general, they have been part of the HIPAA rules, but three have been moved from other parts of the rules to the definition, and wording has been tightened or modified (eg, in (iii), *protected health information* has been substituted for *individually identifiable health information*).[30]

BREACH NOTIFICATION RULE[31]

Statutory Definition of Breach

The HITECH Act provided a statutory definition of a breach[32] as follows:

(1) BREACH.—
  (A) IN GENERAL.—The term "breach" means the unauthorized acquisition, access, use, or disclosure of protected health information which compromises the security or privacy of such information, except where an unauthorized person to whom such information is disclosed would not reasonably have been able to retain such information.
  (B) EXCEPTIONS.—The term "breach" does not include—
    (i) any unintentional acquisition, access, or use of protected health information by an employee or individual acting under the authority of a covered entity or business associate if—
      (I) such acquisition, access, or use was made in good faith and within the course and scope of the employment or other professional relationship of such employee or individual, respectively, with the covered entity or business associate; and
      (II) such information is not further acquired, accessed, used, or disclosed by any person; or
    (ii) any inadvertent disclosure from an individual who is otherwise authorized to access protected health information at a facility operated by a covered entity or business associate to another similarly situated individual at same facility; and
    (iii) any such information received as a result of such disclosure is not further acquired, accessed, used, or disclosed without authorization by any person.

Then, the HITECH Act specified that a breach required notification, which is triggered when there is an incident of "unauthorized acquisition, access, use, or disclosure of unsecured protected health information."[33] Notification must be accomplished "without unreasonable delay and in no case later than 60 calendar days after the discovery of a breach by the covered entity involved (or business associate involved in the case of a notification [to the covered entity following discovery of a breach])."[34]

January 25, 2013, Final Rule Definition of Breach

As required under the HITECH Act, HHS published the Breach Notification for Unsecured Protected Health Information interim final rule in the *Federal Register* on August 24, 2009.[35] The effective date of the interim final rule was September 23, 2009, with enforcement beginning for breaches occurring on or after February 22, 2010. The interim final rule's definition of breach included a "harm standard," which was discussed in the second edition of *HIPAA Plain &*

Simple. Then, on January 25, 2013, HHS published the final rule that modified the definition of breach and provisions related to notification, including eliminating the "harm standard" in favor of a more objective "probability standard." Here is the final rule definition of breach[36] with emphasis added:

> *Breach* means the acquisition, access, use, or disclosure of protected health information in a manner not permitted under subpart E [HIPAA Privacy Rule] of this part [45 CFR 164] which compromises the security or privacy of the protected health information.
>
> (1) Breach excludes:
>
> (i) Any unintentional acquisition, access, or use of protected health information by a workforce member or person acting under the authority of a covered entity or a business associate, if such acquisition, access, or use was made in good faith and within the scope of authority and does not result in further use or disclosure in a manner not permitted under subpart E of this part.
>
> (ii) Any inadvertent disclosure by a person who is authorized to access protected health information at a covered entity or business associate to another person authorized to access protected health information at the same covered entity or business associate, or organized health care arrangement in which the covered entity participates, and the information received as a result of such disclosure is not further used or disclosed in a manner not permitted under subpart E of this part.
>
> (iii) A disclosure of protected health information where a covered entity or business associate has a good faith belief that an unauthorized person to whom the disclosure was made would not reasonably have been able to retain such information.
>
> (2) Except as provided in paragraph (1) of this definition, an acquisition, access, use, or disclosure of protected health information in a manner not permitted under subpart E is presumed to be a breach unless the covered entity or business associate, as applicable, demonstrates that there is a low probability that the protected health information has been compromised based on a risk assessment of a least the following factors:
>
> (i) The nature and extent of the protected health information involved, including the types of identifiers and the likelihood of re-identification;
>
> (ii) The unauthorized person who used the protected health information or to whom the disclosure was made;
>
> (iii) Whether the protected health information was actually acquired or viewed; and
>
> (iv) The extent to which the risk to the protected health information has been mitigated.

In the event of a breach or an "impermissible use or disclosure" of unsecured protected health information that does not fall under one of the exclusions in (1) in the definition above, the language of which did not change from the interim final rule to the final rule, then a covered entity or business associate, as applicable, is obligated to conduct a risk assessment. The burden of proof is on the covered entity or business associate, as applicable, to document and demonstrate why an impermissible use or disclosure would fall under one of the breach exclusions. Based on the definition in the interim final rule, the risk assessment was to determine whether "'compromises the security or privacy of the protected health information' [meant] poses a significant risk of financial, reputational, or other harm to the individual."[37] Under the final rule, which modified and clarified the definition of breach and risk assessment, the purpose of the risk assessment changed to that outlined in paragraph (2) in the definition of breach above, namely, to demonstrate that there is "a low probability that the protected health information has been compromised" based on consideration of the specified factors in (2)(i) to (2)(iv)[38] that were added to the final rule definition of breach.

In the final rule, HHS elaborates on the change from the requirement in the interim final rule[39] [emphasis added]:

> First, we have added language to the definition of breach to clarify that an impermissible use or disclosure of protected health information is presumed to be a breach unless the covered entity or business associate, as applicable, demonstrates that there is a low probability that the protected health information has been compromised. . . . As a result, we have clarified our position that breach notification is necessary in **all situations** except those in which the covered entity or business associate, as applicable, demonstrates that there is a low probability that the protected health information has been compromised (or one of the other exceptions to the definition of breach applies).

A risk assessment is required for all situations involving an impermissible use or disclosure of protected health information to determine whether a breach notification is not necessary. The final rule does note that:

> a covered entity or business associate has the discretion to provide the required notifications following an impermissible use or disclosure of protected health information without performing a risk assessment. Because the final rule clarifies the presumption that a breach has occurred following *every* impermissible use or disclosure of protected health information, entities may decide to notify without evaluation of the probability that the protected health information has been compromised. [emphasis added]

The final rule also notes:

> Second, to further ensure that [the definition of breach and the risk assessment approach] is applied uniformly and objectively by covered entities and business associates, we have removed the [interim final rule] harm standard and modified the risk assessment to focus more objectively on the risk that the protected health information has been compromised. Thus, breach notification is not required under the final rule if a covered entity or business associate, as applicable, demonstrates through a risk assessment that there is a low probability that the protected health information has been compromised, rather than demonstrate that there is no significant risk of harm to the individual as was provided under the interim final rule. **The final rule also identifies the more objective factors covered entities and business associates must consider when performing a risk assessment to determine if the protected health information has been compromised and breach notification is necessary.** [emphasis added]

Limited Data Sets

The interim final rule definition of breach also included a notification exception for limited data sets based on a complicated rationale that we discussed in the second edition of *HIPAA Plain & Simple*. That exception has been removed, as the following from the final rule explains:[40]

> In addition to the removal of the harm standard and the creation of more objective factors to evaluate the probability that protected health information has been compromised, we have removed the exception for limited data sets that do not contain any dates of birth and zip codes. In the final rule, following the impermissible use of disclosure of any limited data set, a covered entity or business associate must perform a risk assessment that evaluates the factors discussed to determine if breach notification is not required.

Breach Notification Requirements

In the event of a breach, whether it be by a covered entity or by a business associate, we recommend that your organization access the OCR Web site titled Breach Notification Rule at http://www.hhs.gov/ocr/privacy/hipaa/administrative/breachnotificationrule/index.html and consult three sections for information: Breach Notification Requirements (including individual notice, media notice, notice to the Secretary, and notification by a business associate); Burden of Proof; and Instructions for Covered Entities to Submit Breach Notifications to the Secretary.

Here we examine briefly several modifications and clarifications related to notification. With regard to notification to individuals, the final rule did not modify the rules, but made the following clarification with respect to the implementation specification at §164.404(d), *Methods of individual notification*:

> In response to questions raised with respect to a breach at or by a business associate, we note that the covered entity ultimately maintains the obligation to notify affected individuals of the breach under §164.404 [*Notification to individuals*], although a covered entity is free to delegate the responsibility to the business associate that suffered the breach or to another of its business associates. . . . Covered entities and business associates should consider which entity is in the best position to provide notice to the individual, which may depend on various circumstances, such as the functions the business associate performs on behalf of the covered entity and which entity has the relationship with the individual.[41]

With regard to notification to media, the final rule made a minor change that aligns the definition of "State" (including American Samoa and Northern Mariana Islands) with HIPAA rules, and pointed out this caution:

> We also emphasize that posting a press release regarding a breach [involving 500 or more residents of a State or jurisdiction] of unsecured protected health information on the home page of the covered entity's Web site will not fulfill the obligation to provide notice to the media (although covered entities are free to post a press release regarding a breach on their Web site). To fulfill this obligation, notification, which may be in the form of a press release, must be provided directly to

prominent media outlets serving the State or jurisdiction where the affected individuals reside.[42]

Finally, with regard to notification to the Secretary of HHS, one modification focuses on breaches "discovered" in a calendar year as opposed to those that "occurred" in a calendar year. "The modification clarifies that covered entities are required to notify the Secretary of all breaches of unsecured protected health information affecting fewer than 500 individuals not later than 60 days after the end of the calendar year in which the breaches were 'discovered,' not in which the breaches 'occurred.'"[43]

HHS provided the following reminder in the final rule: "Although covered entities need only provide notification to the Secretary of breaches involving less than 500 individuals annually, they must still provide notification of such breaches to affected individuals without unreasonable delay and not later than 60 days after discovery of the breach pursuant to §164.404 [*Notification to individuals*]."[44] HHS also included another reminder for large breaches:

> With respect to breaches involving 500 or more individuals, we interpreted the term 'immediately' in the statute to require notification be sent to the Secretary concurrently with the notification sent to the individual under §164.404 (ie, without unreasonable delay but in no case later than 60 calendar days following discovery of a breach).[45]

GUIDANCE ON SECURING PROTECTED HEALTH INFORMATION

As discussed, Section 13402(h)(2) of the HITECH Act[46] required HHS to issue regulations to require covered entities under HIPAA and their business associates to provide notification in the case of breaches of unsecured PHI. HHS included in the August 24, 2009, interim final rule[47] an update of guidance that it had earlier published in the *Federal Register* on April 27, 2009,[48] to conform with HITECH Act provisions, which explained the meaning of "unsecured protected health information."[49] The guidance is related to the HHS and Federal Trade Commission (FTC) breach notification regulations[50] pertaining to unsecured PHI.

Here is the updated August 24, 2009, guidance, which is current as of this writing in late June 2013:

> (B) *Guidance Specifying the Technologies and Methodologies that Render Protected Health Information Unusable, Unreadable, or Indecipherable to Unauthorized Individuals*
>
> Protected health information (PHI) is rendered unusable, unreadable, or indecipherable to unauthorized individuals if one or more of the following applies:
>
> (a) Electronic PHI has been encrypted as specified in the HIPAA Security Rule by "the use of an algorithmic process to transform data into a form in which there is a low probability of assigning meaning without use of a confidential process or key"[51] and such confidential process or key that might enable decryption has not been breached. To avoid a breach of the confidential process or key, these decryption tools should be stored on a device or at a location separate from the data they are used to encrypt or

decrypt. The encryption processes identified below have been tested by the National Institute of Standards and Technology (NIST) and judged to meet this standard.

(i) Valid encryption processes for data at rest are consistent with NIST Special Publication 800-111, *Guide to Storage Encryption Technologies for End User Devices*[52]

(ii) Valid encryption processes for data in motion are those which comply, as appropriate, with NIST Special Publications 800-52, *Guidelines for the Selection and Use of Transport Layer Security (TLS) Implementations;* 800-77, *Guide to IPsec VPNs;* or 800-113, *Guide to SSL VPNs,* or others which are Federal Information Processing Standards (FIPS) 140-2 validated.[53]

(b) The media on which the PHI is stored or recorded has been destroyed in one of the following ways:

(i) Paper, film, or other hard copy media have been shredded or destroyed such that the PHI cannot be read or otherwise cannot be reconstructed. Redaction is specifically excluded as a means of data destruction.

(ii) Electronic media have been cleared, purged, or destroyed consistent with NIST Special Publication 800-88, *Guidelines for Media Sanitization,*[54] such that the PHI cannot be retrieved.

We provide excerpts here from the preamble to the April 27, 2009, guidance that is germane to securing electronic PHI through encryption.

> The term "unsecured protected health information" includes PHI in any form that is not secured through the use of a technology or methodology specified in this guidance. This guidance, however addresses methods for rendering PHI in paper or electronic form unusable, unreadable, or indecipherable to unauthorized individuals.
>
> Data comprising PHI can be vulnerable to a breach in any of the commonly recognized data states: "data in motion" (i.e., data that is moving through a network, including wireless transmission); "data at rest" (i.e., data that resides in databases, file systems, and other structured storage methods); "data in use" (i.e., data in the process of being created, retrieved, updated, or deleted); or "data disposed" (e.g., discarded paper records or recycled electronic media). . . .
>
> Encryption is one method of rendering electronic PHI unusable, unreadable, or indecipherable to unauthorized persons. The successful use of encryption depends upon two main features: The strength of the encryption algorithm and the security of the decryption key or process. The specification of encryption methods in this guidance includes the condition that the processes or keys that might enable decryption have not been breached.[55]

As we discuss in relation to the Security Rule in Chapter 4, and in particular with respect to the two addressable Technical Safeguard encryption implementation specifications, a covered entity or business associate must rely on outcomes of its risk analysis to determine whether encryption is necessary. In that risk analysis, the covered entity or business associate should evaluate potential risks and costs of breach of unsecured ePHI that becomes accessible to unauthorized users outside of the covered entity, whether *data at rest* or *data in motion*, which would trigger the January 25, 2013, final rule's breach notification provisions as previously discussed. If a covered entity or business associate does not encrypt ePHI, then it must document its decision and explain why this implementation specification does not apply. Even in the absence of exposure to an open network, a covered entity should consider, in its risk analysis, the costs and benefits of encrypting ePHI at rest on its closed electronic information system.

With expected increased use of electronic transactions in health care, such as e-prescribing, and electronic communications via e-mail and on mobile devices, such as smart phones and tablets, between a physician practice and a patient, or from physician to physician for treatment, most covered entities will be using open systems and will need encryption tools. We recommend that you contact your electronic information system hardware and software vendors for advice on encryption, and that you also consult the National Institute for Standards and Technology (NIST) Special Publication 800-53, Revision 4, *Security and Privacy Controls for Federal Information Systems and Organizations*, April 2013,[56] and NIST Special Publication 800-66, Revision 1, *An Introductory Resource Guide for Implementing the Health Insurance Portability and Accountability Act (HIPAA) Security Rule*, October 2008.[57] Please refer to Appendix C for additional resources on encryption requirements.

Finally, we close this section with the following from the January 25, 2013, final rule:

> Covered entities and business associates that implement the specified technologies and methodologies with respect to protected health information are not required to provide notifications in the event of a breach of such information—that is, the information is not considered "unsecured" in such cases.[58]
>
> We encourage covered entities and business associates to take advantage of the safe harbor provision of the breach notification rule by encrypting limited data sets and other protected health information pursuant to the Guidance. . . . If protected health information is encrypted pursuant to this guidance, then no breach notification is required following an impermissible use or disclosure of the information."[59]

ENFORCEMENT

On July 27, 2009, HHS Secretary Kathleen Sebelius delegated enforcement of the HIPAA Security Rule to the HHS Office for Civil Rights (OCR), which had HIPAA Privacy Rule enforcement authority since the compliance date of the HIPAA Privacy Rule, April 14, 2003.[60] Then, on October 30, 2009, HHS published in the *Federal Register* its interim final rule[61] that strengthened HIPAA enforcement under the civil financial penalty revisions enacted as part of the HITECH Act on February 17, 2009. These HITECH Act revisions "significantly increase the penalty amounts the Secretary may impose for violations of the HIPAA rules and encourage prompt corrective action," according to the HHS press release.[62] The interim final rule took effect on November 30, 2009, and OCR began to enforce the breach notification rule for notification violations of breaches that were discovered on or after February 22, 2010. Unified enforcement of the HIPAA Privacy Rule, Security Rule, and Breach Notification Rule and higher civil penalties increase the probability and severity of consequences for noncompliance with those rules.

Before enactment of the HITECH Act, civil penalties for HIPAA violations were $100 for each violation or $25,000 for all violations of the same provision in a calendar year.[63] Under the HITECH Act, penalties were markedly raised and have been divided into four tiers, with a maximum penalty of $1.5 million for all violations of an identical provision in a calendar year. That is a 60-fold increase over the previous maximum!

The tiered financial penalties are:

- $100 to $50,000 if the covered entity **did not know** and, by exercising reasonable diligence, would not have known, that it violated such provision.
- $1,000 to $50,000 if the violation was due to **reasonable cause**[64] and not to willful neglect.[65]
- $10,000 to $50,000 if the violation was due to **willful neglect** and was corrected as required.[66]
- $50,000 or more if the violation was due to **willful neglect** and was **not corrected** as required.

According to former OCR director Georgina Verdugo on October 30, 2009, when the interim final rule was published in the *Federal Register*,

> The Department's implementation of these HITECH Act enforcement provisions will strengthen the HIPAA protections and rights related to an individual's health information. . . . This strengthened penalty scheme will encourage health care providers, health plans and other health care entities required to comply with HIPAA to ensure that their compliance programs are effectively designed to prevent, detect and quickly correct violations of the HIPAA rules.[67]

The enforcement provisions were modified in the January 25, 2013, final rule.[68] Section 13410(a) of the HITECH Act [123 STAT. 271] added a new subsection (c) to section 1176 of the Social Security Act:

> (c) Noncompliance Due to Willful Neglect.—
>
> (1) In general.—A violation of a provision of this part due to willful neglect is a violation for which the Secretary is required to impose a penalty under subsection (a)(1) [General Penalty.—In General].
>
> (2) Required investigation.—For purposes of paragraph (1), the Secretary shall formally investigate any complaint of a violation of a provision of this part if a preliminary investigation of the facts of the complaint indicate such a possible violation due to willful neglect.

HHS made four modifications in the January 25, 2013, final rule to buttress investigations and imposition of penalties for willful neglect [78 Federal Register 5578]:

- *Complaint investigations.* The October 30, 2009, Enforcement Rule, at 45 CFR 160.306(c), "currently provides the Secretary with discretion to investigate HIPAA complaints through the use of the word 'may.' As a practical matter, however, the Department currently conducts a preliminary review of every complaint received and proceeds with the investigation in every eligible case where its preliminary review of the facts indicates a possible violation of the HIPAA Rules. Nonetheless, to implement section 1176(c)(2) [above], the Department [added] a new paragraph (1) [above] . . . to make clear that the Secretary **will investigate** any complaint filed under this section when a preliminary review of the facts indicates a possible violation due to willful neglect. [emphasis added] Under . . . §160.306(c)(2), the Secretary [has] continued discretion with respect to investigating any other complaints."

- *Compliance reviews.* "The Department [modified] §160.308 by adding a new paragraph (a) to provide that the Secretary will conduct a compliance review to determine whether a covered entity or business associate is complying with the applicable administrative simplification provision when a preliminary review of the facts indicates a possible violation due to willful neglect. Like §160.306(c) with respect to complaints [discussed above], the current §160.308(c) provides the Secretary with discretion to conduct compliance reviews. While section 13410(a) of the HITECH Act specifically mentions complaints and not compliance reviews with respect to willful neglect, the Department proposed to treat compliance reviews in the same manner because it believed doing so would strengthen enforcement with respect to potential violations of willful neglect and would ensure that investigations, whether or not initiated by a complaint, would be handled in a consistent manner. Under . . . §160.308(b), the Secretary [will] continue to have discretion to conduct compliance reviews in circumstances not indicating willful neglect."
- *Resolving investigations or compliance reviews.* "[G]iven the HITECH Act's requirement that the Secretary impose a penalty for any violation due to willful neglect, the Department proposed changes to §160.312, which [had required] the Secretary to attempt to resolve investigations or compliance reviews indicating noncompliance by informal means. The [July 14, 2010, Notice of Proposed Rule Making (NPRM)[69] provided] instead in §160.312(a) that the Secretary 'may' rather than 'will' attempt to resolve investigations or compliance reviews indicating noncompliance by informal means. This [modification in the final rule permits] the Department to proceed with a willful neglect violation determination as appropriate, while also permitting the Department to seek resolution of complaints and compliance reviews that did not indicate willful neglect violations by informal means (eg, where the covered entity or business associate did not know and by exercising reasonable diligence would not have known of a violation, or where the violation is due to reasonable cause)."[70]
- *Compliance cooperation.* "The Department proposed a conforming change to §160.304(a), which [had required] the Secretary to seek, to the extent practicable, the cooperation of covered entities in obtaining compliance with the HIPAA Rules. The [July 14, 2010,] NPRM [clarified] that the Secretary would continue to do so 'consistent with the provisions of this subpart' in recognition of the new HITECH Act requirement to impose a

civil money penalty for a violation due to willful neglect. While the Secretary often will still seek to correct indications of noncompliance through voluntary corrective action, there may be circumstances (such as circumstances indicating willful neglect), where the Secretary may proceed directly to formal enforcement."[71]

The final rule also spells out the factors considered in determining the amount of a civil money penalty.[72] At a high level, there are five primary factors, with subsidiary factors "consideration of which may include but is not limited to" spelled out at 45 CFR 160.408. The five primary factors are:

1. The nature and extent of the violation.
2. The nature and extent of the harm resulting from the violation.
3. The history of prior compliance with the administrative simplification provisions, including violations, by the covered entity or business associate.
4. The financial condition of the covered entity or business associate.
5. Such other matters as justice may require.

To see how these factors have been applied, examine the OCR Web site titled "Case Examples and Resolution Agreements" at http://www.hhs.gov/ocr/privacy/hipaa/enforcement/examples/index.html, and in the resolution agreements available at this site, pay particular to the consequences of noncompliance described in the corrective action plans.

Finally, with regard to enforcement, the HITECH Act granted state attorneys general the authority to enforce HIPAA rules by bringing civil actions on behalf of state residents in federal district court. Detailed information is available on the OCR Web site titled State Attorneys General at http://www.hhs.gov/ocr/privacy/hipaa/enforcement/sag.

The following discussion about a modification to 45 CFR 160.310(c)(3), adopted in the January 25, 2013, final rule, is relevant to the enforcement role of state attorneys general:[73]

> Section 160.310 requires that covered entities make information available to and cooperate with the Secretary during complaint investigations and compliance reviews. Section 160.310(c)(3) provides that any protected health information obtained by the Secretary in connection with an investigation or compliance review will not be disclosed by the Secretary, except as necessary for determining and enforcing compliance with the HIPAA Rules or as otherwise required by law. In the proposed rule, we proposed to modify this paragraph to also allow the Secretary to disclose protected health information if permitted under the Privacy Act at 5 U.S.C. 552a(b)(7). Section 5 U.S.C. 552a(b)(7) permits the disclosure of a record on an individual contained within a government system of records protected under the Privacy Act to another agency or instrumentality of any governmental jurisdiction within or under the control of the United States for a civil or criminal law enforcement activity if the activity is authorized by law and if the agency has made a written request to the agency that maintains the record. The proposed change would permit the Secretary to coordinate with other law enforcement agencies, such as the State Attorneys General pursuing civil actions to enforce the HIPAA Rules on behalf of State residents pursuant to section 13410(e) of the Act. . . .

> To facilitate cooperation between the Department and other law enforcement agencies, the final rule adopts the modifications to §160.310(c)(3) as proposed in the NPRM. . . . Further, the Department will be working closely with State Attorneys General to coordinate enforcement in appropriate cases, as provided under section 13410(e) of the HITECH Act. The Department will continue to update its web site as necessary and appropriate to maintain transparency with the public and the regulated community about these coordinated activities and its other enforcement actions and activities.

The OCR Web site titled State Attorneys General, referenced above, elaborates further:

> This new enforcement authority granted to State Attorneys General (SAG) by section 13410(e) of the HITECH Act will require significant coordination between OCR and SAG. OCR welcomes collaboration with SAG seeking to bring civil actions to enforce the HIPAA Privacy and Security Rules, and OCR will assist SAG in the exercise of this new enforcement authority. OCR will provide information upon request about pending or concluded OCR actions against covered entities or business associates related to SAG investigations. OCR will also provide guidance regarding the HIPAA statute, the HITECH Act, and the HIPAA Privacy, Security, and Enforcement Rules as well as the Breach Notification Rule.

Lastly, a companion OCR Web site, HIPAA Enforcement Training for State Attorneys General,[74] provides information on HIPAA training for state attorneys general. The OCR notes:

> OCR developed HIPAA Enforcement Training to help State Attorneys General and their staff use their new authority to enforce the HIPAA Privacy and Security Rules. The training course will aid State Attorneys General in investigating and seeking damages for HIPAA violations that affect residents of their states.[75]

We recommend that readers periodically visit the OCR enforcement Web site, http://www.hhs.gov/ocr/privacy/hipaa/enforcement/index.html, for additional information and updates.

IMPORTANCE OF ACHIEVING COMPLIANCE

As you begin to examine in the following chapters the details of the HIPAA administrative simplification transaction and code set standards and the Privacy Rule and Security Rule modified by the HITECH Act in the January 25, 2013, final rule, we would like you to always keep in mind the three fundamental properties[76] of privacy and security of PHI in oral, hard copy, or electronic form:

- *Confidentiality* is the property that data or information is not made available or disclosed to unauthorized persons or processes.
- *Integrity* is the property that data or information has not been altered or destroyed in an unauthorized manner.
- *Availability* is the property that data or information is accessible and usable upon demand by an authorized person.

We also would like you to keep in mind that in the years ahead, there will be additional regulatory activity related to enabling the administrative simplification provisions of the HITECH Act, the Patient Protection and Affordable Care Act (discussed at the end of Chapter 2), and perhaps other federal legislative initiatives. You also should be alert to any changes in the guidance pertaining to encryption methods for *data at rest* and *data in motion*, and to destruction methods of electronic and hard copy media for securing PHI. You can do so by visiting the OCR Web site titled Guidance to Render Protected Health Information Unusable, Unreadable, or Indecipherable to Unauthorized Individuals at http://www.hhs.gov/ocr/privacy/hipaa/administrative/breachnotificationrule/brguidance.html.

In addition, practices should prepare and expect to be busy with clinical initiatives relating to the HITECH Act, such as the financial incentives for adoption and meaningful use of certified electronic health record (EHR) technology.[77] Both the meaningful use criteria and the EHR certification programs are works in progress, and current information is available at the Centers for Medicare & Medicaid Services (CMS) Web site at http://www.cms.gov/Regulations-and-Guidance/Legislation/EHRIncentivePrograms/index.html.

One of the meaningful use objectives is "Protect electronic health information created or maintained by the certified EHR technology through the implementation of appropriate technical capabilities," and the meaningful use measure is "Conduct or review a security risk analysis per 45 CFR 164.308(a)(1) [discussed in Chapter 4] and implement security updates as necessary and correct identified security deficiencies as part of its risk management process."[78] In addition to conducting a risk assessment, there are eight security-related criteria within the objective-measure category that mirror provisions in the HIPAA Security Rule and with which eligible professionals must attest compliance as part of the qualification process for receiving incentive payments for adoption of certified EHR technology.[79] We recommend that practices pay particular attention to these criteria as part of their overall compliance with the HIPAA Security Rule.

Finally, as outlined above in the discussion on guidance, there are available technologies and methods for securing hard copy and/or electronic PHI, which will provide a safe harbor from breach notification requirements and avoid potential reputational, financial, and other costs associated with having to publicly report a breach due to loss, theft, or other misuse of PHI. The Ponemon Institute *2013 Cost of Data Breach Study: Global Analysis*, released in May 2013, estimates that the health care industry's breach cost is $233 per record compromised.[80] One breach of 500 records would cost an average of $116,500, which would seriously dent any return on investment. We have reproduced from this study as Figure 1.2 a depiction of cost centers from breach discovery through mitigation as required under HIPAA rules. In a June 2013 interview, Larry Ponemon of the Ponemon Institute stated: "We also know it helps an organization, from a structure point of view, that regulations like HIPAA and some of the financial-service regulations provide prescriptive guidance—steps that you can take. And as organizations learn to do this, they probably become even better and more efficient at managing the cost of the data breach."[81] The following chapters on transaction and code set, privacy, and security standards will give your organization the information it needs to understand what is required to achieve compliance and mitigate the likelihood of experiencing potentially costly noncompliant electronic transactions, privacy breaches, or security incidents.

FIGURE 1-2

Ponemon Institute Depiction of Breach Cost Centers

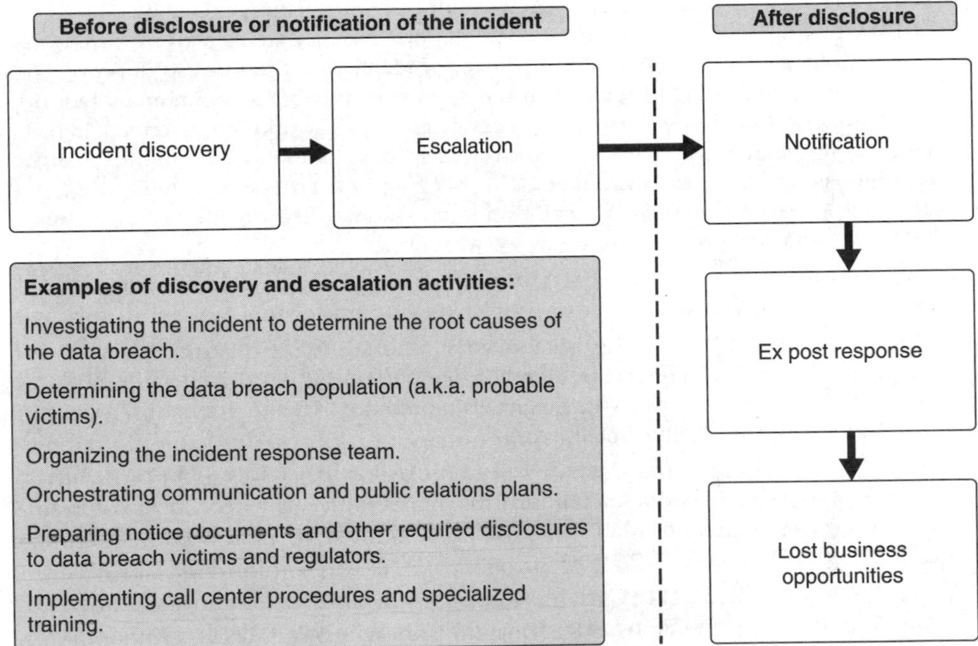

The Ponemon study identified three types of costs associated with cost centers:

- "Direct cost-direct expense outlay to accomplish a given activity
- "Indirect cost—amount of time, effort, and other organizational resources spent, but not as a direct cash outlay
- "Opportunity cost—cost resulting from lost business opportunities as a consequence of negative reputation effects after the breach has been reported to victims (and publicly revealed to the media."

Reproduced with permission from Ponemon Institute, Figure 21 from *2013 Cost of Data Breach Study: Global Analysis*, May 2013, p.22. Benchmark research sponsored by Symantec, independently conducted by the Ponemon Institute, Traverse City, MI.

ENDNOTES

1. Hartman, M., et al., National Health Spending In 2011: Overall Growth Remains Low, But Some Payers and Services Show Signs of Acceleration, *Health Affairs*, January 2013, v. 32, n. 1, pp. 87-99. Also, see the May 2013 "Tackling the Cost Conundrum" issue of *Health Affairs* (v. 32, n. 5) at http://www.healthaffairs.org.
2. Today, WEDI is a vibrant organization of more than 400 members that continues to work through these issues to further the adoption of electronic technology and to achieve greater efficiency for electronic health care information exchange. In early 2013, WEDI initiated the *2013 WEDI Report* project, a 20th anniversary update of its original report (see note 3), and a roadmap for identifying priorities to improve health care delivery and lower cost in the years ahead. Using a common analytical framework, the work of the project is conducted in four workgroups: enhancing patient engagement, alternative payment models, data harmonization and exchange, and innovative electronic encounters. The *2013 WEDI Report* is expected to be released in December 2013. You can find information on the organization and the *2013 WEDI Report* project at http://www.wedi.org.
3. The *1993 WEDI Report* is available at http://www.wedi.org/docs/public-policy/1993-wedi-report.pdf?sfvrsn=0.
4. When we refer to HIPAA in this book, we are referring to the relatively short 14-page Subtitle F, Administrative Simplification, of Title II of Public Law 104–191, enacted on August 21, 1996, which is available at http://www.hhs.gov/ocr/privacy/hipaa/administrative/statute/index.html.
5. Please see the discussion in Chapter 2 about enhanced objectives and new operating rule provisions regarding administrative simplification that were included in the Patient Protection and Affordable Care Act, enacted on March 23, 2010, as Public Law 111–148 (124 STAT. 119-1024).
6. Since passage of the HITECH Act, enacted on February 17, 2009, as part of the American Recovery and Reinvestment Act (the "stimulus bill"), the federal government has relied more on interim final rules in an effort to enable the privacy and security provisions of the HITECH Act more quickly than the typical Notice of Proposed Rulemaking and Final Rule procedures of the federal Administrative Procedure Act.
7. A standard is a requirement, and a rule is a document that includes the standards in the context of HIPAA administrative simplification.
8. The ASC X12N Insurance Subcommittee prepared documentation on the transaction standards. We identify the documentation in use since January 1, 2012 (Version 5010 Technical Reports Type 3), in Chapter 2. Washington Publishing Company (WPC) publishes the Version 5010 documentation, which can be accessed at http://www.wpc-edi.com.
9. To learn more about the DSMO process, visit http://www.hipaa-dsmo.org/.
10. For information on how the Final Rule modified business associate agreement provisions, see the Office for Civil Rights (OCR) Web site, published January 25, 2013, titled Business Associate Contracts: Sample Business Associate Agreement Provisions, at http://www.hhs.gov/ocr/privacy/hipaa/understanding/coveredentities/contractprov.html.
11. The one exception is that if your practice chooses to secure its ePHI through encryption, it must use the encryption technologies and methodologies specified in

the guidance issued by HHS in the August 24, 2009, interim final rule pertaining to Breach Notification published in the *Federal Register*. We discuss this further later in this chapter and, with respect to two Technical Safeguard encryption implementation specifications, in Chapter 4.

12. The Employer Identification Number (EIN), issued by the Internal Revenue Service (IRS), was selected as the identifier for employers.
13. Small health plans had an additional year to comply, until August 1, 2005.
14. The National Provider Identifier (NPI) is a unique identification number for covered health care providers. Covered health care providers and all health plans and health care clearinghouses must use NPIs in administrative and financial transactions adopted under HIPAA. The NPI is a 10-digit, intelligence-free numeric identifier (10-digit number), meaning that NPIs do not carry other information about health care providers, such as states in which they live or their medical specialties. NPIs must be used in lieu of legacy provider identifiers in the HIPAA transaction standards. Covered providers also must share their NPI with other providers, health plans, clearinghouses, and any entity that may need it for billing purposes. A September 5, 2012, final rule extended the NPI: "This final rule also specifies the circumstances under which an organization covered health care provider must require certain non-covered individual health care providers who are prescribers to obtain and disclose a National Provider Identifier (NPI)." See Table 1.1 note xxi for source citation (77 *Federal Register* 54664).
15. Small health plans had an additional year to comply, until May 23, 2008.
16. Please see the discussion in Chapter 2 about administrative simplification provisions of the Patient Protection and Affordable Care Act, enacted on March 23, 2010, with the statutory effective date deadline of October 1, 2012, for the *unique health plan identifier*. A September 5, 2012, final rule adopted a standard for the health plan identifier: "This final rule adopts the standard for a national unique health plan identifier (HPID) and establishes requirements for the implementation of the HPID. In addition, it adopts a data element that will serve as another entity identifier (OEID), or an identifier for entities that are not health plans, health care providers, or individuals, but that need to be identified in standard transactions." See Table 1.1 note xxi for source citation (77 *Federal Register* 54664). Also, see the Centers for Medicare and Medicaid Services (CMS) document titled Health Plan (HPID) and Other Entity Identifier (OEID) applications available in the Health Plan and Other Entity Enumeration System (HPOES) beginning March 29, 2013! that is available at http://www.cms.gov/Regulations-and-Guidance/HIPAA-Administrative-Simplification/Affordable-Care-Act/Health-Plan-Identifier.html.
17. Small health plans have until November 5, 2015, to comply.
18. The National Individual Identifier is controversial. Congress has a long-standing hold on any regulatory action on this identifier. Prior to enactment of HIPAA, the de facto individual identifier had been the Social Security number—which is the source of controversy about requiring it as a standard. Since the enactment of HIPAA, a number of states have restricted the use of the Social Security number as an identifier in matters other than Social Security, and large health plans have developed unique individual identifiers for their members as a workaround.
19. Visit the National Archives site for more information on the E-Government Act at http://www.archives.gov/about/laws/egov-act-section-207.html.

20. HHS, "HHS Launches New Efforts to Promote Paperless Healthcare System," news release, July 1, 2003, which is available at http://archive.hhs.gov/news/press/2003pres/20030701.html.
21. HHS, "Secretary Thompson, Seeking Fastest Possible Results, Names First Health Information Technology Coordinator," news release, May 6, 2004, which is available at http://archive.hhs.gov/news/press/2004pres/20040506.html.
22. HHS, The Decade of Health Information Technology: Delivering Consumer-Centric and Information-Rich Healthcare, fact sheet, Wednesday, July 21, 2004. Available at http://archive.hhs.gov/news/press/2004pres/20040721.html.
23. See C. P. Hartley and E. D. Jones III, EHR Implementation: A Step-by-Step Guide for the Medical Practice, 2nd ed., Chicago, IL: American Medical Association, 2012.
24. ARRA, as signed by President Obama, is available at http://www.gpo.gov:80/fdsys/pkg/PLAW-111publ5/pdf/PLAW-111publ5.pdf.
25. Application of the Security Rule to business associates of covered entities is a significant compliance change. Prior to the change, if a covered entity was aware of a breach involving a business associate, then the covered entity could just terminate the contract if the breach was not remedied. Responsibility and liability rested with the covered entity. Now, with the change in the HITECH Act privacy provisions, the business associate, as well as the covered entity, has responsibility and direct liability for a breach.
26. HHS, Office of the Secretary, 45 CFR Parts 160 and 164: Modifications to the HIPAA Privacy, Security, Enforcement, and Breach Notification Rules Under the Health Information Technology for Economic and Clinical Health Act and the Genetic Information Nondiscrimination Act; Other Modifications to the HIPAA Rules; Final Rule, *Federal Register*, v. 78, n. 17, January 25, 2013, pp. 5566-5702. Citations to this document hereafter are in the standard reference format of 78 *Federal Register* <page(s)> (eg, 78 *Federal Register* 5566). This document is available at http://www.gpo.gov/fdsys/pkg/FR-2013-01-25/pdf/2013-01073.pdf.
27. 45 CFR 160.103, at 78 *Federal Register* 5688.
28. For information on how the Final Rule modified business associate agreement provisions, see the Office for Civil Rights (OCR) Web site, published January 25, 2013, titled Business Associate Contracts: Sample Business Associate Agreement Provisions, at http://www.hhs.gov/ocr/privacy/hipaa/understanding/coveredentities/contractprov.html.
29. An analysis of (3)(i) and (3)(ii) can be found in the February 11, 2013, and February 12, 2013, postings, respectively, at http://www.hipaa.com (Ed Jones, HIPAA Final Rule: Modification of Business Associate Definition, Part (3), February 11, 2013, and HIPAA Final Rule: Modification of Business Associate Definition, Part (4)—Personal Health Record Vendor, February 12, 2013).
30. 78 *Federal Register* 5574. For further explanation, see the February 14, 2013, posting at http://www.hipaa.com (Ed Jones, HIPAA Final Rule: Modification of Business Associate Definition, Part (6)—Exceptions).
31. 123 STAT. 258. Additional information and updates on breach notification are available at the OCR Web site at http://www.hhs.gov/ocr/privacy/hipaa/administrative/breachnotificationrule/index.html.
32. 123 STAT. 258.
33. See 123 STAT. 260-263.

34. 123 STAT. 261.

35. Department of Health and Human Services, Office of the Secretary, 45 Parts 160 and 164: Breach Notification for Unsecured Protected Health Information; Interim Final Rule, *Federal Register*, v. 74, n. 162, August 24, 2009, pp. 42740-42770. Citations to this document hereafter are in the standard reference format of 74 *Federal Register* <page(s)> (eg, 74 *Federal Register* 42740).

36. 45 CFR 164.402, at 78 *Federal Register* 5695.

37. 78 *Federal Register* 5639.

38. A detailed examination of these risk assessment factors is available in the January 29, 2013, posting by Ed Jones titled HIPAA Final Rule: Breach Risk Assessment Factors for 'Probability Standard' at http://www.hipaa.com.

39. 78 *Federal Register* 5641, 5643.

40. 78 *Federal Register* 5644.

41. 78 *Federal Register* 5650-5651.

42. 78 *Federal Register* 5653.

43. 78 *Federal Register* 5654.

44. Ibid.

45. 78 *Federal Register* 5653.

46. 123 STAT. 263.

47. 74 *Federal Register* 42740-42770.

48. Department of Health and Human Services, Office of the Secretary, 45 CFR Parts 160 and 164: Guidance Specifying the Technologies and Methodologies That Render Protected Health Information Unusable, Unreadable, or Indecipherable to Unauthorized Individuals for Purposes of the Breach Notification Requirements under Section 13402 of Title XIII (Health Information Technology for Economic and Clinical Health Act) of the American Recovery and Reinvestment Act of 2009; Guidance and Request for Information, *Federal Register*, v. 74, n. 79, April 27, 2009, pp. 19006-19010.

49. This definition was modified in the January 25, 2013, final rule: "Unsecured protected health information means protected health information that is not rendered unusable, unreadable, or indecipherable to unauthorized persons through the use of a technology or methodology specified by the Secretary in the guidance issued under section 13402(h)(2) of Public Law 111-5." 45 CFR 164.402, at 78 *Federal Register* 5695.

50. Federal Trade Commission, 16 CFR Part 318; Health Breach Notification Rule: Final Rule, *Federal Register*, v. 74, n. 163, August 25, 2009, pp. 42962-42982. "The rule requires vendors of personal health records and related entities to notify consumers when the security of their individually identifiable health information has been breached." 74 *Federal Register* 42962. Full compliance was required by February 22, 2010.

51. 45 CFR 164.304, definition of "encryption."

52. Available at http://csrc.nist.gov; NIST Roadmap plans include the development of security guidelines for enterprise-level storage devices, and such guidelines will be considered in updates to this guidance, when available.

53. Available at http://csrc.nist.gov.

54. Ibid.

55. 74 *Federal Register* 19008-19009.
56. Available at http://nvlpubs.nist.gov/nistpubs/SpecialPublications/NIST.SP.800-53r4.pdf; includes updates as of May 7, 2013.
57. Available at http://csrc.nist.gov/publications/nistpubs/800-66-Rev1/SP-800-66-Revision1.pdf.
58. 78 *Federal Register* 5639.
59. 78 *Federal Register* 5644.
60. Department of Health and Human Services, Office of the Secretary, Office for Civil Rights; Delegation of Authority, *Federal Register*, v. 74, n. 148, August 4, 2009, p. 38630. Available at http://www.hhs.gov/ocr/privacy/hipaa/administrative/security-rule/srdelegation.pdf.
61. Department of Health and Human Services, Office of the Secretary, 45 CFR Part 160: HIPAA Administrative Simplification: Enforcement; Interim Final Rule, *Federal Register*, v. 74, n. 209, October 30, 2009, pp. 56123-56131. Available at http://www.hhs.gov/ocr/privacy/hipaa/administrative/enforcementrule/enfifr.pdf.
62. HHS Strengthens HIPAA Enforcement, press release, October 30, 2009, which is available at http://www.hhs.gov/news/press/2009pres/10/20091030a.html.
63. 74 *Federal Register* 56131.
64. Reasonable cause is defined as "an act or omission in which a covered entity or business associate knew, or by exercising reasonable diligence would have known, that the act or omission violated an administrative simplification provision, but in which the covered entity or business associate did not act with willful neglect." 45 CFR 160.401, at 78 *Federal Register* 5691.
65. Willful neglect is defined as "conscious, intentional failure or reckless indifference to the obligation to comply with the administrative simplification provision violated." 45 CFR 160.401.
66. "For a violation in which it is established that the violation was due to willful neglect and was corrected during the 30-day period beginning on the first date the covered entity liable for the penalty knew, or by exercising reasonable diligence, would have known that the violation occurred." 74 *Federal Register* 56131.
67. HHS Strengthens HIPAA Enforcement, press release, October 30, 2009, which is available at http://www.hhs.gov/news/press/2009pres/10/20091030a.html.
68. 78 *Federal Register* 5578.
69. Department of Health and Human Services, Office of the Secretary, 45 CFR Parts 160 and 164: Modifications to the HIPAA Privacy, Security, and Enforcement Rules Under the Health Information Technology for Economic and Clinical Health Act; Notice of Proposed Rulemaking, Federal Register, v. 75, n. 134, July 14, 2010, pp. 40867-40924. This document is available at http://edocket.access.gpo.gov/2010/pdf/2010-16718.pdf.
70. 78 *Federal Register* 5578.
71. Ibid.
72. 45 CFR 160.408, at 78 *Federal Register* 5691.
73. 78 *Federal Register* 5579.
74. See http://www.hhs.gov/ocr/privacy/hipaa/enforcement/sag/sagmoreinfo.html.
75. OCR, "State Attorneys General," available at http://www.hhs.gov/ocr/privacy/hipaa/enforcement/sag.

76. These definitions are from 45 CFR 164.304.

77. On July 28, 2010, HHS published two final rules in the *Federal Register* pertaining to the HITECH Act EHR incentive programs and EHR certification standards and criteria: Department of Health and Human Services, Centers for Medicare & Medicaid Services (CMS), 42 CFR Parts 412, 413, 422, and 495: Medicare and Medicaid Programs; Electronic Health Record Incentive Program; Final Rule, *Federal Register*, v. 75, n. 144, July 28, 2010, pp. 44313-44588, which is available at http://edocket.access.gpo.gov/2010/pdf/2010-17207.pdf, and Department of Health and Human Services, Office of the Secretary (on behalf of the Office of the National Coordinator for Health Information Technology [ONC]), 45 CFR Part 170: Health Information Technology: Initial Set of Standards, Implementation Specifications, and Certification Criteria for Electronic Health Record Technology; Final Rule, *Federal Register*, v. 75, n. 144, July 28, 2010, pp. 44589-44654, which is available at http://edocket.access.gpo.gov/2010/pdf/2010-17210.pdf. Citations to these documents hereafter are in the standard reference format of 75 *Federal Register* <page(s)> (eg, 75 *Federal Register* 44313).

78. 75 *Federal Register* 44617.

79. See 45 CFR 170.302(o)-(v) and discussion related to those security certification criteria at 75 *Federal Register* 44652 and 44616-44623, respectively.

80. The 2013 Ponemon study is available at https://www4.symantec.com/mktginfo/whitepaper/053013_GL_NA_WP_Ponemon-2013-Cost-of-a-Data-Breach-Report_daiNA_cta72382.pdf. The health care industry cost estimate on page 6 of this report is close in magnitude to estimates we reported in the second edition of *HIPAA Plain & Simple*.

81. Eric Chabrow, Regulations' Impact on Data Breach Costs: Analyzing Latest Ponemon/Symantec Cost of Data Breach Study, June 11, 2013, which is available at http://www.bankinfosecurity.com/interviews/data-breach-i-1953.

chapter 2

Transactions and Code Sets

This chapter describes the HIPAA transaction standards and code sets in effect for covered entities from mid-September 2013 and those that will be modified in the next several years, including the code set conversion from the *International Classification of Diseases, Ninth Revision, Clinical Modification* (ICD-9-CM) to the *International Classification of Diseases, Tenth Revision, Clinical Modification* (ICD-10-CM) and *International Classification of Diseases, Tenth Revision, Procedure Coding System* (ICD-10-PCS) for diagnostic codes for all covered entities and for procedure codes for inpatient encounters on October 1, 2014, and the systematic conversion of standard transactions to operating rules through December 31, 2015. We also highlight the Accredited Standards Committee (ASC) X12N Version 5010 transaction standard, with which compliance has been required since January 1, 2012. It is imperative that physician practices prepare now for implementation of forthcoming transaction and ICD-10-CM/PCS changes by developing an implementation strategy with their software vendors and health care clearinghouses for testing standard electronic transaction operating rules and ICD-10-CM diagnostic codes with trading partners. Physician practices will continue to use Current Procedural Terminology, 4th Edition (CPT-4) and Healthcare Common Procedure Coding System (HCPCS) codes for procedures.

What You Will Learn in This Chapter

In this chapter you will learn about the Version 5010 transaction standards, with which compliance was required by January 1, 2012, and where to acquire related documentation. You also will learn that there are two broad categories of external code sets used in the standard transactions: medical and nonmedical. You will see a brief description of each. Many of these code sets are used in more than one of the ASC X12N standard transactions. You are not expected to memorize these external code sets, but it is important to know what they are, how they are defined and used, and where to find them. In Table 2.3, you will see a cross-tabulation of code sets by transaction standard for Version 5010. ICD-10-CM external codes are included, but physician practices and other covered entities are not required to comply with them until October 1, 2014. The Department of Health and Human Services (HHS) has indicated that there will be no tolerance for ICD-10-CM noncompliance after the compliance date of October 1, 2014.

Key Terms

- Code set
- Code set maintaining organization
- Compliance date
- Data content
- Data element
- Data set
- Descriptor
- Operating rules
- Standard transaction

HIPAA Administrative Simplification was enacted in August 1996. In the years that followed, the federal government promulgated transaction standards and code sets, as well as privacy, security, identifier, claim attachment, and enforcement standards, which we briefly discussed in Chapter 1. In this chapter, we examine in detail transaction standards and code sets and how they apply to the physician practice.

We discussed the 4010/4010A transaction and code set standards in our earlier books, including the first and second editions of *HIPAA Plain & Simple.*[1] In this book, we outline the Version 5010 transaction and code set standards, with which compliance was required on January 1, 2012, and the ICD-10-CM standard, with which compliance will be required on October 1, 2014.

TRANSACTION STANDARDS AND CODE SET STANDARDS

The Centers for Medicare and Medicaid Services (CMS) provides an explanation of transaction standards and code set standards, which was last updated on April 17, 2013:

> Transactions are electronic exchanges involving the transfer of information between two parties for specific purposes. For example, a health care provider will send a claim to a health plan to request payment for medical services. The Health Insurance Portability & Accountability Act of 1996 (HIPAA) named certain types of organizations as covered entities, including health plans, health care clearinghouses, and certain health care providers. In the HIPAA regulations, the Secretary of Health and Human Services (HHS) adopted certain standard transactions for Electronic Data Interchange (EDI) of health care data. These transactions are: claims and encounter information, payment and remittance advice, claims status, eligibility, enrollment and disenrollment, referrals and authorizations, coordination of benefits and premium payment. Under HIPAA, if a covered entity conducts one of the adopted transactions electronically, it must use the adopted standard—either from ASC X12N or NCPDP (for certain pharmacy transactions). Covered entities must adhere to the content and format requirements of each transaction. Under HIPAA, HHS also adopted specific code sets for diagnoses and procedures to be used in all transactions. The HCPCS (Ancillary Services/Procedures), CPT-4 (Physician Procedures), CDT (Dental Terminology), ICD-9-CM (Diagnosis and Hospital Inpatient

Procedures), ICD-10-CM/PCS (as of October 1, 2014), and NDC (National Drug Code) codes, with which providers and health plans are familiar, are the adopted code sets for procedures, diagnoses, and drugs. Finally, HHS adopted standards for unique identifiers for employers and providers, which also must be used in all transactions.[2]

TRANSACTION STANDARDS

The overarching message with regard to HIPAA transaction standards is that if a covered entity is sending or receiving *administrative* electronic transactions that relate to the claims process, it must use a standard format.

What this means to health plans is:

- Health plans must send and receive standard transactions when requested by a covered entity.
- Health plans may not delay or reject any standard transaction solely because it is standard.
- Health plans may not reject standard transactions that contain situational data elements not used by the health plan.
- Health plans may use clearinghouses as business associates to accept standard transactions from other covered entities.

What this means to physician practices is:

- If your practice conducts business using electronic transactions, you must use the applicable standard transactions.[3]

Compliance with the transaction and code set standard was required on October 16, 2003.[4] In understanding the HHS requirement for Version 5010 compliance on January 1, 2012, and ICD-10-CM compliance on October 1, 2014, it is important to look at what happened before and after the 2003 compliance date. In July 2003, CMS determined that covered entities likely would not be compliant by the October 16, 2003, date.[5] On August 4, 2005, CMS announced that it "[would] not process incoming non-HIPAA-compliant electronic Medicare claims" after October 1, 2005. In its announcement, it reported:

> As of June 2005 only about 0.5 percent of Medicare fee-for-service providers submitted non-HIPAA-compliant electronic claims. The highest rate of non-complaint claims as of May [2005] was from clinical laboratories, 1.72 percent. Only 1.45 percent of claims from hospitals were non-compliant and 0.45 percent from physicians. The high percentage among all provider types and sizes shows that everyone can become compliant. . . . The law required all payers to conduct HIPAA-compliant transactions no later than Oct. 16, 2003. However, only about 31 percent of Medicare claims were compliant at that time. Other payers had even lower numbers of compliant claims.[6]

As you will see in the discussion of Version 5010 and ICD-10-CM that follows, HHS believes that there is—and has been since 2003—sufficient time for covered entities to increase the use of the electronic transaction standards and code sets and to achieve compliance.

Need for Transaction and Code Set Modifications

On September 26, 2007, the National Committee on Vital and Health Statistics (NCVHS) made the following recommendations to then HHS Secretary Michael Leavitt: "The Secretary should expedite the development and issuance of a Notice of Proposed Rulemaking (NPRM) to adopt the ASC X12N Version 5010 suite of transactions."[7] The NPRM was published in the *Federal Register* on August 22, 2008,[8] allowing 60 days for public comment, and the final rule was published in the *Federal Register* on January 16, 2009.[9] You will see in the next section that the proposed and final rules for ICD-10-CM were contiguous to the proposed and final Version 5010 rules, respectively, because the use of ICD-10-CM requires Version 5010. Below, we discuss both the proposed and final ICD-10-CM rulings.

The final Version 5010 rule required all covered entities to use Version 5010 standards:

> Except as otherwise provided in this part, if a covered entity conducts, with another covered entity that is required to comply with a transaction standard adopted under this part (or within the same covered entity), using electronic media, a transaction for which the Secretary has adopted a standard under this part, the covered entity must conduct the transaction as a standard transaction.[10]

For physician practices, these six typical electronic transaction standards are covered:

- Health Care Claim: Professional (837)[11]
- Health Care Eligibility Benefit Inquiry and Response (270/271)[12]
- Health Care Services Review—Request for Review and Response (278)[13]
- Health Care Claim Status Request and Response (276/277)[14]
- Health Care Claim Payment/Advice (835)[15]
- Coordination of Benefits Information[16]

The NPRM explained why the transaction standards that were in place since October 2003 were being modified:

> In addition to technical issues and business developments necessitating consideration of the new versions of the standards, there remain a number of unresolved issues that had been identified by the industry early in the implementation period for the first set of standards, and those issues were never addressed through regulation.[17]

The focus in the following discussion is on the effect of those concerns on two modified standards because they have implications for policies and procedures in your practice that, over the next five years, may substantially enhance cash flow and reduce cost.[18] These two standards are:

- Health Care Claim Payment/Advice (835)
- Health Care Claim Status Request and Response (276/277)

Think about the effect on your practice of receiving your remittances and payments more quickly in electronic formats and having them automatically posted to your practice management system without human intervention. Also, think about making automated claim status inquiries based on rules embedded in your software, without human intervention, thus eliminating the need for your workforce to spend time on the telephone with representatives of health plans.[19] The regulatory impact analysis that is part of the Version 5010 NPRM indicates that both health care providers and health plans receive a net gain in implementing electronic standards for remittance and payments processing and claims status.[20]

What does the NPRM suggest as specific improvements underlying the modifications of the remittance and payments processing and claims status standards? Remember, unlike mandated policies and procedures required by other rules—such as the Security Rule, discussed in Chapter 4—your practice has a choice to jettison paper transactions and adopt Version 5010–based policies and procedures regarding how it processes remittances and payments from and how it makes claim status inquiries to health plan payers, based on business decisions. Your practice's software vendor(s) will play a key role in helping your practice address these business policy and procedure issues. Be sure to ask your software vendor(s) how your practice can prepare the information that will be needed to address these issues. Consider any expenditure of preparation time or money as an investment in your practice's future as a business, especially if your practice has waited until now to adopt electronic transactions.

Health Care Claim Payment/Advice (835)

According to the NPRM, "[m]any of the enhancements in Version 5010 involve the Front Matter section of the Technical Report Type 3, which contains expanded instructions for accurately processing a compliant 835 transaction. Version 5010 provides refined terminology for using a standard, and enhances the data content to promote clarity."[21] The NPRM highlights the following potential benefits of the refinements:

- More accurate use of the standard
- Reduction of manual intervention
- Motivation for vendors and billing services to provide more cost-effective solutions for electronic remittance advice transactions

  The NPRM goes on to highlight other changes:
- Tightened business rules and fewer code value options in Version 5010. The previous version "lacks standard definitions and procedures for translating remittance information and payments from various health plans to a provider, which makes automatic remittance posting difficult."
- New instructions for handling certain business situations in Version 5010. "Version 5010 instructs providers on how to negate a payment that may be incorrect and post a correction."
- Inclusion of a new Medical Policy segment in Version 5010:
  - This segment "provides more up-to-date information on payer policies and helps in detail management, appeals, and reduces telephone and written inquiries to payers."

- □ This segment also "helps providers locate related published medical policies that are used to determine benefits by virtue of the addition of a segment for a payer's URL [Universal Resource Locator] for easy access to a plan's medical policies."

- Elimination of Not Advised codes in Version 5010. For example, In Version 4010/4010A, there was confusion in a payment context on the use of the code "debit," which was marked "Not Advised." In Version 5010, it is treated "as situational, with instructions on how and when to use the code."
- Clarification for use of claim status indicator codes. In Version 4010/4010A, there were "status codes that indicate a primary, secondary, or tertiary claim, but no instruction for the use of these codes," which "creates confusion when a claim is partially processed, or when a claim is processed but there is no payment."[22]

In general, these changes provide a practice more convenient access to health plan information that will facilitate submission of claims, thereby expediting remittance processing and payment. The Version 5010 final rule concurred with the NPRM claims, noting that "[c]orrect implementation of the X12 835 will reduce phone calls to health plans, reduce appeals due to incomplete information, eliminate unnecessary customer support, and reduce the cost of sending and processing paper remittance advices."[23] Finally, the NPRM estimates that costs savings for claim and remittance processing with the modification to standards for the claim (837) and remittance (835) components will amount to $0.55 per claim for providers and $0.18 for health plans, for a total of $0.73 per claim.[24]

Health Care Claim Status Request and Response (276/277)

Unlike the 835 claim payment/advice standard transaction, which was estimated in 2008 to be accepted by about 60% of all covered entities, the 276/277 claim status request and response standard transaction[25] was estimated in 2008 to be accepted by only about 10% of all covered entities.[26] Version 5010 addresses the following issues in order to increase the percentage of acceptance:

- Identification of prescription numbers to determine which "prescription numbers are paid or not paid at the claim level" of the transaction. "The ability to identify a prescription by the prescription number is important for pharmacy providers when identifying claims data in their systems."
- Elimination of some sensitive personal information that is extraneous to the purpose of checking claim status and that raises privacy and minimum necessary data issues under the HIPAA Privacy Rule, which is discussed in Chapter 3. For example, the previous standard "require[d] the subscriber's date of birth and insurance policy number, which often is a Social Security number," which "is not needed to identify the subscriber because the policy number recorded for the patient already uniquely identifies the subscriber."

- Clarification of *situational data element* rules in order to "reduce reliance on *companion guides*,[27] . . . ensure consistency in the use of the Implementation Guides," and "reduce multiple interpretations." A physician practice's reliance on identifying different interpretations of situational fields and data elements for properly submitting claims to their patients' multiple health plans is time consuming and costly. "For example, Version 5010 clarifies the relationships between dependents and subscribers, and makes a clear distinction between the term 'covered status' (whether the particular service is covered under the benefit package) and 'covered beneficiary' (the individual who is eligible for services)."
- Implementation of consistent rules across all standards "regarding the requirement to include both patient and subscriber information in the transaction." If a dependent patient "can be uniquely identified with an individual identification number," then the subscriber identification is not necessary in the transaction, and "to include the subscriber information with the dependent member information for a uniquely identifiable dependent is an administrative burden for the provider."

Benefits of Improvements to Transaction Standards

The Version 5010 Health Care Claim Payment/Advice (835) and Health Care Claim Status Request and Response (276/277) transaction standards have been the focus in this discussion of transaction standards for implementation by the physician practice because improvements in the implementation specifications have the potential to reduce time and cost regarding the receipt of payment from health plans for services rendered. In 2005, the Medical Group Management Association indicated that "it takes 45 days for a doctor to get an average payment."[28] With patient coinsurance at the front end of an encounter and health plan processing of a claim and a final payment from the patient, if any, after the delivery of service, it may actually take considerably longer for an account receivable to be reconciled and for a claim to be paid in full and closed.[29] Improvements to the Version 5010 Health Care Claim Payment/Advice (835) and Health Care Claim Status Request and Response (276/277) transaction standards have the potential to markedly speed up payment, which could favorably affect practice cash flow and claim and remittance processing costs.

CRITICAL POINT

We recommend that you periodically visit the CMS "Electronic Billing & EDI Transactions" Web site for additional information on the transactions discussed above, other transactions, and related links.[30]

HIPAA Transaction Standards: Final Rule

On January 16, 2009, less than five months after publication of the NPRM—a very short period if calculated in "HIPAA time"—the office of the Secretary of

HHS published in the *Federal Register* final rules pertaining to Version 5010 and ICD-10-CM/PCS. In part, the timing was due to the upcoming change from the Bush administration to the Obama administration. The Version 5010 final rule is discussed below, and the ICD-10-CM/PCS rule, in the next section. Please note that the discussion pertaining to the Version 5010/National Council for Prescription Drug Programs (NCPDP) D.0 and ICD-10-CM/PCS NPRMs, except where noted, is unaffected by changes in the final rules.

The Version 5010 final rule adopted Accredited Standards Committee (ASC) X12 Version 5010 and NCPDP Version D.0, Version 3.0, and Version 5.1 standards for electronic transactions, as shown in Table 2.1 (reproduced here from Table 1 in the final rule).[31]

Most of the transaction standards reflect updates. The Medicaid subrogation standard was newly adopted, and two standards were adopted for retail pharmacy supplies and professional services. Excluding the Medicaid pharmacy subrogation standard, Table 2.2 compares the previous transaction standard versions with modified or new transaction standard versions with which compliance by covered entities was required beginning January 1, 2012.

Effective Dates of Final Rule

There were two effective dates for the final transaction rule. For all standards except the Medicaid pharmacy subrogation transaction standard, the effective date was March 17, 2009. For the Medicaid pharmacy subrogation transaction standard, the effective date was January 1, 2010. "The effective date is the date that the policies set forth in this final rule take effect, and new policies are considered to be officially adopted."[32]

TABLE 2.1

HIPAA Standards for Electronic Transactions

Standard	Transaction
ASC X12 837D	Health care claims—Dental
ASC X12 837P	Health care claims—Professional
ASC X12 837I	Health care claims—Institutional
NCPDP D.0	Health care claims—Retail pharmacy drug
ASC X12 837P and NCPDP D.0	Health care claims—Retail pharmacy supplies and professional services
NCPDP D.0	Coordination of benefits—Retail pharmacy drug
ASC X12 837D	Coordination of benefits—Dental
ASC X12 837P	Coordination of benefits—Professional
ASC X12 837I	Coordination of benefits—Institutional
ASC X12 270/271	Eligibility for a health plan (request and response)—Dental, professional, and institutional
NCPDP D.0	Eligibility for a health plan (request and response)—Retail pharmacy drugs

Standard	Transaction
ASC X12 276/277	Health care claim status (request and response)
ASC X12 834	Enrollment and disenrollment in a health plan
ASC X12 835	Health care payment and remittance advice
ASC X12 820	Health plan premium payment
ASC X12 278	Referral certification and authorization (request and response)
NCPDP D.0	Referral certification and authorization (request and response)—Retail pharmacy drugs
NCPDP 5.1 and NCPDP D.0	Retail pharmacy drug claims (telecommunication and batch standards)
NCPDP 3.0	Medicaid pharmacy subrogation (batch standard)

TABLE 2.2

Comparison of Previous and Current Standard Transaction Versions

Standard	Transaction	Through December 31, 2011	From January 1, 2012
Health Care Claims or Equivalent Encounter Information Transaction	Retail pharmacy drug claims	NCPDP Telecommunication Standard Implementation Guide, Version 5, Release 1 (Version 5.1), Sept. 1999, and equivalent NCPDP Batch Implementation Guide, Version 1, Release 1 (Version 1.1), Jan. 2000, in support of Telecommunication Standard Implementation Guide, Version 5.1, for the NCPDP Data Record in the Detail Data Record	Telecommunication Standard Implementation Guide Version D, Release 0 (Version D.0), Aug. 2007 and equivalent Batch Standard Implementation Guide, Version 1, Release 2 (Version 1.2), NCPDP
	Dental health care claims	Accredited Standards Committee (ASC) X12N 837, Healthcare Claim: Dental, Version 4010, May 2000, WPC, 004010X097, and Addenda to Healthcare Claim: Dental, Version 4010, Oct. 2002, WPC, 004010X097A1	ASC X12 Standards for Electronic Data Interchange Technical Report Type 3, Health Care Claim: Dental (837), May 2006, WPC, 005010X224, and Type 1 Errata to Health Care Claim: Dental (837), ASC X12 Standards for Electronic Data Interchange Technical Report Type 3, Oct. 2007, WPC, 005010X224A1

Continued

TABLE 2.2 (continued)

Comparison of Previous and Current Standard Transaction Versions

Standard	Transaction	Through December 31, 2011	From January 1, 2012
	Professional health care claims	ASC X12N 837, Healthcare Claim: Professional, Volumes 1 and 2, Version 4010, May 2000, WPC, 004010X098, and Addenda to Healthcare Claim: Professional, Volumes 1 and 2, Version 4010, Oct. 2002, WPC, 004010X098A1	ASC X12 Standards for Electronic Data Interchange Technical Report Type 3, Health Care Claim: Professional (837), May 2006, WPC, 005010X222
	Institutional health care claims	ASC X12N 837, Healthcare Claim: Institutional, Volumes 1 and 2, Version 4010, May 2000, WPC, 004010X096, and Addenda to Healthcare Claim: Institutional, Volumes 1 and 2, Version 4010, Oct. 2002, WPC, 004010X096A1	ASC X12 Standards for Electronic Data Interchange Technical Report Type 3, Health Care Claim: Institutional (837), May 2006, WPC, 005010X223, and Type 1 Errata to Health Care Claim: Institutional (837), ASC X12 Standards for Electronic Data Interchange Technical Report Type 3, Oct. 2007, WPC, 005010X223A1
	Retail pharmacy supplies and professional services claims		Telecommunication Standard Implementation Guide Version D, Release 0 (Version D.0), Aug. 2007, and equivalent Batch Standard Implementation Guide, Version 1, Release 2 (Version 1.2), NCPDP; and ASC X12 Standards for Electronic Data Interchange Technical Report Type 3, Health Care Claim: Professional (837), May 2006, WPC, 005010X222
Eligibility for a Health Plan	Retail pharmacy drugs	NCPDP Telecommunication Standard Implementation Guide, Version 5, Release 1 (Version 5.1), Sept. 1999, and equivalent NCPDP Batch Implementation Guide, Version 1, Release 1 (Version 1.1), Jan. 2000, in support of Telecommunication Standard Implementation Guide, Version 5.1, for the NCPDP Data Record in the Detail Data Record	Telecommunication Standard Implementation Guide Version D, Release 0 (Version D.0), Aug. 2007, and equivalent Batch Standard Implementation Guide, Version 1, Release 2 (Version 1.2), NCPDP

TABLE 2.2 (continued)

Comparison of Previous and Current Standard Transaction Versions

Standard	Transaction	Through December 31, 2011	From January 1, 2012
	Dental, professional, and institutional health care eligibility benefit inquiry and response	ASC X12N 270/271, Healthcare Eligibility Benefit Inquiry and Response, Version 4010, May 2000, WPC, 004010X092, and Addenda to Healthcare Eligibility Benefit Inquiry and Response, Version 4010, Oct. 2002, WPC, 004010X092A1	ASC X12 Standards for Electronic Data Interchange Technical Report Type 3, Health Care Eligibility Benefit Inquiry and Response (270/271), April 2008, WPC, 005010X279
Referral Certification and Authorization	Retail pharmacy drugs	NCPDP Telecommunication Standard Implementation Guide, Version 5, Release 1 (Version 5.1), Sept. 1999, and equivalent NCPDP Batch Implementation Guide, Version 1, Release 1 (Version 1.1), Jan. 2000, in support of Telecommunication Standard Implementation Guide, Version 5.1, for the NCPDP Data Record in the Detail Data Record	Telecommunication Standard Implementation Guide Version D, Release 0 (Version D.0), Aug. 2007, and equivalent Batch Standard Implementation Guide, Version 1, Release 2 (Version 1.2), NCPDP
	Dental, professional, and institutional request for review and response	ASC X12N 278, Health Care Services Review—Request for Review and Response, Version 4010, May 2000, WPC, 004010X094, and Addenda to Health Care Services Review—Request for Review and Response, Version 4010, Oct. 2002, WPC, 004010X094A1	ASC X12 Standards for Electronic Data Interchange Technical Report Type 3, Health Care Services Review—Request for Review and Response (278), May 2006, WPC, 005010X217, and Type 1 Errata to Health Care Services Review—Request for Review and Response (278), ASC X12 Standards for Electronic Data Interchange Technical Report Type 3, April 2008, WPC, 005010X217E1
Health Care Claim Status	Dental, professional, institutional, and pharmacy	ASC X12N 276/277, Healthcare Claim Status Request and Response, Version 4010, May 2000, WPC, 004010X093, and Addenda to Healthcare Claim Status Request and Response, Version 4010, Oct. 2002, WPC, 004010X093A1	ASC X12 Standards for Electronic Data Interchange Technical Report Type 3, Health Care Claim Status Request and Response (276/277), Aug. 2006, WPC, 005010X212, and Type 1 Errata to Health Care Claim Status Request and Response (276/277), ASC X12 Standards for Electronic Data Interchange Technical Report Type 3, April 2008, WPC, 005010X212E1

Continued

TABLE 2.2 (continued)

Comparison of Previous and Current Standard Transaction Versions

Standard	Transaction	Through December 31, 2011	From January 1, 2012
Enrollment and Disenrollment in a Health Plan		ASC X12N 834, Benefit Enrollment and Maintenance, Version 4010, May 2000, WPC, 004010X095, and Addenda to Benefit Enrollment and Maintenance, Version 4010, Oct. 2002, WPC, 004010X095A1	ASC X12 Standards for Electronic Data Interchange Technical Report Type 3, Benefit Enrollment and Maintenance (834), Aug. 2006, WPC, 005010X220
Health Care Payment and Remittance Advice	Dental, professional, institutional, and pharmacy	ASC X12N 835, Healthcare Claim Payment/Advice, Version 4010, May 2000, WPC, 004010X091, and Addenda to Healthcare Claim Payment/Advice, Version 4010, Oct. 2002, WPC, 004010X091A1	ASC X12 Standards for Electronic Data Interchange Technical Report Type 3, Health Care Claim Payment/Advice (835), April 2006, WPC, 005010X221
Health Plan Premium Payments		ASC X12N 820, Payroll Deducted and Other Group Premium Payment for Insurance Products, Version 4010, May 2000, WPC, 004010X061, and Addenda to Payroll Deducted and Other Group Premium Payment for Insurance Products, Version 4010, Oct. 2002, WPC, 004010X061A1	ASC X12 Standards for Electronic Data Interchange Technical Report Type 3, Payroll Deducted and Other Group Premium Payment for Insurance Products (820), Feb. 2007, WPC, 005010X218
Coordination of Benefits Information	Retail pharmacy drug claims	NCPDP Telecommunication Standard Implementation Guide, Version 5, Release 1 (Version 5.1), Sept. 1999, and equivalent NCPDP Batch Implementation Guide, Version 1, Release 1 (Version 1.1), Jan. 2000, in support of Telecommunication Standard Implementation Guide, Version 5.1, for the NCPDP Data Record in the Detail Data Record	Telecommunication Standard Implementation Guide Version D, Release 0 (Version D.0), Aug. 2007 and equivalent Batch Standard Implementation Guide, Version 1, Release 2 (Version 1.2), NCPDP

Continued

TABLE 2.2 (continued)

Comparison of Previous and Current Standard Transaction Versions

Standard	Transaction	Through December 31, 2011	From January 1, 2012
	Dental health care claims	Accredited Standards Committee (ASC) X12N 837, Healthcare Claim: Dental, Version 4010, May 2000, WPC, 004010X097, and Addenda to Healthcare Claim: Dental, Version 4010, Oct. 2002, WPC, 004010X097A1	ASC X12 Standards for Electronic Data Interchange Technical Report Type 3, Health Care Claim: Dental (837), May 2006, WPC, 005010X224, and Type 1 Errata to Health Care Claim: Dental (837) ASC X12 Standards for Electronic Data Interchange Technical Report Type 3, Oct. 2007, WPC, 005010X224A1
	Professional health care claims	ASC X12N 837, Healthcare Claim: Professional, Volumes 1 and 2, Version 4010, May 2000, WPC, 004010X098, and Addenda to Healthcare Claim: Professional, Volumes 1 and 2, Version 4010, Oct. 2002, WPC, 004010X098A1	ASC X12 Standards for Electronic Data Interchange Technical Report Type 3, Health Care Claim: Professional (837), May 2006, WPC, 005010X222
	Institutional health care claims	ASC X12N 837, Healthcare Claim: Institutional, Volumes 1 and 2, Version 4010, May 2000, WPC, 004010X096, and Addenda to Healthcare Claim: Institutional, Volumes 1 and 2, Version 4010, Oct. 2002, WPC, 004010X096A1	ASC X12 Standards for Electronic Data Interchange Technical Report Type 3, Health Care Claim: Institutional (837), May 2006, WPC, 005010X223, and Type 1 Errata to Health Care Claim: Institutional (837), ASC X12 Standards for Electronic Data Interchange Technical Report Type 3, Oct. 2007, WPC, 005010X223A1

Compliance Dates for Final Rule

With one exception, all covered entities had to comply with the standards in the final rule by January 1, 2012. The exception is that small health plans had an additional year, to January 1, 2013, to comply with the Medicaid pharmacy subrogation transaction standard. Note the following discussion in the preamble to the final rule (emphasis added):

> Covered entities are urged to begin preparations *now*, to incorporate effective planning, collaboration and testing in their implementation strategies, and to identify and mitigate barriers long before the deadline. *While we have authorized contingency plans in the past,*[33] *we do not intend to do so in this case, as such an action would likely adversely impact ICD-10 implementation activities.* HIPAA gives us [HHS] authority to invoke civil money penalties against covered entities who do not

> comply with the standards, and we have been encouraged by industry to use our authority on a wider scale.[34]

Nevertheless, on November 17, 2011, CMS announced that "[w]hile enforcement action will not be taken [from January 1 to March 31, 2012], OESS [its Office of E-Health Standards and Services] will continue to accept complaints associated with compliance with Version 5010, NCPDP D.0 and NCPDP 3.0 transaction standards during the 90-day period. . . . If requested by OESS, covered entities that are the subject of complaints (known as 'filed-against entities') *must produce evidence of either compliance or a good faith effort to become compliant* with the new HIPAA [transaction] standards during the 90-day period" (emphasis added).[35]

Testing Requirements and Dates in Final Rule

Again, referring to the preamble of the final rule, HHS outlined *expectations* for covered entities to conduct two levels of testing of the standard transactions.[36] To facilitate testing from the effective date (March 17, 2009) until the compliance date (January 1, 2012) of the final rule, HHS permitted, subject to trading partner agreement, "dual use of standards during that timeframe, so that either Version 4010/4010A1 or Version 5010, and either Version 5.1 or D.0, may be used."[37]

Two levels of testing were required under the final rule.

> The Level 1 testing period is the period during which covered entities perform all of their internal readiness activities in preparation for testing the new versions of the standards with their trading partners. When we refer to compliance with Level 1, we mean that a covered entity can demonstrably create and receive compliant transactions, resulting from the completion of all design/build activities and internal testing.[38]

By the end of 2010, covered entities should have completed internal testing (sending and receiving compliant transactions) for Versions 5010 and D.0.

> The Level 2 testing period is the period during which covered entities are preparing to reach full production readiness with all trading partners. When a covered entity is in compliance with Level 2, it has completed end-to-end testing with each of its trading partners, and is able to operate in production mode with the new versions of the standards by the end of that period. By "production mode," we mean that covered entities can successfully exchange (accept and/or send) standard transactions and, as appropriate, be able to process them successfully.[39]

It was expected that by January 1, 2012, "all covered entities will have reached Level 2 compliance, and must be fully compliant in using Versions 5010 and D.0 exclusively."[40] Even though this testing period has passed, it is worth noting, especially in the discussion below regarding both ICD-10-CM and operating rule readiness, that testing is not a last-minute exercise but rather takes considerable time when dealing with multiple trading partners involving electronic exchange of information.

CODE SETS

"Each year, in the United States, health care insurers process over 5 billion claims for payment. For Medicare and other health insurance programs to ensure that these claims are processed in an orderly and consistent manner, standardized coding systems are essential."[41]

A *code set* is a body of information used to encode data elements that is created and maintained by a code set maintaining organization. A code set has predetermined values, which are distinguished from data elements that are based on values drawn, for example, from information about a person, such as age.

An example of a code set that is easily recognized is the zip code system. A zip code directory, created and maintained by the US Postal Service, is a code set from which you would select a predetermined value based on the location of a particular address. For example, if you knew an address in Charleston, South Carolina, you could go to the zip code directory, look up the street name, and find the zip code.[42] We learn zip code values from a directory or computer file and write them in correspondence in addresses and return addresses. In contrast, age is a value based on personal knowledge that is self-reported or otherwise imparted to you. We learn values that define the numeric characteristic of age at an early age, based on a common understanding of implicit rules. Everybody uses zip codes and everybody defines the numeric characteristic of age in round numbers, but we get the values from different sources. Both types of values are critical to implementation of standards and populating underlying data elements.

External code sets are integral to the establishment and use of standard transactions. You are not expected to know vast bodies of information that will facilitate an exchange of information in a transaction. You also are not expected to develop your own description of a place or an event; if you did, the other party to the transaction might not understand your description. Think about what would happen if, instead of using a zip code, each person used his or her own location rule. Usually, an outside body that is recognized as an authority and has expertise in a particular area or ability defines and constructs a common system of rules and values that will be widely used, either by acceptance or mandate.

Code sets such as zip codes and implicit rules such as age are both subject to explicit rules on how they are used in HIPAA transaction standards.

Code Sets in the Physician's Office

If you work in a physician practice, you may only use a small subset of procedure codes, with which you will become familiar over time. Similarly, a back-office coder in a physician's office or in a payer's office will develop a working knowledge of these code sets over time. Within the physician practice, it is important that the service rendered be translated into the appropriate procedure code and that procedure code be accurately reflected in the data set that constitutes the standard transaction for a claim.[43] Knowledge of the rules of how procedure codes are handled in electronic standard transactions (eg, the claim transaction) will enhance the likelihood that transactions are transmitted error free from the physician's practice. Doing so will speed up the response from the payer and will minimize time spent in the practice correcting errors and resubmitting claims or other transactions, such as eligibility or claim status inquiries.

CRITICAL POINT
Knowledge of the rules of how procedure codes are handled in electronic standard transactions in the practice will enhance the likelihood that transaction standards are transmitted error free, elicit a faster response from the payer, and minimize time spent correcting errors and resubmitting claims.

Whether you are in a practice or in a health plan payment environment, you also will want to ensure that your software vendor is knowledgeable about the code sets and the rules that define how they are used in the transaction standards. Remember, as covered entities, the health care provider and health plan are responsible for compliant transactions, so the vendor's activities are your responsibility.[44]

Code Set Categories

There are two categories of code sets:

- Medical data code sets that are *specified* in the Transaction Standards and Code Sets final rule and in the implementation guides
- Nonmedical data code sets, which are *described* in the implementation guides

  Each of these types of code sets is discussed here.

Medical Data Code Sets

Each of the standard transactions involves an exchange of information between a health care provider and a health plan regarding the delivery of health care or the financing of health care or health care benefits. To make the exchange meaningful and understandable, each party to the exchange has to be able to interpret precisely what the other is conveying. To encompass the complexity and variety of actions in the health care field, the common language consists of four broad types of medical data code sets:

- Diseases, impairments, and other health-related problems
- Causes of injury, disease, impairment, and other health-related problems
- Actions taken to prevent, diagnose, treat, or manage diseases, injuries, and impairments
- Any substances, equipment, supplies, or other items used to perform these actions

HHS has adopted these specified code sets that correspond with the four types of medical data code sets identified above.[45]

- *International Classification of Diseases, Ninth Revision, Clinical Modification* (ICD-9-CM), Volumes 1 and 2, as updated and distributed by HHS, for the following:
  - ☐ Diseases
  - ☐ Injuries
  - ☐ Impairments
  - ☐ Other health-related problems and their manifestations
  - ☐ Causes of injury, disease, impairment, and other health-related problems.
- *International Classification of Diseases, Ninth Revision, Clinical Modification* (ICD-9-CM), Volume 3 (Procedures), as updated and distributed by HHS, for procedures or actions taken for diseases, injuries, and impairments of *hospital* inpatients and reported by hospitals, such as actions related to the following:
  - ☐ Prevention
  - ☐ Diagnosis
  - ☐ Treatment
  - ☐ Management
- The National Drug Code (NDC), as maintained and distributed by HHS, for reporting by retail pharmacies on drugs and biologics.[46]
- The Code on Dental Procedures and Nomenclature, as maintained and distributed by the American Dental Association, for dental services.[47]
- The combination of the Healthcare Common Procedure Coding System (HCPCS), as maintained and distributed by HHS, and the Current Procedural Terminology (CPT®) coding system, as maintained and distributed by the American Medical Association (AMA), for physician and other health care services, including but not limited to the following:
  - ☐ Physician services
  - ☐ Physical and occupational therapy services
  - ☐ Radiologic procedures
  - ☐ Clinical laboratory tests
  - ☐ Other medical diagnostic procedures
  - ☐ Transportation services, including ambulance
- HCPCS Level II,[48] as maintained and distributed by HHS, for all other substances, equipment, supplies, and other items used in health care services, with the exception of drugs and biologics, including but not limited to the following:
  - ☐ Medical supplies
  - ☐ Orthodontic and prosthetic devices
  - ☐ Durable medical equipment

An issue regarding use of NDC and HCPCS codes was resolved with publication of the modification to the final rule on February 20, 2003, namely, the adoption of the NDC standard for retail pharmacy transactions and no standard for nonretail pharmacy transactions.[49] In the final transaction and code set standard rule published on August 17, 2000, retail pharmacy and nonretail professional, institutional, and dental pharmacy transactions had to use the NDC.[50] In the proposed modification published on May 31, 2002, the NDC would be the standard code only for retail pharmacy transactions, with no standard for nonretail pharmacy transactions. However, HHS also solicited comments from the public on whether HCPCS should be the standard for nonretail pharmacy transactions in lieu of having no standard for those transactions.[51]

In its decision-making process, HHS considered a variety of comments from the public.[52] HHS noted that "the NDC and HCPCS remain two of the most prevalent and useful code sets for reporting drugs and biologics in nonretail pharmacy transactions" and that in the absence of a standard, "the selection of the code set to be used would likely be specified by health plans via trading partner agreements, as long as the Implementation Guides permitted that selection."[53] Implementation Guides permit the use of the NDC or HCPCS in nonretail pharmacy transactions.

Another important factor in the decision-making process was fostering development of new code sets:

> [A]nother significant advantage to repealing the adoption of the NDC for reporting drugs and biologics in non-retail pharmacy standard transactions and not adopting a replacement standard code set at this time is that the industry and HHS will have time to explore the development of a new drug coding system to meet current and future needs of this sector of the health care industry.[54]

Any new code set would have to be included in the implementation guides, which would involve, as a first step, proposing the code set and supporting its business case as part of the Designated Standard Maintenance Organization (DSMO) process.[55]

Another important issue with regard to code sets concerned the use of HCPCS Level III, which includes codes used on a local basis. Health care delivery is essentially local, so over time codes evolved for alterations or modifications to procedures that had a local or regional character. Local or regional private payers or state payers such as Medicaid could accommodate these codes in a nonstandard, proprietary electronic environment in which both the health care provider and payer recognized the codes. However, with national standards, local codes should not be used. As a result, HIPAA administrative simplification transaction standards do not permit their use. If users can justify on business grounds the use of new national codes, they can apply to CMS for HCPCS and AMA for CPT® consideration of the new codes, which would then go through the DSMO process for validation of business need. We shall see later in this chapter how ICD-10-CM/PCS codes will supplant ICD-9-CM codes beginning on October 1, 2014.

Nonmedical Data Code Sets

To conduct any of the standard transactions, a variety of nonmedical data code sets must accompany the exchange of medical information. For example, in identifying the location of a physical address, all standard transactions require the use of a zip code, which is a commonly known nonmedical data code set. A less well-known code set is the US Department of Defense (DOD) pay grade, known as DOD2, which is used only in the Health Care Eligibility Benefit Inquiry and Response (270/271) transaction standard.

How to Read Code Sets

Nonmedical and medical data code sets are listed in Appendix A: External Code Sources, of each of the ASC X12N Version 5010 implementation guides.[56] Table 2.3 lists the external data code sets and shows their applicability for each of the ASC X12N transaction standards that an implementation guide represents.

Appendix A: External Code Sources in each of the Technical Reports Type 3 identifies each code set by a *code source number* and *code set name*, and categorizes each code set in four ways:

- Simple data element/code references
- Source
- Available from
- Abstract[57]

Two examples from Appendix A of the ASC X12N implementation guide, *Health Care Services Review—Request for Review and Response (278)*, ASC X12N/005010X217, May 2006, are reproduced here.[58]

TABLE 2.3

Version 5010 External Codes

External Set	212	217	218	220	221	222	223	224	279
4 ABA Routing Number			X		X				
5 Countries, Currencies and Funds		X	X	X	X	X	X	X	X
16 D-U-N-S Number			X						
22 States and Provinces		X	X	X	X	X	X	X	X
51 Zip Code		X	X	X	X	X	X	X	X
60 (DFI) Identification Code			X		X				
91 Canadian Financial Institution Branch and Institution Number			X		X				
94 International Organization for Standardization (Date and Time)				X					
102 Languages				X					
121 Health Industry Number					X				

Continued

TABLE 2.3 (continued)

Version 5010 External Codes

External Set	212	217	218	220	221	222	223	224	279
130 Healthcare Common Procedure Coding System	X	X			X	X	X		X
131 International Classification of Diseases, Ninth Revision, Clinical Modification (ICD-9-CM)		X		X		X	X	X	X
132 National Uniform Billing Committee (NUBC) Codes	X				X	X	X		
133 Current Procedural Terminology (CPT) Codes									X
135 American Dental Association	X	X			X			X	X
139 Claim Adjustment Reason Code					X	X	X	X	
206 Government Bill of Lading Office Code				X					X
229 Diagnosis Related Group Number		X			X		X		
230 Admission Source Code		X					X		
231 Admission Type Code		X					X		
235 Claim Frequency Type Code		X			X	X	X	X	
236 Uniform Billing Claim Form Bill Type		X					X		
237 Place of Service Codes for Professional Claims		X				X		X	X
239 Patient Status Code		X					X		
240 National Drug Code by Format	X	X			X	X	X		X
245 National Association of Insurance Commissioners (NAIC)					X	X	X	X	
284 Nature of Injury Code									X
307 National Council for Prescription Drug Programs Pharmacy Number				X	X				X
327 Society for Worldwide Interbank Financial Telecommunication (SWIFT)			X						
359 Treatment Codes							X		
407 Occupational Injury and Illness Classification Manual									X
411 Remittance Advice Remark Codes					X	X	X	X	

Continued

TABLE 2.3 (continued)

Version 5010 External Codes

External Set	212	217	218	220	221	222	223	224	279
457 NISO Z39.53 Language Code List				X					
468 Ambulatory Payment Classification					X				
507 Health Care Claim Status Category Code	X								
508 Health Care Claim Status Code	X								
513 Home Infusion EDI Coalition (HIEC) Product/Service Code List	X	X			X	X	X		X
530 National Council for Prescription Drug Programs Reject/Payment Codes	X				X				
537 Centers for Medicare and Medicaid Services (CMS) National Provider Identifier	X	X		X	X	X	X	X	X
540 CMS Plan ID	X	X	X	X	X	X	X	X	X
576 Workers Compensation Specific Procedure and Supply Codes	X				X	X	X	X	
582 CMS Durable Medical Equipment Regional Carrier (DMERC) Certificate of Medical Necessity (CMN) Forms						X			
656 Form Type Codes						X			
663 Logical Observation Identifier Names and Codes (LOINC)		X							
682 Health Care Provider Taxonomy		X				X	X	X	X
716 Health Insurance Prospective Payment System (HIPPS) Rate Code for Skilled Nursing Facilities	X				X		X		
843 Advanced Billing Concepts (ABC) Codes	X	X			X	X	X		
844 Eligibility Category									X
859 Classification of Race or Ethnicity				X					
860 Race or Ethnicity Collection Code				X					
886 Health Care Service Review Decision Reason Codes		X							

Continued

TABLE 2.3 (continued)

Version 5010 External Codes

External Set	212	217	218	220	221	222	223	224	279
896 International Classification of Diseases, 10th Revision, Procedure Coding System (ICD-10-PCS)				x			x		x
897 International Classification of Diseases, 10th Revision, Clinical Modification (ICD-10-CM)		x				x	x	x	x
932 Universal Postal Codes		x	x	x	x	x	x	x	x
DOD1 Military Rank and Health Care Service Region									x
DOD2 Pay grade									x

Legend

212: Health Care Claim Status Request and Response (276/277), WPC, August 2006.

217: Health Care Services Review—Request for Review and Response (278), WPC, May 2006.

218: Payroll Deducted and Other Group Premium Payment for Insurance Products (820), WPC, February 2007.

220: Benefit Enrollment and Maintenance (834), WPC, August 2006.

221: Health Care Claim Payment/Advice (835), WPC, April 2006.

222: Health Care Claim: Professional (837), WPC, May 2006.

223: Health Care Claim: Institutional (837), WPC, May 2006.

224: Health Care Claim: Dental (837), WPC, May 2006.

279: Health Care Eligibility Benefit Inquiry and Response (270/271), WPC, April 2008.

Source

Accredited Standards Committee (ASC) X12, Insurance Subcommittee, ASC X12N. Appendix A: External Code Sources of documents referenced in legend. Washington Publishing Company (WPC), www.wpc-edi.com.

Code Source Number 51: Code Set Name: Zip Code

- *Simple Data Element/Code References*[59]
  - 116, 66/16, 309/PQ, 309/PR, 309/PS, 771/010
- *Source*
  - National Zip Code and Post Office Directory, Publication 65, The USPS Domestic Mail Manual
- *Available from*
  - US Postal Service, Washington, DC 20260; New Orders, Superintendent of Documents, P.O. Box 371954, Pittsburgh, PA 15250–7954
- *Abstract*

The zip code is a geographic identifier of areas within the United States and its territories for purposes of expediting mail distribution by the US Postal Service. It is five or nine numeric digits. The zip code structure divides the US into ten large groups of states. The leftmost digit identifies one of these groups. The next two digits identify a smaller geographic area within the large group. The two rightmost digits identify a local delivery area. In the nine-digit zip code, the four digits that follow the hyphen further subdivide the delivery area. The two leftmost digits identify a sector, which may consist of several large buildings, blocks, or groups of streets. The rightmost digits divide the sector into segments such as a street, a block, a floor of a building, or a cluster of mailboxes.

The USPS Domestic Mail Manual includes information on the use of the new 11-digit zip code.

Code Source Number 897: Code Set Name: International Classification of Diseases, 10th Revision, Clinical Modification (ICD-10-CM)

- *Simple Data Element/Code References*
  - 235/DC, 1270/ABF, 1270/ABJ, 1270/ABK, 1270/ABN, 1270/ABU, 1270/ABV, 1270/ADD, 1270/APR, 1270/ASD, 1270/ATD
- *Source*
  - *International Classification of Diseases*, 10th Revision, *Clinical Modification* (ICD-10-CM)
- *Available from*
  OCD/Classifications and Public Health Data Standards
  National Center for Health Statistics
  3311 Toledo Road
  Hyattsville, MD 20782
- *Abstract*
  - *The International Classification of Diseases*, 10th Revision, *Clinical Modification* (ICD-10-CM), describes the classification of morbidity and mortality information for statistical purposes and for the indexing of hospital records by diseases.

Zip code is used with each of the transaction standards, except *Health* Care Claim Status Request and Response (276/277) (ASC X12N/005010X212). ICD-10-CM will be used with the following transactions when compliance with its use for diagnosis by physician practices[60] is required on October 1, 2014:

- Health Care Services Review—Request for Review and Response (278) (ASC X12N/005010X217)
- Health Care Claim: Professional (837) (ASC X12N/005010X222)
- Health Care Claim: Institutional (837) (ASC X12N/005010X223)
- Health Care Claim: Dental (837) (ASC X12N/005010X224)
- Health Care Eligibility Benefit Inquiry and Response (270/271) (ASC X12N/005010X279)

When checking on any external code, it is important to examine which standard transactions it is used in and where it is used. The "where" is found in the *Simple Data Element/Code References* category, and the entries are the same across standard transactions in which a specified code set is used.

ICD-10-CM/PCS: Code Set Standards Modification

Introduction

The Notice of Proposed Rulemaking (NPRM) for ICD-10-CM/PCS was published in the *Federal Register* on August 22, 2008,[61] the same day that the NPRM for Version 5010 was published in the *Federal Register*. Then, on January 16, 2009, the final ICD-10-CM/PCS rule was published,[62] again on the same day as the final rule for Version 5010. These two rules go together: ICD-10-CM/PCS cannot work with the existing Version 4010/4010A transaction standards, and Version 5010 needs to be in place to accommodate the different ICD-10-CM/PCS data element character length. Below, we discuss both the proposed and final ICD-10-CM/PCS rulings.

The ICD-10-CM/PCS rule comprises two parts:

- *International Classification of Diseases, Tenth Revision, Clinical Modification* (ICD-10-CM) for diagnosis coding
- *International Classification of Diseases, Tenth Revision, Procedure Coding System* (ICD-10-PCS) for inpatient hospital procedure coding only[63]

Only ICD-10-CM is germane to transactions generated by physician practices. However, physicians that practice in hospitals, on staff or privileged, will have to have acquaintance with the structure of the ICD-10-PCS procedural codes.

The currently used ICD-9-CM diagnosis codes were "adopted as a HIPAA [code set] standard in 2000 for reporting diagnoses, injuries, impairments, and other health problems and their manifestations, and causes of injury, disease, impairment or other health problems in standard transactions."[64] ICD-9-CM diagnosis codes, of which there are approximately 13,000,[65] are three to five digits in length. The ICD-9-CM code set functionality "has been exhausted" and "is nearing the end of its useful life."[66] In addition to assignable code limitations, there are three other key reasons to replace it:[67]

- **Effects of workarounds on structural hierarchy.** Some parts of ICD-9-CM are full, so new codes "must be assigned to other topically unrelated chapters," making the codes sometimes difficult to find.
- **Lack of detail.** "[I]n an age of electronic health records, it does not make sense to use a coding system that lacks specificity and does not lend itself well to updates. . . . Emerging health care technologies, new and advanced terminologies, and the need for interoperability amid the increase in electronic health records (EHRs) and personal health records (PHRs) require a standard code set that is expandable and sufficiently detailed to accurately capture current and future health care information."
- **Obsolescence.** The *International Classification of Diseases, Ninth Revision*, on which ICD-9-CM is based, is no longer supported or maintained by the World Health Organization: "As we [the United States] become a global community, it is vital that our health care data represent current medical conditions and technologies, and that they are compatible with the international version of ICD-10."

In contrast to ICD-9-CM, "ICD-10-CM diagnosis codes are three to seven alphanumeric characters," and "the number of ICD-10-CM codes is approximately 68,000. The ICD-10-CM code set provides much more information and detail within the codes than ICD-9-CM, facilitating timely electronic processing of claims by reducing requests for additional information."[68] This last point is very important: in conjunction with the Version 5010 transaction standard modifications, ICD-10-CM will facilitate better information exchange between health care stakeholders, thereby leading to more efficient processing of claims and payments. Looking to the future, the ICD-10-CM/PCS NPRM concludes that "ICD-10 code sets provide a standard coding convention that is flexible, providing unique codes for all substantially different procedures or health conditions and allowing new procedures and diagnoses to be easily incorporated as new codes for both existing and future clinical protocols."[69]

The ICD-10-CM/PCS NPRM provided a compliance date of October 1, 2011, for use of ICD-10-CM in physician practices and by other covered entities. During the public comment period, the Workgroup for Electronic Data Interchange (WEDI), in its advisory role to HHS under the HIPAA administrative simplification legislation and enabling regulations, submitted comments on the ICD-10-CM/PCS NPRM to HHS, indicating that the compliance date did not provide sufficient time for a successful implementation in the health care industry.[70] Instead, WEDI "recommends that a minimum of four years will be needed after completion of transaction upgrades and a total of six years after publication of the final rules for upgrades of transactions and medical code sets (October 1 after the anniversary of the sixth year)."[71] That would make the compliance date near or several years after the end of the "Decade of Health Information Technology" in 2014. By taking so long, the US health care industry would be unable to achieve in a timely manner the objectives of implementing EHRs[72] and ensuring interoperability, which cannot be done without updating the code sets. As we shall see in the discussion of the final ICD-10-CM/PCS rule below, the compliance date was originally October 1, 2013, just prior to the completion of the Decade of Health Information Technology, but it was subsequently delayed to October 1, 2014.

In 2005, Linda Kloss, CEO of the American Health Information Management Association (AHIMA), made the following statement:

> The full benefits of an EHR can only be realized if we improve the quality of data that EHRs are designed to manage. The current classification coding system used in the US, ICD-9-CM, is a 30-year-old system and can no longer accurately describe today's practice of medicine. Continuing to use this system jeopardizes the ability to effectively collect and use accurate, detailed healthcare data and information for the betterment of domestic and global healthcare. By failing to upgrade, we could find ourselves building an infrastructure that does not provide the information necessary to meet the healthcare demands of the 21st century.[73]

On November 5, 2003, the National Committee on Vital and Health Statistics (NCVHS) recommended in a letter to then Secretary of HHS, Tommy Thompson, that ICD-10-CM be adopted as a HIPAA administrative simplification code set standard.[74] NCVHS made the following observation in its letter:

> Benefits are harder to quantify, but appear to outweigh the costs. They include facilitating improvements to the quality of care and patient safety, fewer rejected claims, improved information for disease management, and more accurate reimbursement rates for emerging technologies. These costs and benefits and related issues also have been substantially documented in testimony before the Subcommittee, as well as in a cost/benefit study by the RAND Corporation[75] that was specially commissioned by NCVHS.

The ICD-10-CM/PCS NPRM highlights projected benefits:[76]

- More accurate payments for new procedures
- Fewer rejected claims
- Fewer improper claims
- Better understanding of new procedures
- Improved disease management
- Better understanding of health conditions and health care outcomes

For physician practices, the NPRM analysis estimates that, on average, practices will experience costs of 0.04 percent of revenue/receipts, which "include a portion of the coding training costs and productivity losses in addition to costs directly allocated to physicians and practice expenses."[77]

The costs and benefits will have to be determined by each practice. However, it appears reasonable to assume that if ICD-9-CM is "exhausted" and benefits would accrue through use of ICD-10-CM, in contrast to WEDI's recommendation of further delay to the future, the federal government and the health care industry may wish to proceed with all deliberate speed in a concentrated effort to implement ICD-10-CM sooner rather than later. The original October 1, 2013, compliance date was a step in the right direction.

ICD-10-CM/PCS Final Rule

The final rule, published in the *Federal Register* on January 16, 2009, adopted modifications to two code set standards in the Transaction Standards and Code Sets final rule that required compliance by covered entities on or after October 16, 2003. This new final rule modified standard medical data code sets for coding diagnoses (ICD-10-CM)[78] and inpatient hospital procedures (ICD-10-PCS).[79] Noninpatient (ambulatory) procedures continue to be coded using CPT-4 and HCPCS. Table 2.4 compares code sets under the existing and modified rules.

TABLE 2.4

Modification of Transaction and Code Set Diagnosis and Procedure Code Rules

	Current Code Set Rule	Modified Code Set Rule
All diagnoses	*International Classification of Diseases, Ninth Revision, Clinical Modification* (ICD-9-CM), Volumes 1 and 2, including the Official ICD-9-CM Guidelines for Coding and Reporting	ICD-10-CM
Inpatient procedures	*International Classification of Diseases, Ninth Revision, Clinical Modification* (ICD-9-CM), Volume 3, including the Official ICD-9-CM Guidelines for Coding and Reporting	ICD-10-PCS
Noninpatient (ambulatory) procedures	CPT-4 and HCPCS	CPT-4 and HCPCS

Effective Date

The effective date of the ICD-10-CM/PCS final rule was March 17, 2009. "The effective date is the date that the policies herein take effect, and new policies are considered to be officially adopted."[80]

Compliance Date

The compliance date for the modification of the diagnosis and procedure code sets from ICD-9-CM to ICD-10-CM/PCS in the final rule was October 1, 2013, later changed to October 1, 2014.[81] "The compliance date . . . is the date on which entities are required to have implemented the policies adopted in this rule."[82]

October 1 was chosen to coincide with the effective date of the annual Medicare Inpatient Prospective Payment System. The ICD-10-CM/PCS compliance date is 21 months after the compliance date for the Version 5010 rule. Based on health care industry input, "it appears that 24 months (2 years) is the minimum amount of time that the industry needs to achieve compliance with ICD-10 once Version 5010 has moved into external (Level 2) testing,"[83] which commenced January 1, 2011 (33 months before the original ICD-10-CM/PCS compliance date).

> [HHS has] concluded that it would be in the health care industry's best interests if *all entities* [emphasis added] were to comply with the ICD-10 code set standards at the same time to ensure the accuracy and timeliness of claims and transaction processing. . . . The availability and use of crosswalks, mappings and guidelines should assist entities in making the switchover from ICD-9 to ICD-10 code sets on October 1, 2013, without the need for the concurrent use of both code sets [ICD-9 and ICD-10] in claims processing, medical record and related systems with respect to claims for services provided on the same day. . . . [HHS believes] that different compliance dates based on the size of a health plan would also be problematic since a provider has no way of knowing if a health plan qualifies as a small health plan or not.[84]

Note that coding of procedures that occur before, on, or after the compliance date is based on the *date of discharge*.

On September 5, 2012, HHS published in the *Federal Register* the change in the compliance date from October 1, 2013, to October 1, 2014.[85] HHS provided in the rule the reason for the delay of the compliance date:

> According to a recent survey conducted by the Centers for Medicare & Medicaid Services (CMS), up to one quarter of health care providers believe they will not be ready for an October 1, 2013 compliance date. While the survey found no significant differences among practice settings regarding the likelihood of achieving compliance before the deadline, based on recent industry feedback we believe that larger health career plans and providers generally are more prepared than smaller entities. The uncertainty about provider readiness is confirmed in another recent readiness survey [conducted by WEDI] in which nearly 50 percent of the 2,140 provider respondents did not know when they would complete their impact assessment of the ICD-10 transition. By delaying the compliance date of ICD-10 from October 1, 2013 to October 1, 2014, we are allowing more time for covered entities to prepare for the transition to ICD-10 and to conduct thorough testing. By allowing more time to prepare, covered entities may be able to avoid costly obstacles that would otherwise emerge while in production.[86]

Testing

"[HHS has] not established dates for Level 1 and Level 2 testing compliance for ICD-10 implementation. We encourage all industry segments to be ready to test their systems with ICD-10 as soon as it is feasible."[87] Recall the definitions of Level 1 and 2 testing from the Version 5010 final rule:

> The Level 1 testing period is the period during which covered entities perform all of their internal readiness activities in preparation for testing the new versions of the standards with their trading partners. When we refer to compliance with Level 1, we mean that a covered entity can demonstrably create and receive compliant transactions, resulting from the completion of all design/build activities and internal testing.[88]
>
> The Level 2 testing period is the period during which covered entities are preparing to reach full production readiness with all trading partners. When a covered entity is in compliance with Level 2, it has completed end-to-end testing with each of its trading partners, and is able to operate in production mode with the new versions of the standards by the end of that period. By 'production mode,' we mean that covered entities can successfully exchange (accept and/or send) standard transactions and as appropriate, be able to process them successfully.[89]

Crosswalks

HHS acknowledges that crosswalks or mappings of data element code values between ICD-9-CM and ICD-10-CM/PCS "will be critical."[90] The HIPAA administrative simplification act requires under Section 1174(b)(2)(B)(ii) that:

> if a code set is modified under this subsection, the modified code set shall include instructions on how data elements of health information that were encoded prior to the modification may be converted or translated so as to preserve the informational value of the data elements that existed before the modification . . . [and] in a manner that minimizes the disruption and cost of complying with such modification.[91]

Bidirectional crosswalks that can translate from the old code set to the new one or from the new code set to the old one are referred to as General Equivalence Mapping (GEM) files.

The *International Classification of Diseases* (ICD) is developed and maintained by the World Health Organization. The National Center for Health Statistics (NCHS), part of the Centers for Disease Control and Prevention (CDC), has responsibility for implementation of the ICD in the United States and developed ICD-9-CM, the clinical adaptation for US use. We reproduce here detail from the NCHS ICD-10-CM Web site (http://www.cdc.gov/nchs/icd/icd10cm.htm; current as of June 19, 2013, the date of the last update prior to this writing):

> The ICD-10 is copyrighted by the World Health Organization (WHO), which owns and publishes the classification. WHO has authorized the development of an adaptation of ICD-10 for use in the United States for U.S. government purposes. As agreed, all modifications to the ICD-10 must conform to WHO conventions for the ICD. ICD-10-CM was developed following a thorough evaluation by a Technical Advisory Panel and extensive additional consultation with physician groups, clinical coders, and others to assure clinical accuracy and utility.
>
> The entire draft of the Tabular List of ICD-10-CM, and the preliminary crosswalk between ICD-9-CM and ICD-10-CM were made available on the NCHS web site for public comment. The public comment period ran from December 1997 through February 1998. The American Hospital Association [AHA] and the American Health Information Management Association [AHIMA] conducted a field test for ICD-10-CM in the summer of 2003, [with a subsequent] report [of their findings].[92] All comments and suggestions from the open comment period and the field test were reviewed, and additional modifications to ICD-10-CM were made based on these comments and suggestions. Additionally, new concepts have been added to ICD-10-CM based on the established update process for ICD-9-CM (the ICD-9-CM Coordination and Maintenance Committee) and the World Health Organization's ICD-10 (the Update and Revision Committee). This represents ICD-9-CM modifications from 2003–2011 and ICD-10 modifications from 2002–2010.
>
> The clinical modification represents a significant improvement over ICD-9-CM and ICD-10. Specific improvements include: the addition of information relevant to ambulatory and managed care encounters; expanded injury codes; the creation of combination diagnosis/symptom codes to reduce the number of codes needed to fully describe a condition; the addition of sixth and seventh characters; incorporation of common 4th and 5th digit subclassifications; laterality; and greater specificity in code assignment. The new structure will allow further expansion than was possible with ICD-9-CM. . . .
>
> **2014 Release of ICD-10-CM**
> **Note: This replaces the July 2012 release.**
>
> [The] files linked below are the 2014 update of the ICD-10-CM. Content changes to the full ICD-10-CM files are described in the respective addenda files. This year in addition to PDF (Adobe) files XML format is also being made available. Most files are provided in compressed zip format for ease in downloading. . . .

> *Although this release of ICD-10-CM is now available for public viewing, the codes in ICD-10-CM are not currently valid for any purpose or use. The effective implementation date for ICD-10-CM (and ICD-10-PCS) is October 1, 2014. Updates to this version of ICD-10-CM are anticipated prior to its implementation.* [Emphasis added]
>
> The 2014 General Equivalence Mappings (GEMs) will be posted in October 2013.[93]

The 2014 files that currently are available on the NCHS ICD-10-CM Web site are the following:

- ICD-10-CM PDF Format
- ICD-10-CM XML Format
- ICD-10-CM 2013 Addenda
- ICD-10-CM List of Codes and Descriptions

We recommend that you refer to the ICD-10-CM files periodically—and in particular the GEM files—to keep abreast of changes in ICD-10-CM before the implementation date of October 1, 2014, and to be familiar with the way ICD-10-CM differs from ICD-9-CM in format and content.

CMS also has a useful ICD-10 Provider Resources Web site at http://www.cms.gov/Medicare/Coding/ICD10/ProviderResources.html. This Web site provides guidance for practices that are preparing to implement ICD-10 and links to useful downloads. For reference, we recommend that you visit the CMS Web site 2013 ICD-10-CM and GEMs (http://www.cms.gov/Medicare/Coding/ICD10/2013-ICD-10-CM-and-GEMs.html), and explore the downloads referenced therein. These downloads contain information on the ICD-10-CM diagnosis coding system. This page is accessible from a link at the CMS Provider Resources Web site on the left side of the page.

Finally, for small and medium practices, we reproduce two important figures from the Provider Resources Web site. Figure 2.1 shows what should be accomplished and when from January 2013 through the October 1, 2014, compliance date. Figure 2.2 breaks down actions into three time frames: planning, communication, and assessment, to be done immediately; transition and testing, to be accomplished between March 2013 and September 2014; and complete transition/full compliance, to be achieved by October 1, 2014. Be sure to download the implementation guide for small and medium practices at the Provider Resources Web site. While we focus on small and medium practices here, similar resources for large practices and small hospitals are available at the same Web site.

FIGURE 2.1

ICD-10 Timeline for Small-Medium Practices at a Glance

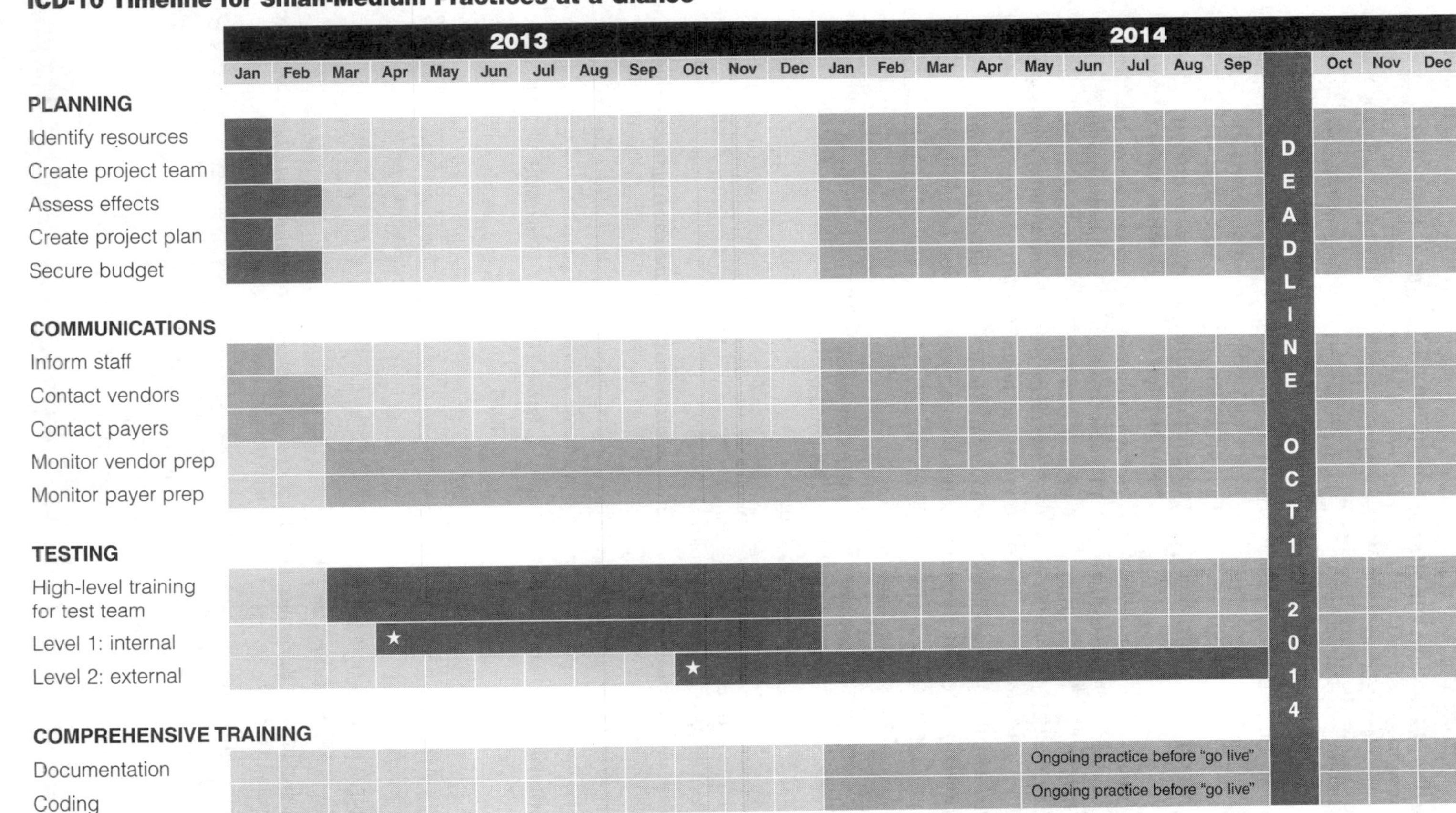

Source: Centers for Medicare and Medicaid Services (CMS). Provider Resources. http://www.cms.gov/Medicare/Coding/ICD10/ProviderResources.html.

FIGURE 2.2

Small and Medium Practices: ICD-10 Transition Checklist

The following is a checklist of ICD-10 tasks, including estimated timeframes for each task. Depending on your organization, many of these tasks can be performed on a compressed timeline or performed at the same time as other tasks.

This checklist is designed to provide a viable path forward for organizations just beginning to prepare for ICD-10. CMS encourages those who are ahead of this schedule to continue their progress forward.

PLANNING, COMMUNICATION, AND ASSESSMENT

Actions to Take Immediately

To prepare for testing, make sure you have completed the following activities. If you have already completed these tasks, review the information to make sure you did not overlook an important step.

- ☐ **Review ICD-10 resources** from CMS, trade associations, payers, and vendors
- ☐ **Inform your staff colleagues** of upcoming changes (1 month)
- ☐ Create an **ICD-10 project team** (1-2 days)
- ☐ Identify **how ICD-10 can affect your practice** (1-2 months)
  - ☐ How will ICD-10 affect your people and processes? To find out, ask all staff members how/where they use/see ICD-9
  - ☐ Include ICD-10 as you plan for projects like meaningful use of electronic health records
- ☐ Develop and complete an **ICD-10 project plan** for your practice (1-2 weeks)
  - ☐ Identify each task, including deadline and who is responsible
  - ☐ Develop plan for communicating with staff and business partners about ICD-10
- ☐ Estimate and **secure budget** (potential costs include updates to practice management systems, new coding guides and superbills, staff training) (2 months)
- ☐ **Ask your payers and vendors—software systems, clearinghouses, billing services—about ICD-10 readiness** (2 months)
  - ☐ Review trading partner agreements
  - ☐ Ask about systems changes, a timeline, costs, and testing plans
  - ☐ Ask when they will start testing, how long they will need, and how you and other clients will be involved
  - ☐ Select/retain vendor(s)
- ☐ Review **changes in documentation requirements** and educate staff by looking at frequently used ICD-9 codes and new ICD-10 codes (ongoing)

TRANSITION AND TESTING

March 2013 to September 2014

- ☐ **March 1, 2013 – December 31, 2013:** Conduct **high-level training on ICD-10** for clinicians and coders to prepare for testing (eg, clinical documentation, software updates) (ongoing)
- ☐ **April – June 2013:** Start testing ICD-10 codes and systems with your practice's coding, billing, and clinical staff (9 months)
  - ☐ Use ICD-10 codes for diagnoses your practice sees most often
  - ☐ Test data and reports for accuracy
- ☐ Monitor vendor and payer preparedness, identify and address gaps (ongoing)

- ☐ **October 2013 – January 2014:** Begin testing claims and other transactions using ICD-10 codes with business trading partners such as payers, clearinghouses, and billing services (10 months minimum)
- ☐ **January 1, 2014 – April 1, 2014:** Review coder and clinician preparation; begin detailed ICD-10 coding training (6-9 months)
- ☐ Work with vendors to complete transition to production-ready ICD-10 systems

COMPLETE TRANSITION/FULL COMPLIANCE

October 1, 2014

- ☐ Complete ICD-10 transition for full compliance
  - ☐ ICD-9 codes continue to be used for services provided before October 1, 2014
  - ☐ ICD-10 codes required for services provided on or after October 1, 2014
  - ☐ Monitor systems and correct errors if needed

CMS consulted resources from the American Medical Association (AMA), the American Health Information Management Association (AHIMA), the North Carolina Healthcare Information & Communications Alliance (NCHICA) and the Workgroup for Electronic Data Interchange (WEDI) in developing this timeline.

Source: Centers for Medicare and Medicaid Services (CMS). Provider Resources. http://www.cms.gov/Medicare/Coding/ICD10/ProviderResources.html.

What 5010 and ICD-10-CM Mean to Your Practice

The clock is ticking! Accordingly, your practice should be thinking about how the ICD-10-CM diagnosis coding changes will impact your practice, especially your business-related policies and procedures. You will want help from your information technology (IT) vendor because ICD-10-CM modifications will have significant impacts on your software related to standard transactions and how you identify diagnoses in your EHR systems.

The ICD-10-CM code set rule modifications will have a significant impact on your practice's *administrative* policies and procedures. Again, the time from today to the October 1, 2014, compliance date will go by quickly—less than 15 months from the time of this writing. Furthermore, the federal health information technology initiatives will compound your workload as your practice examines how your *clinical* workflows, policies, and procedures will change as you introduce more and more electronic tools and records for collecting, compiling, analyzing, and reporting data. If you haven't already, ask your software vendors *now* how they plan to handle ICD-10-CM by the compliance date, including testing, and get answers and milestones of accomplishment with respect to achieving compliance, in writing, especially in any contract that you execute for software.

Although your first concern needs to be the looming ICD-10-CM/PCS compliance date, you also must be aware of future additions and enhancements to administrative simplification standards outlined in the Patient Protection and Affordable Care Act, which we discuss next.

Health Insurance Reform: Administrative Simplification

On March 23, 2010, President Obama signed into law the Patient Protection and Affordable Care Act (HR 3590) as Public Law 111–148.[94] One week later, on March 30, 2010, President Obama signed into law the follow-on Health Care and Education Reconciliation Act of 2010 as Public Law 111–152.[95] The focus here is on two sections of Public Law 111–148:

- Section 1104 (Administrative Simplification) in Subtitle B—Immediate Actions to Preserve and Expand Coverage of Title I—Quality, Affordable Health Care for All Americans[96]
- Section 10109 (Development of Standards for Financial and Administrative Transactions) in Subtitle A—Provisions Relating to Title I of Title X—Strengthening Quality, Affordable Health Care for All Americans[97]

Section 1104

The effective date of Section 1104, Administrative Simplification, was the date of enactment, March 23, 2010.[98] Section 1104(a) amends part of the purpose of administrative simplification as specified in the HIPAA statute in two places, as indicated in bold:

> To improve . . . efficiency and effectiveness of the health care system, by encouraging the development of a health information system through the **establishment of uniform standards and requirements** for the electronic transmission of certain health information and to **reduce the clerical burden on patients, health care providers, and health plans.**[99]

Based on years of experience implementing HIPAA administrative simplification, the amendments focused on moving toward minimization or elimination of variance in the application and use of standards by requiring uniform standards, and, coincident with the need for uniformity and further adoption of electronic business processes in lieu of paper-based transactions, minimization or elimination of nonproductive workflows experienced by the health care workforce.

Section 1104(b) contains the substantive details for accomplishing the amended purpose, namely, using operating rules for health information transactions.[100] Operating rules are defined as "the necessary business rules and guidelines for the electronic exchange of information that are not defined by a standard or its implementation specifications as adopted for purposes of this part."[101]

Section 1104(b) also specifies a new standard—electronic funds transfers—in addition to discussing conversion of existing standards to operating rules, and lays out the requirements for financial and administrative transactions:

> (A) In General—The standards and associated operating rules adopted by the Secretary shall—
>
> (i) to the extent feasible and appropriate, enable determinations of an individual's eligibility and financial responsibility for specific services prior to or at the point of care;

(ii) be comprehensive, requiring minimal augmentation by paper or other communications;

(iii) provide for timely acknowledgment, response, and status reporting that supports a transparent claims and denial management process (including adjudication and appeals); and

(iv) describe all data elements (including reason and remark codes) in unambiguous terms, require that such data elements be required or conditioned upon set values in other fields, and prohibit additional conditions (except where necessary to implement State or Federal law, or to protect against fraud and abuse).[102]

Following the specification of requirements, Section 1104(b) outlines provisions relating to:

- Procedures for development of operating rules
- Review and recommendations from the National Committee on Vital and Health Statistics (NCVHS)[103] to the Secretary of HHS for their adoption[104]
- Adoption, effective, and compliance date deadlines, as shown in Table 2.5
- Compliance with operating rules, including health plan certification and documentation requirements
- Review and modification of operating rules based on usage
- Penalties for noncompliance

TABLE 2.5

Adoption, Effective, and Compliance Dates for Operating Rules

Standard	Adoption Date[i]	Effective Date[i]	Health Plan Compliance Date[ii]
Eligibility for a health plan[iii]	7/1/2011	1/1/2013	12/31/2012
Health claim status[iii]	7/1/2011	1/1/2013	12/31/2012
Electronic funds transfers[iv]	7/1/2012	1/1/2014	12/31/2013
Health care payment and remittance advice[iv]	7/1/2012	1/1/2014	12/31/2013
Health claims or equivalent encounter information	7/1/2014	1/1/2016	12/31/2015
Enrollment and disenrollment in a health plan	7/1/2014	1/1/2016	12/31/2015
Health plan premium payments	7/1/2014	1/1/2016	12/31/2015
Referral certification and authorization	7/1/2014	1/1/2016	12/31/2015

[i] Not later than.

[ii] Not later than. Requires written certification of compliance provided to the Secretary of HHS. Note also that the compliance dates for the first two entries—"Eligibility for a health plan" and "Health claim status"—reflect the language of provision (h)(5)(b): "Date of Compliance—A health plan shall comply with such requirements not later than the effective date of the applicable standard or operating rule [124 STAT. 150]," rather than the date specified for these transactions in (h)(1)(A) [124 STAT. 149].

[iii] On July 8, 2011, HHS issued an interim final rule for these operating rules. See Department of Health and Human Services, Office of the Secretary, 45 CFR Parts 160 and 162: Administrative Simplification: Adoption of Operating Rules for Eligibility for a Health Plan and Health Care Claim Status Transactions; Interim Final Rule, *Federal Register*, v. 76, n. 131, July 8, 2011, pp. 40458-40496, which is available at http://www.gpo.gov/fdsys/pkg/FR-2011-07-08/pdf/2011-16834.pdf. "On December 7, 2011, CMS notified the health care industry that the interim final rule was now a final rule: "After careful review and consideration of all comments, we have decided not to change any of the policies established in [the interim final rule]." See CMS, CMS-0032-IFC Notice to Industry Wednesday, December 7, 2011, at https://www.cms.gov/Regulations-and-Guidance/HIPAA-Administrative-Simplification/Affordable-Care-Act/CMS-0032-IFC.pdf. For information on the operating rules mandate for eligibility and health claim status transactions, including a copy of the operating rules, visit the Council for Affordable Quality Health Care (CAQH) Web site at http://www.caqh.org/ORMandate_Eligibility.php.

[iv] On January 10, 2012, HHS issued an interim final rule for adoption of standards for these operating rules. See Department of Health and Human Services, Office of the Secretary, 45 CFR Parts 160 and 162: Administrative Simplification: Adoption of Standards for Health Care Electronic Funds Transfers (EFTs) and Remittance Advice, Interim Final Rule, *Federal Register*, v. 77, n. 6, January 10, 2012, pp. 1556-1590, which is available at http://www.gpo.gov/fdsys/pkg/FR-2012-01-10/pdf/2012-132.pdf. On August 10, 2012, HHS issued an interim final rule for implementing these operating rules. See Department of Health and Human Services, Office of the Secretary, 45 CFR Part 162: Administrative Simplification: Adoption of Operating Rules for Health Care Electronic Funds Transfers (EFT) and Remittance Advice Transactions; Interim Final Rule, *Federal Register*, v. 77, n. 155, August 10, 2012, pp. 48008-48044, which is available at http://www.gpo.gov/fdsys/pkg/FR-2012-08-10/pdf/2012-19557.pdf. On April 19, 2013, CMS notified the health care industry that the interim final rule was now a final rule: "[W]e have decided not to change any polices established in the EFT & ERA Operating Rule Set [the interim final rule]." See CMS, Health Care Electronic Funds Transfers (EFT) and Remittance Advice Transactions Interim Final Rule, at http://www.caqh.org/pdf/CMSEFTERAFinalRuleAnnouncement.pdf. For information on the operating rules mandate for electronic funds transfers and remittance advice transactions, including a copy of the operating rules, visit the CAQH Web site at http://www.caqh.org/ORMandate_EFT.php.

Finally, Section 1104(c) provides for promulgation of three new final rules:[105]

- **Unique Health Plan Identifier.** "To be effective not later than October 1, 2012," which "[t]he Secretary may do . . . on an interim final basis."
- **Electronic Funds Transfer.** To be adopted "not later than January 1, 2012, in a manner ensuring that such standard is effective not later than January 1, 2014," which may be "on an interim final basis."
- **Health Claims Attachments.** To "establish a transaction standard and a single set of associate operating rules . . . that is consistent with the X12 Version 5010 transaction standards," to be adopted, "not later than January 1, 2014, in a manner ensuring that such standard is effective not later than January 1, 2016," which may be "on an interim final basis."[106]

Section 10109

Section 10109 outlines in three subsections considerations relating to development of standards for financial and administrative transactions. Section 10109(a) requires the Secretary of HHS to solicit "not later than January 1, 2012, and not less than every three years thereafter, input from [NCVHS,[107] the Health Information Technology Policy Committee,[108] the Health Information Technology Standards Committee,[109] standard setting organizations, and health care stakeholders] whether there could be greater uniformity in financial and administrative activities . . . and whether such activities should be considered financial and administrative transactions for which the adoption of standards and operating rules would improve the operation of the health care system and reduce administrative costs."[110]

Section 10109(b) outlines five areas for initial evaluation by January 1, 2012, of "activities and items" pertaining to "greater uniformity and/or consideration as operating rules and transaction standards."[111] They are the following:

- Application process for enrollment of health care providers by health plans
- Health care transactions of automobile insurance
- Financial audits required by health plans, federal and state agencies, and others determined by the Secretary of HHS
- Greater transparency and consistency of methodologies and processes used to establish claim edits used by health plans
- Health plan publication of rules about timeliness of payment

Finally, Section 10109(c) requires the Secretary of HHS to "task the ICD-9-CM Coordination and Maintenance Committee[112] to convene a meeting, not later than January 1, 2011,[113] to receive input from appropriate stakeholders (including health plans, health care providers, and clinicians) regarding the crosswalk between ICD-9 and ICD-10 that is posted on the CMS Web site, and make recommendations about appropriate revisions to it." [114] Such revisions would be posted on the CMS Web site, the revised crosswalk would be deemed a code set standard, and any subsequent revised crosswalks would be posted on the CMS Web site prior to "implementation of such subsequent revision."[115]

SUMMARY

In this chapter we have reviewed administrative simplification transaction and code set standards and their modifications, which went into effect on January 1, 2012 (Version 5010/D.0) and will go into effect on October 1, 2014 (ICD-10-CM/PCS), and new operating rules and a new standard for electronic funds transfers that is outlined in the Patient Protection and Affordable Care Act. It is important for your practice to carefully follow regulatory initiatives and developments related to these administrative simplification transactions and code sets in the coming years. To keep your practice informed, we recommend that you subscribe—at no cost—to the California HealthCare Foundation's excellent daily electronic newsletter, *iHealthBeat*, which is available at http://www.ihealthbeat.org. Your practice can also follow federal regulatory initiatives and developments that will affect your practice at http://www.cms.hhs.gov, http://www.healthit.gov, http://www.ama-assn.org, and http://www.hipaa.com.

We also recommend that your practice develop a game plan and have periodic meetings with the workforce to discuss administrative and clinical aspects of moving further toward electronic business tools in your practice. As a first step, if you have not done so already, have your software vendor attend your meetings and outline its plan for enabling ICD-10-CM/PCS code set standards in your software. Plan to meet monthly to check progress, and make sure that key workforce members in your practice read and understand the final rules. We have discussed how to go about planning for these changes and assessing their affects in other chapters of this book, in our other books cited earlier in this chapter, and in *EHR Implementation: A Step-by-Step Guide for the Medical Practice*, 2nd ed.[116]

ENDNOTES

1. C. P. Hartley and E. D. Jones III. Chicago, IL: American Medical Association, 2004; 2011.
2. Centers for Medicare and Medicaid Services (CMS). Transaction & Code Sets Standards. http://www.cms.hhs.gov/TransactionCodeSetsStands/. We recommend that you visit this Web site periodically for updates.
3. "Under HIPAA, if a covered entity conducts one of the adopted transactions electronically, they must use the adopted standard." (See note 2.) This means that they must adhere to the content and format requirements of each standard.
4. The final rule was published in the *Federal Register* on August 17, 2000, and is cited in the references to Table 1.1 in Chapter 1. The history of the enabling regulations for the transaction and code set standards is covered in our other books cited in this chapter. A modification to the final rule was published on February 20, 2003, and that is the document used for the discussion that follows. See Department of Health and Human Services, Office of the Secretary, 45 Part 162: Health Insurance Reform: Modifications to Electronic Data Transaction Standards and Code Sets; Final Rule, *Federal Register*, v. 68, n. 34, February 20, 2003, pp. 8381-8399. Hereafter, citations will be in the standard format 68 *Federal Register* <page(s)> (eg, 68 *Federal Register* 8381).
5. C. P. Hartley and E. D. Jones III. Appendix. *HIPAA Transactions: A Nontechnical Business Guide for Health Care*. Chicago, IL: American Medical Association, 2004, pp. 108-110.
6. See CMS Ending Contingency for Non-HIPAA-Compliant Medicare Claims, CMS Press Release, August 4, 2005, which is available at http://cms.hhs.gov/Newsroom/MediaReleaseDatabase/Press-Releases/2005-Press-Releases-Items/2005-08-04.html.
7. Letter from Simon P. Cohn, MD, MPH, Chair, National Committee on Vital and Health Statistics (NCVHS), to Michael O. Leavitt, Secretary, US Department of Health and Human Services, Revisions to HIPAA Transactions Standards Urgently Needed, September 26, 2007. Available at http://www.ncvhs.hhs.gov/070926lt.pdf.
8. Department of Health and Human Services, Office of the Secretary, 45 CFR Part 162: Health Insurance Reform; Modifications to the Health Insurance Portability and Accountability Act (HIPAA) Electronic Transaction Standards; Proposed Rule, *Federal Register*, v. 73, n. 164, August 22, 2008, pp. 49741–49793. Hereafter, citations will be in the standard format 73 *Federal Register* <page(s)> (eg, 73 *Federal Register* 49741).
9. Department of Health and Human Services, Office of the Secretary, 45 CFR Part 162: Health Insurance Reform; Modifications to the Health Insurance Portability and Accountability Act (HIPAA) Electronic Transaction Standards; Final Rule, *Federal Register*, v. 74, n. 11, January 16, 2009, pp. 3295-3328. Hereafter, citations will be in the standard format 74 *Federal Register* <page(s)> (eg, 74 *Federal Register* 3295).
10. 74 *Federal Register* 3325 and 45 CFR 162.923(a).
11. Accredited Standards Committee X12, Insurance Subcommittee, ASC X12N. *Health Care Claim: Professional (837)*. ASC Standards for Electronic Data Interchange Technical Report Type 3 (ASC X12N/005010X222). May 2006. Washington Publishing Company.

12. Accredited Standards Committee X12, Insurance Subcommittee, ASC X12N. *Health Care Eligibility Benefit Inquiry and Response (270/271).* ASC Standards for Electronic Data Interchange Technical Report Type 3 (ASC X12N/005010X279). April 2008. Washington Publishing Company.
13. Accredited Standards Committee X12, Insurance Subcommittee, ASC X12N. *Health Care Services Review—Request for Review and Response (278).* ASC Standards for Electronic Data Interchange Technical Report Type 3 (ASC X12N/005010X217), May 2006. Washington Publishing Company. This standard covers three types of transactions: "(a) A request from a health care provider to a health plan for the review of health care to obtain an authorization for the health care. (b) A request from a health care provider to a health plan to obtain authorization for referring an individual to another health care provider. (c) A response from a health plan to a health care provider to a request described in paragraph (a) or (b) of this section." 73 *Federal Register* 49791.
14. Accredited Standards Committee X12, Insurance Subcommittee, ASC X12N. *Health Care Claim Status Request and Response (276/277).* ASC Standards for Electronic Data Interchange Technical Report Type 3 (ASC X12N/005010X212). August 2006. Washington Publishing Company.
15. Accredited Standards Committee X12, Insurance Subcommittee, ASC X12N. *Health Care Claim Payment/Advice (835).* ASC Standards for Electronic Data Interchange Technical Report Type 3 (ASC X12N/005010X221). April 2006. Washington Publishing Company.
16. See note 11. The ASC X12 transaction standard for the health care claim and for coordination of benefits is the same (837).
17. 73 *Federal Register* 49743.
18. In the first edition of this book, we introduced the concepts of raising the bridge and lowering the river. "*Raising the bridge* means generating more revenue per unit of service. *Lowering the river* means lowering costs per unit of service. Either, controlling for the other, will increase net revenue. Both will increase it even more." See C. P. Hartley and E. D. Jones III, *HIPAA Plain & Simple: A Compliance Guide for Health Care Professionals*, Chicago, IL: American Medical Association, 2004, pp. 193-194.
19. Do you know how much time your practice allocates to handling remittance, payment, and claims status issues with health plans, and the cost of the workforce resources required to handle these issues?
20. 73 *Federal Register* 49757-49768, especially 49767-49768. The conclusion was confirmed in the final Version 5010 rule. See 74 *Federal Register* 3316-3317.
21. The NPRM discussion of this transaction standard is at 73 *Federal Register* 49748.
22. This and preceding quotations in the section on the 835 transaction standard are from 73 *Federal Register* 49748.
23. 74 *Federal Register* 3298.
24. 73 *Federal Register* 49765.
25. The NPRM discussion of the 276/277 transaction standard, including the quotations in this section, is at 73 *Federal Register* 49750.
26. 73 *Federal Register* 49763.
27. "These deficiencies in the current implementation specifications have caused much of the industry to rely on 'companion guides' created by health plans to address

areas of Version 4010/4010A that are not specific enough or require work-around solutions to address business needs. These companion guides are unique, plan-specific implementation instructions for the situational use of certain fields and/or data elements that are needed to support current business operations." 73 *Federal Register* 49746.

28. R. Lieber, "Asking Your Doc for Discounts: New Health Plans Mean It's Not as Farfetched as It Sounds," *Wall Street Journal,* October 29, 2005, p. B1.
29. With compliance required by covered entity health care providers on September 23, 2013, and thereafter, a patient who pays . . . for purposes of carrying out treatment, and a health care provider *must* comply [emphasis added]. 45 CFR 164.522(a)(1)(vi) at 78 *Federal Register* 5701. It is unclear what the incidence of this HITECH Act requirement will be on patients paying out of pocket in full at time of service.
30. The CMS Electronic Billing & EDI Transactions Web site is available at http://www.cms.gov/Medicare/Billing/ElectronicBillingEDITrans/index.html?redirect=/electronicbillingeditrans.
31. 74 *Federal Register* 3296-3297.
32. 74 *Federal Register* 3302.
33. See the discussion earlier in this chapter about the contingency plan regarding the October 2003 transaction and code set compliance date.
34. 74 *Federal Register* 3303.
35. See CMS, Centers for Medicare & Medicaid Services' Office of E-Health Standards and Services Announces 90-Day Period of Enforcement Discretion for Compliance With New HIPAA Transaction Standards, November 17, 2011, which is available at http://www.cms.gov/Medicare/Coding/ICD10/downloads/CMSStatement5010EnforcementDiscretion111711.pdf.
36. 74 *Federal Register* 3302-3303.
37. 74 *Federal Register* 3306.
38. 74 *Federal Register* 3302.
39. 74 *Federal Register* 3302-3303.
40. 74 *Federal Register* 3303.
41. See CMS, HCPCS - General Information, which is available at http://www.cms.gov/MedHCPCSGENInfo/.
42. At http://www.usps.com, you can click on "Find a Zip Code," enter the street address, city, and state, and receive a zip+4 code (the five-digit zip code plus four additional digits) in response. This is an example of accessing an external code set. You will learn in Chapter 3 that zip code is one of 18 protected health information (PHI) identifiers when it is used in conjunction with other PHI identifiers.
43. With increasing deployment of electronic health record (EHR) systems and their integration or interface with practice management systems in the coming decade, the appropriate procedure code(s) will be automatically determined by the entries in the EHR that characterize the services rendered by the physician during the encounter.
44. Your practice's software vendor or clearinghouse, in a business associate role, may be subject to civil penalties for violations of standard transaction rules beginning September 23, 2013, when business associates, as required by the HITECH Act, are

regulated directly by the federal government rather than indirectly by covered entities with respect to the HIPAA Security Rule and certain provisions of the HIPAA Privacy Rule, including breach notification. Such violations could be discovered during a security or privacy compliance audit or complaint investigation, conducted by the HHS Office for Civil Rights (OCR), and referred to CMS, which has responsibility for enforcing compliance with standard transaction and code set rules.

45. See CMS, Transaction & Code Sets Standards, which is available at http://www.cms.hhs.gov/TransactionCodeSetsStands/.
46. See US Food and Drug Administration (FDA), National Drug Code Directory, which is available at http://www.fda.gov/Drugs/InformationOnDrugs/ucm142438.htm.
47. See American Dental Association, Code on Dental Procedures and Nomenclature (CDT), which is available at http://www.ada.org/3827.aspx. Information on the current code, CDT 2013, is available at http://www.ada.org/3836.aspx.
48. For information on HCPCS Level II coding procedures, see CMS, Alpha-Numeric HCPCS, which is available at http://www.cms.gov/Medicare/Coding/HCPCSReleaseCodeSets/Alpha-Numeric-HCPCS.html.
49. 68 *Federal Register* 8381-8399.
50. Department of Health and Human Services, Office of the Secretary, 45 CFR Parts 160 and 162: Health Insurance Reform: Standards for Electronic Transactions; Announcement of Designated Standard Maintenance Organizations; Final Rule and Notice, *Federal Register*, v. 65, n. 160, August 17, 2000, p. 50370.
51. Department of Health and Human Services, Office of the Secretary, 45 CFR Part 160 162: Health Insurance Reform: Modifications to Standards for Electronic Transactions and Code Sets; Proposed Rule, *Federal Register*, v. 67, n. 105, May 31, 2002, pp. 38044-38050.
52. 68 *Federal Register* 8385-8387.
53. 68 *Federal Register* 8386.
54. 68 *Federal Register* 8387.
55. While it is beyond the scope of the discussion here, information on the DSMO process is available at 68 *Federal Register* 8382. Also, see HIPAA-DSMO Transaction Change Request System, which is available at http://www.hipaa-dsmo:org/Main.asp.
56. Compliance with these external code sources was required on January 1, 2012, when Version 5010 transaction standards had to be used. A similar table for external code sources in use through December 31, 2011, can be found in Table 4.1 (pp. 65-67) of Edward D. Jones III and Carolyn P. Hartley, *HIPAA Transactions: A Nontechnical Business Guide for Health Care*, Chicago, IL: American Medical Association, 2004.
57. The abstract is the descriptor of a code set.
58. Accredited Standards Committee X12, Insurance Subcommittee, ASC X12N, as referenced in text. For more information, visit the Web site for Washington Publishing Company at http://www.wpc-edi.com.
59. The category, Simple Data Element/Code References, identifies where in the transaction the code set is used.

60. Physicians will be required to use ICD-10-CM on and after October 1, 2014, to code diagnoses, but they will not be required to use ICD-10-PCS procedure codes in an ambulatory setting.
61. Department of Health and Human Services, Office of the Secretary, 45 CFR Parts 160 and 162: HIPAA Administrative Simplification: Modification to Medical Data Code Set Standards to Adopt ICD-10-CM and ICD-10-PCS; Proposed Rule, *Federal Register*, v. 73, n. 164, August 22, 2008, pp. 49795-49832. Hereafter, citations will be in the standard format 73 *Federal Register* <page(s)>.
62. Department of Health and Human Services, Office of the Secretary, 45 CFR Part 162: HIPAA Administrative Simplification: Modifications to Medical Data Code Set Standards to Adopt ICD-10-CM and ICD-10-PCS; Final Rule, *Federal Register*, v. 74, n. 11, January 16, 2009, pp. 3328-3362. Hereafter, citations will be in the standard format 74 *Federal Register* <page(s)> (eg, 74 *Federal Register* 3328).
63. Noninpatient (ambulatory) providers will continue to use CPT-4 and HCPCS codes for coding procedures.
64. 73 *Federal Register* 49798.
65. 73 *Federal Register* 49799.
66. Ibid.
67. 73 *Federal Register* 49800.
68. 73 *Federal Register* 49801.
69. 73 *Federal Register* 49800.
70. Letter from Jim Whicker, Chairman, WEDI, to CMS, October 20, 2008. Available upon written request to WEDI at the mailing address provided at http://www.wedi.org.
71. Ibid.
72. See CMS, EHR Incentive Programs: The Official Web Site for the Medicare and Medicaid Electronic Health Records (EHR) Incentive Programs, at http://www.cms.gov/Regulations-and-Guidance/Legislation/EHRIncentivePrograms/index.html?redirect=/ehrincentiveprograms.
73. Linda Kloss, "The Promise of ICD-10-CM," *Health Management Technology*, July 2005, p. 48.
74. This letter is available at http://www.ncvhs.hhs.gov/031105lt.htm.
75. The referenced RAND study is M. C. Libicki and I. T. Brahmakulam, *The Costs and Benefits of Moving to the ICD-10 Code Sets* (TR-132-DHS), Santa Monica, CA: RAND Corporation, March 2004. This report is available at http://www.rand.org/pubs/technical_reports/TR132.html.
76. 73 *Federal Register* 49821.
77. 73 *Federal Register* 49820.
78. ICD-10-CM means the *International Classification of Diseases, Tenth Revision, Clinical Modification* for diagnosis coding, including the Official ICD-10-CM Guidelines for Coding and Reporting, as maintained and distributed by HHS.
79. ICD-10-PCS means the *International Classification of Diseases, Tenth Revision, Procedure Coding System* for inpatient hospital procedure coding, including the Official ICD-10-PCS Guidelines for Coding and Reporting, as maintained and distributed by HHS.
80. 74 *Federal Register* 3328.

81. Department of Health and Human Services, Office of the Secretary, 45 CFR Part 162: Administrative Simplification: Adoption of a Standard for a Unique Health Plan Identifier; Addition to the National Provider Identifier Requirements; and a Change to the Compliance Date for the International Classification of Diseases, 10th Edition (ICD-10-CM and ICD-10-PCS) Medical Data Code Sets; Final Rule, *Federal Register*, v. 77, n. 172, September 5, 2012, pp. 54664-54720. Hereafter, citations will be in the standard format 77 *Federal Register* pages (eg, 77 *Federal Register* 54664).
82. 74 *Federal Register* 3328.
83. 74 *Federal Register* 3334.
84. 74 *Federal Register* 3335.
85. 77 *Federal Register* 54720.
86. 77 *Federal Register* 54665-54666.
87. 74 *Federal Register* 3336.
88. 74 *Federal Register* 3302.
89. 74 *Federal Register* 3302-3303.
90. 74 *Federal Register* 3337.
91. Ibid.
92. American Hospital Association (AHA) and American Health Information Management Association (AHIMA). *ICD-10-CM Field Testing Project: Report on Findings*. September 23, 2013. http://www.ahima.org/downloads/pdfs/resources/FinalStudy.pdf.
93. The 2013 GEMs are currently available on the same Web site (http://www.cdc.gov/nchs/icd/icd10cm.htm) under the heading "2013 release of ICD-10-CM."
94. Public Law 111–148, published as 124 STAT. 119–1024, is available at http://www.gpo.gov/fdsys/pkg/PLAW-111publ148/pdf/PLAW-111publ148.pdf.
95. Public Law 111–152, published as 124 STAT. 1029–1083, is available at http://www.gpo.gov:80/fdsys/pkg/PLAW-111publ152/pdf/PLAW-111publ152.pdf.
96. 124 STAT. 146–154.
97. 124 STAT. 915–917.
98. Section 1105, 124 STAT. 154.
99. The purpose is in Section 261 of Subtitle F—Administrative Simplification—of HIPAA, which is available at http://www.hhs.gov/ocr/privacy/hipaa/administrative/statute/index.html#261. Section 1104(a) is at 124 STAT. 146.
100. 124 STAT. 146–153.
101. 124 STAT. 147. Additional information on operating rules as they relate to the Committee on Operating Rules for Informational Exchange (CORE) is available online at: http://www.caqh.org/CORE_rules.php.
102. 124 STAT. 147.
103. NCVHS is the public advisory body to the Secretary of HHS.
104. The Secretary of HHS is directed to issue final rules by certain dates with discretion to use interim final rules, if necessary. 124 STAT. 151.
105. 124 STAT. 153.

106. Be aware that the Secretary of HHS issued a NPRM for a claim attachment on September 23, 2005 (70 *Federal Register* 55989-56025), which was withdrawn on January 25, 2010 (75 *Federal Register* 21804).
107. See the NCVHS Web site (http://www.ncvhs.hhs.gov).
108. See the Office of the National Coordinator for Health Information Technology Web site (http://healthit.hhs.gov).
109. Ibid.
110. 124 STAT. 916.
111. Ibid.
112. See the CDC Web site (http://www.cdc.gov/nchs/icd/icd9cm_maintenance.htm).
113. The meeting occurred on September 15, 2010. For additional information pertaining to the meeting, see NHIC Corp., "Meeting on ACA Requirements for ICD-10 Crosswalk Revisions (CMS Message 201007-57)," August 6, 2010, at http://www.medicarenhic.com/dme/articles/080610_201007-57.pdf.
114. 124 STAT. 916–917.
115. 124 STAT. 917.
116. C. P. Hartley and Edward D. Jones III. Chicago, IL: American Medical Association, 2012.

chapter 3

The Privacy Team

Respecting a patient's privacy and confidentiality has always been part of the culture of a physician's practice. Initially, the rules and enforcement activities surrounding privacy practices seemed to be an affront to many workforce members. But you completed the tasks, consulted legal advisers, created your Notice of Privacy Practices (NPP), implemented authorization and consent forms, and built new habits. As a result of the final rule published in the Federal Register on January 25, 2013, "Modifications to the HIPAA Privacy, Security, Enforcement, and Breach Notification Rules Under the Health Information Technology for Economic and Clinical Health Act and the Genetic Information Nondiscrimination Act; Other Modifications to the HIPAA Rules; Final Rule,"[1] often called the HIPAA Omnibus Rule because of the wide, sweeping changes it makes. Some privacy practices will change and are likely to require new workflows, while other standards did not change and are still in effect. (For simplicity, we refer to this rule as the HIPAA Omnibus Rule throughout the chapter.) The HIPAA Omnibus Rule uses the terms patient and individual interchangeably, as we do here.

The health information technology (health IT) landscape has changed exponentially since the privacy rule went into effect. The electronic environment has become comonplace, not only for individuals but also for health care providers.

- Electronic health record (EHR) systems are replacing paper charts, and the Centers for Medicare and Medicaid Services (CMS) now provides incentive funds up to $44,000 per physician to support the transition.[2]
- Regional health information organizations (RHIOs) provide a secure network for providers, payers, and patients to exchange electronic protected health information (ePHI).
- Social networking sites provide a means for individuals to exchange updates on their health progress or the progress of a family member and, if they wish, their own confidential health information. (Individuals are not covered entities.)
- Employers are supporting employees in wellness activities and in-house clinics.
- E-prescribing networks store individuals' prescriptions and send automatic patient alerts to avoid interactions and allergies while reconciling medications the patient has picked up from the pharmacy.

- A SIM (subscriber identity module) card that once stored telephone numbers in a mobile phone now integrates with other functions to synchronize stored information into servers and computers. Providers can access patient records from anywhere in the world, if service is available.

In an effort to stay current with and forecast emerging technology while also creating incentives for physicians to adopt technology, regulations safeguarding protected health information (PHI) had to be updated as well.

What You Will Learn in This Chapter

This chapter, loaded with lists, charts, diagrams, and insider tips on how to manage patient privacy, gives you step-by-step instructions on current HIPAA privacy regulations. The updates for your privacy implementation are divided into 10 steps.

Step 1: Build a foundation for privacy, including provisions from the HIPAA Omnibus Rule.

Step 2: Learn when you are permitted to use and disclose PHI without authorization.

Step 3: Identify uses and disclosures of PHI that require authorizations. This includes guidelines on what you can share with family and friends, disaster relief agencies, and enforcement agencies.

Step 4: Identify personal identity authentication issues, such as verification of personal representatives, guidance on custody agreements, and guidance about how to deny a use or disclosure to someone you think may cause substantial harm to the patient.

Step 5: Update Your HIPAA Privacy Safeguards.

Step 6: Update new patient rights, including rights provided in the HITECH (Health Information Technology for Economic and Clinical Health) Act and the Breach Notification Rule.

Step 7: Update business associates' contracts in light of their new compliance status.

Step 8: Revise and protect marketing activities with rules that close loopholes in prior marketing activities.

Step 9: Train your staff on new issues, including requirements specified in the HIPAA Omnibus Rule.

Step 10: Implement your updated plan, and safeguard your assets by preparing for an audit.

With each step, you'll find "What to Do" and "How to Do It" sections to use as a foundation for writing simple policies and procedures for a small to mid-size physician practice. Real scenarios show you how the situation may look so that you can see why the policy or procedure is necessary.

Key Terms

In this chapter, we will introduce terms, many of which have been updated in the HIPAA Omnibus Rule. Here, you will see a list of terms, and in the Glossary, you'll find definitions for each.

- Breach
- Business associate
- Designated record set
- Disclosure
- Electronic media
- Electronic protected health information (ePHI)
- Genetic information
- Health and Human Services (HHS), Department of
- Health care operations
- Incidental use and disclosure
- Individual
- Marketing
- Minimum necessary
- Office for Civil Rights (OCR)
- Patient safety organizations
- Payment
- Personal representative
- Protected health information (PHI)
- Subcontractor
- Treatment
- Use

WHAT CHANGED IN THE HIPAA OMNIBUS RULE, AND WHAT DIDN'T CHANGE?

As health care expanded its electronic capabilities and data increasingly became readily exchanged between covered entities and their business associates, the federal government made a promise to individuals that their health information would be governed by stronger privacy and security measures. The enhancements were necessary to build trust and also relieve some of the burden covered entities have undertaken since 2003 to ensure that their business associates complied with federal privacy and security regulations.

Effective September 23, 2013, business associates will be under the jurisdiction of the Office for Civil Rights (OCR) and face federal penalties for failures to comply with the HIPAA Security Rule, and certain provisions of the HIPAA Privacy Rule. No longer is the covered entity totally responsible for the actions of the business associate. Instead, the business associate must now meet requirements in the HIPAA Security Rule, discussed in Chapter 4, as well as some components of the Privacy Rule. Since the Breach Notification interim final rule of August 24, 2009, business associates have been under the jurisdiction of OCR for purposes of breach notification enforcement.

As a result of the HIPAA Omnibus Rule, you will be required to complete the following, each of which is discussed in this chapter:

- Modify your NPP as needed and redistribute it beginning on its effective date. If your current NPP is consistent with the HIPAA Omnibus Rule and individuals coming into the practice have been informed of all material revisions made to the NPP, then you are not required to revise and redistribute the NPP.[3] (See Appendix A for a sample Acknowledgment of Receipt of HIPAA Privacy Policies and Procedures form.)
- Update your HIPAA privacy and security policies and procedures. The majority of the necessary updates focus on privacy.
- Update or revise all business associate agreements so that you are not held responsible for a breach caused by a business associate.
- Revise your procedures for release of school immunization records, which are now considered a "public health disclosure."

The HIPAA Omnibus Rule actually contains four final rules, identified in Table 3.1.

TABLE 3.1

HIPAA Omnibus Rule Contents

Rule	What's Inside the Rule	What This Means to You
1. Final modifications to the HIPAA Privacy Rule, Security Rule, and Enforcement Rule mandated in the HITECH Act	Makes business associates directly liable for compliance	■ Review and update all previously signed business associate agreements to reduce and manage your liability for the business associate's actions. Business Associate Agreements (BAA) in place on January 25, 2013, may be updated not later than September 23, 2014. BAAs scheduled for update after January 25, 2013 cannot be grandfathered into this extended period.
	Places stronger limitations on marketing and fundraising activities	■ Update policies and procedures on marketing and fundraising activities. ■ Update authorization forms. ■ Include policies in Notice of Privacy Practices (NPP). ■ Prohibit sale of protected health information (PHI) without authorization.
	Expands individual rights	■ Update policies and procedures with new individual rights. ■ Include new rights in updated NPP. ■ Train all workforce members on new rights.

Rule	What's Inside the Rule	What This Means to You
	Requires practices to modify and redistribute NPP	■ Modify NPP. ■ Once you determine the new NPP's effective date, distribute to all existing patients when they come into the practice. Continue to provide NPP as you did before to all new patients.
	Modifies individual authorization for a child's immunization records to enable health research	■ Modify NPP. ■ Modify authorization forms.
	Enables family members of deceased to access records	■ Modify NPP. ■ Modify policies and procedures.
	Defines provisions for non-compliance, such as for willful neglect	■ Implement HIPAA privacy and security regulations and regularly update policies and procedures.
2. HIPAA Enforcement Rule	Incorporates increased and tiered civil monetary penalties	■ Ensure updated privacy and security policies and procedures are in place and workforce is trained on policies. ■ Ensure risk assessment reflects new risks, and assign risk managers to manage new risks, if applicable. ■ Ensure the practice has an audit response plan in place. ■ Defines "willful neglect" and associated penalties for workforce members.
3. Breach Notification for Unsecured Protected Health Information	Changes the "harm" threshold to a "probability" threshold with four objective standards. Supplants interim final rule and makes penalties enforceable.	■ Presumes breach notification required in absence of demonstration of "low probability" of impermissible use or disclosure of PHI. Avoid breach notification by security PHI with appropriate NIST-defined encryption of PHI.
4. Genetic Information Nondiscrimination Act (GINA)	Prevents most payers from using genetic information for underwriting purposes	■ Physicians are not subject to GINA, but questions will likely come up. Add patient rights to NPP.

The remainder of this chapter provides step-by-step measures to evaluate your current privacy strategy. Highlighted in each section are HIPAA Omnibus Rule additions and clarifications.

STEP 1: BUILD THE FOUNDATION FOR PRIVACY MANAGEMENT

The HIPAA Privacy Rule establishes the foundation upon which layers of electronic transactions can be built. Technology already exists whereby physicians can order a CBC (complete blood count) panel and within moments receive lab results, even if the blood is drawn at a hospital across town. To set the stage for your electronic exchange, begin by identifying a privacy official.

There are 10 implementation specifications in the privacy management component of the HIPAA Privacy Rule. We'll discuss each one and provide guidance on how to complete each specification.

Step 1A: Identify a Privacy Official

Since April 14, 2003, your organization has been required to identify a privacy official who is responsible for developing and implementing your privacy policies and procedures. If your privacy official has taken another position elsewhere, you must name another person to manage this job.

CRITICAL POINT

If the original privacy official is no longer with the practice, failure to appoint and train another privacy official leaves the practice exposed without anyone guiding the privacy strategy. More than ever, you must be sure one person takes on this role and stays abreast of changes to the rules.

The privacy official is also the contact person responsible for receiving complaints and providing individuals with further information about matters contained in the organization's NPP.

Privacy officials must continually update their knowledge of the Privacy Rule guidelines, updates, and new regulations and must train the workforce on these requirements. The privacy official also is responsible for ensuring that the workforce adheres to those policies and procedures, including imposing sanctions on workforce members that breach an individual's privacy.

Privacy officials must have the support of the organization's leadership, and in many cases, the privacy official reports directly to the president, board of directors, or managing partner.

While the privacy official is responsible for privacy management, he or she may delegate responsibilities to others within the organization if they are trained and communicate promptly with the privacy official on these matters.

Standard	Code of Federal Regulations	Privacy Management
Personnel designations (privacy official)	45 CFR 164.530(a)	Administrative requirements

What to Do:

Assign an individual to be your privacy official.

How to Do It:

1. The practice's management team creates a job description for the privacy official. A job description is included in Figure 3.1.

FIGURE 3.1

Privacy Official Job Description

The Privacy Official

The privacy official will report directly to the managing partner of the practice and will be responsible for the implementation and day-to-day administration and oversight of our HIPAA Privacy Rule compliance program. The privacy officer is also responsible for coordinating HIPAA Privacy Rule activities with HIPAA Security Rule and Breach Notification activities.

Critical Functions

Our privacy official is responsible for the following activities:

- Maintain an inventory of how we use and disclose all protected health information (PHI).
- Identify how PHI is created, stored, used, and disclosed in paper and electronic format. Critical to the electronic health record (EHR) environment is identifying PHI in a hybrid chart, one that is part paper and part EHR, or stored in one EHR system while the practice is migrating to another separate EHR or practice management system.
- Update the NPP, acknowledgment forms, authorizations, consents, and other forms as required.
- Establish policies and procedures to ensure that individual rights guaranteed by HIPAA and the Breach Notification Rule are upheld, including a complaint process and sanctions.
- Distribute the NPP to all new patients. Once you determine the effective date of your updated NPP, you must begin to notify all patients seeking services from your practice of the changes to your NPP. For example, if the effective date of your updated NPP is September 21, 2013, then all patients, including new patients, must be notified of your updated NPP beginning September 21, 2013, when they come into the practice. Also post the updated NPP on your Web site.
- Develop a training program.
- Review all business associate agreements to determine the practice's liability under old business associate agreements. If you have any doubt, consult legal counsel to determine whether you must draft amended and/or new agreements that address business associate compliance requirements under the HIPAA Security Rule, Breach Notification Rule, and Privacy Rule as appropriate to the service performed for the practice.
- Keep up to date on the latest privacy and security developments and federal and state laws and regulations.
- Coordinate privacy safeguards with the practice's security officer to ensure consistency in development, documentation, and training for security and privacy requirements.
- Serve as the practice's resource for regulatory and accrediting bodies on matters relating to privacy and security.
- Coordinate and communicate to practice leaders any audits of the Office for Civil Rights (OCR) or any other governmental or accrediting organization concerning state or federal privacy laws or regulations.

Continued

FIGURE 3.1 (continued)

Privacy Official Job Description

- Notify individuals when health information has been used or disclosed in violation of our privacy practices.
- Regularly communicate the status of legal complaints, risks, and sanctions imposed on workforce members with the managing partner(s) of this practice.
- Consistently apply sanctions, in accordance with the practice's policies and procedures approved by the managing partners.
- Work with health information systems and portable technologies.
- Effectively communicate technical and legal information to nontechnical and nonlegal staff for employee training.
- Ensure devices containing electronic protected health information (ePHI) are encrypted as required by the HIPAA Security Rule and Breach Notification Rule.
- (For a larger practice) The privacy official will report directly to the practice administrator or, if one is available, the organization's risk manager, and will make presentations as necessary to large audiences.

The privacy official will meet the following qualifications:

- Bachelor's degree in management, information systems, human resources, health administration, or other relevant field
- Minimum five years' experience in health care
- Familiar with regulatory development and compliance, including federal and state laws and regulations concerning information security and privacy
- Familiar with business functions and operations of a larger institution
- Have strong organizational and problem-solving skills, and work effectively in a team environment
- Have the ability to communicate with clarity both orally and in writing
- Ideally maintain a privacy designation from an accredited college, university, or health information management organization

2. Determine the research and communications skills needed. The privacy official must be familiar with the clinical and administrative functions of the office; be willing to take on new responsibility, including fast-track learning of HIPAA content; be highly ethical; exhibit strong organizational and communication skills; and work well with management and staff.
3. Establish a reporting structure. The office manager and the privacy official, even though they may be the same person, may report to two different supervisors.
4. Discuss salary or bonuses for the new privacy official or the employee taking on the additional responsibilities. The salary for privacy officials in medical offices typically ranges from $50,000 to $85,000, depending on the size of the practice and the responsibilities of the position.
5. Document the level of independent decision-making authority given to the privacy official. The privacy official needs authority to oversee some activities but should consult the management team for approval on others.

6. Consult with an attorney to review documentation that you believe may be called into question should a breach or OCR audit occur. Much of HIPAA compliance is about documentation, but keep in mind that your documentation could become evidence in a criminal or civil enforcement proceeding. See Step 1E for more guidance on documentation.

Designate a Privacy Team

The privacy official cannot handle privacy implementation independently. There is too much work to be done. In addition, the privacy official cannot be the "privacy watchdog" for the office. Privacy is a team activity and requires support from many levels. Consider the following as candidates for the privacy team: your head nurse, billing supervisor, receptionist, management, and insurance clerk.

Develop a Budget and Time-and-Task Chart

How big should your budget be? That depends on when you started and how fast you moved through the compliance process. If you've been working on compliance since 2003, most of your work on privacy has been completed and your HIPAA Omnibus Rule updates will be better managed. But if you have not kept accurate records of HIPAA forms, such as authorizations, accounting of disclosures, and sanctions, start now. These are consistently requested in OCR audits.[4] Also see Step 1E.

Include costs for legal counsel to determine whether your NPP is consistent with the final HIPAA Omnibus Rule, and review your updated NPP.

Step 1B: Revisit Your Notice of Privacy Practices

Standard	Code of Federal Regulations	Privacy Management
Notice of privacy practices	45 CFR 164.520; 45 CFR 164.530(i)(4)	Notice of privacy practices for PHI; changes to privacy practices stated in the notice

What to Do:

Revise your NPP. Your legal counsel can advise you whether updates to the Breach Notification Rule, Security Rule, and Privacy Rule are significant to warrant a new NPP.

New patient rights include the following new rights discussed in Chapter 1:

- The right to restrict disclosure of PHI to a health plan for a specific treatment for which the patient has paid in full and out of pocket.
- If your organization has adopted EHRs, the patient can now request an accounting of electronic disclosures. To achieve certified EHR technology (CEHRT) status,[5] an EHR system is not required to demonstrate that it can electronically collate an accounting of electronic and paper disclosures. Therefore, a patient's request for an accounting of disclosures still comes with a 30-day response time,

with a one-time 30-day extension allowed per request to complete this task. The HIPAA Omnibus Rule does not require disclosures for treatment, payment, and health care operations to be included in the electronic accounting of disclosures, as was previously proposed.

How to Do It:

Your NPP is a legal document and should be developed under the advice of legal counsel. You are required to provide the NPP to individuals the first time they seek health care from providers in your organization. You also are required to post your updated NPP in a public viewing area, and also on your Web site, if one exists. Required elements in your NPP include the following:

- Describe how you may use and disclose PHI.
- State your duty to protect privacy, provide a notice of privacy practices, and abide by the terms of the current notice.
- Describe the individual's rights, including the right to complain to HHS's Office for Civil Rights and to the covered entity.
- Include a statement that authorization will be, in most cases, required before the practice

  uses and discloses psychotherapy notes (where appropriate),

  uses and discloses protected health information for marketing and fundraising purposes, and

  makes disclosures that constitute a sale of PHI (these require authorization, as well as a statement on how to opt out or opt in for marketing purposes).
- Under Title VI of the Civil Rights Act of 1964, the covered entity must take reasonable steps to ensure meaningful access for individuals with limited English proficiency.[6]

Every workforce member should understand the content of your NPP, including new individual rights updated in the HIPAA Omnibus Rule.This will help field complaints internally so that you can mitigate privacy concerns before they are filed with an outside organization, such as HHS.

When providing the NPP to patients, you are required to:

- Provide the NPP upon the patient's first visit to your facility. You also are required to redistribute the revised NPP when the existing patient revisits the office.[7]
- Ask the patient to acknowledge receipt of the NPP. This can be done using an electronic signature pad.
- Provide the NPP to any individual or a personal representative acting on behalf of a patient who requests it.

If you maintain a Web site, you may provide the NPP on the site. You also may e-mail the NPP to an existing patient, but only if the individual agrees to an electronic notice and that agreement has not been withdrawn.

Step 1C: Consistent with Other Documentation

Standard	Code of Federal Regulations	Privacy Management
Consistent with notice of privacy practices	45 CFR 164.502(i)	Uses and disclosures of protected health information: general rules

What to Do:

Your NPP must be consistent with other documents, including your HIPAA privacy and security policies and procedures, the Breach Notification Rule, and HITECH rules. If state privacy laws conflict with HIPAA, more stringent state laws take precedence.

How to Do It:

In small organizations, the privacy and security officials may be the same person. In larger organizations, responsibilities for privacy and security officials are significantly expanded, so officials must tightly coordinate documentation to avoid conflict and confusion.

In updating or rebuilding your privacy and security policies and procedures (including those that reflect state laws), your NPP, and the Breach Notification Rule, make sure the language of these items is not in conflict.

Step 1D: Develop Policies and Procedures

Standard	Code of Federal Regulations	Privacy Management
Policies and procedures	45 CFR 164.530(i)	Administrative requirements

What to Do:

A covered entity must develop and implement written privacy policies and procedures that are consistent with the HIPAA Privacy Rule and the Breach Notification Rule.

How to Do It:

All covered entities must update policies and procedures to reflect the changes in the Privacy Rule and Breach Notification Rule. Security Rule updates are provided in Chapter 4.

As a covered entity, your organization must develop and implement written policies and procedures that are consistent with the HIPAA Privacy Rule, the Breach Notification Rule, and state law.

While the privacy official is responsible for the development of policies and procedures, the task can be daunting if completed by one person.

Therefore, the development of privacy policies and procedures can be simplified using one of three strategies:

1. Form a team to review the Privacy Rule published in the Federal Register and build your policies and procedures.
2. If you purchased a set of policies and procedures from a reputable organization, customize them according to the size of your organization.
3. Consult and contract with a privacy expert or attorney to customize your policies and procedures for your organization.

Provide hard-copy or electronic versions of your policies and procedures to all workforce members with an additional copy to be placed in your library.

As liability can now be extended to employers and workforce members, each workforce member must also receive a copy of your updated policies and procedures and sign an acknowledgment form stating that he or she understands the policies and procedures and will comply with them. Retain these forms for six years.

CRITICAL POINT

If your organization allows workforce members to be seen as a patient in the same organization, the only workforce members that may access that patient's record are those immediately engaged in the patient's care. Unauthorized access to a patient's chart by a fellow employee not involved in the patient's care is a breach, and the patient has a right to file a complaint with HHS.

Step 1E: Policies and Procedures

Standard	Code of Federal Regulations	Privacy Management
Policies and procedures	45 CFR 164.530(j)	Administrative requirements

What to Do:

Maintain HIPAA documentation for six years after whichever comes later: the date of its creation or its last effective date. Documents to maintain include but are not limited to:

- Privacy policies and procedures
- NPPs
- Authorizations
- Patient requests, such as access requests, or requests to withhold information from a payer if the patient pays in full for the specified treatment
- Disposition of complaints and documentation of other actions
- Documentation of activities and designations that the Privacy Rule requires to be documented

How to Do It:

For practices moving to an electronic format, you will find storing HIPAA forms to be part of your scanning or electronic workflow.

Maintain all acknowledgments signed by workforce members and patients. Medical practices often implement an electronic signature pad to capture patient approvals within the patient chart.

Maintain all hard-copy documentation in a secure storage facility, and back up any electronic documentation off site.

Permit an agent of HHS to access your facilities, books, records, accounts, and other information during your practice's normal business hours in response to a compliance audit or complaint investigation. If HHS determines that special circumstances warrant further access, such as in the case of hidden or destroyed files, your practice must allow HHS access at any time.

Document when a parent requests immunizations records for a patient. Even though immunization requests no longer require written authorization if immunization records are required by state or local authorities as an entrance requirement, you must still maintain documentation, eg, (log) on when they were requested and when they were sent. Parents may request these records by phone (orally), by e-mail, or in person.[8]

Privacy documents may be maintained in hard-copy or electronic format provided they are in a secure storage facility.

Step 1F: Training

Standard	Code of Federal Regulations	Privacy Management
Training	45 CFR 164.530(b)	Administrative requirements

What to Do:

Train all workforce members[9] on privacy and breach notification policies and procedures, as necessary and appropriate for them to carry out their functions.

You must apply appropriate sanctions against workforce members who violate privacy policies and procedures or the Privacy Rule may require retraining as part of your organization's Sanctions policy (discussed in Step 1G). Should your organization be audited by HHS or a state attorney general, or required to post notice of a breach, it may be required to produce documentation that you trained workforce members or retrained violators.

Business associates are not covered entities, but they are under the direct authority of OCR. You are not required to train business associates, or their subcontractors, as they now must train their own workforce on their HIPAA Security Rule[10] and Breach Notification Rule compliance policies and procedures. Business associates also must train their workforce to safeguard the PHI that they manage or transmit on behalf of a covered entity.

How to Do It:

Privacy, security, and breach notification training must be completed both formally (once yearly) and in an ongoing and informal way. Retraining must be part of your sanctions policy as a method of remediation for workforce members needing reminders of your privacy policies and procedures.

All workforce members, including physicians, must participate in retraining on privacy policies and procedures related to the HITECH Act and the Breach Notification Rule, as well as new security regulations related to the safeguarding of PHI.[11]

Your privacy official will determine who needs additional training, the type of training that is appropriate, and the frequency with which such training will occur. New employees must participate in training within 30 days following their first date of service.

Privacy topics to be included in updated training include:

- New patient rights
- Electronic communication with a patient, such as reminders to access the patient portal (Covered entities are permitted to send individuals unencrypted e-mail if they have advised the individual of the risk and the individual still prefers unencrypted e-mail.[12] Include the individual's permission in your documentation. Fundraising and marketing activities by e-mail, however, do not fall under this patient right. See Step 8.)
- Accounting of electronic disclosures
- The right to restrict disclosures if a specific service is paid in full (For example, if an individual requests a blood test to measure the increased risk of heart disease or to run a series of genetic tests, and makes a formal request in writing that neither the cost of the tests nor the results go to the payer, you must comply with the individual's wishes.)
- Penalties imposed on workforce members and employers
- New business associate requirements
- New enforcement activities, including:
  - Empowerment of state attorneys general to investigate privacy violations (Generally, state attorneys general get involved in privacy complaints if the complaint involves criminal action and have resisted involvement on civil complaints.)
  - Increased financial penalties
  - OCR audits
- Coordination of administrative, physical, and technical safeguards with your security official for training on content included in the Breach Notification Rule, such as your encryption policy (discussed in Chapter 4)

Upon completing training, each member of your workforce will sign an acknowledgment of attendance form[13] stating that he or she participated in training and is aware of and understands the practice's privacy policies and procedures.

If retraining is the result of a sanction, maintain a copy of the workforce member's acknowledgment form in your records.

Step 1G: Sanctions

Standard	Code of Federal Regulations	Privacy Management
Sanctions	45 CFR 164.530(e)	Administrative requirements

What to Do:

A covered entity must have a sanctions policy and apply appropriate sanctions against workforce members who violate its privacy policies and procedures or the Privacy Rule. The rule does not exempt medical staff from sanctions; however, your policies and procedures must define how practice owners will be sanctioned for repeated offenses or a breach. For example, your sanctions policy may indicate that a repeated offense may lead to termination. However, the practice could suffer from the loss of a noncompliant physician. Rather than dismissing the physician, the practice's leadership may instead impose direct costs of a breach, including legal fees and reputational damage, onto the physician. The American Health Information Management Assocation (AHIMA) addresses consistency of sanctions policies in a guidance tool available online.[14]

How to Do It:

Be cautious about applying sanctions without first researching details to verify what really happened.

The privacy official or another person designated by the privacy official must first review the privacy violation.

For repeat privacy violations, consider the following sanctions:

First violation: The privacy official provides a verbal reminder.

Second violation: A reminder is provided, and the workforce member is required to participate in privacy retraining.

Third violation: A reminder is placed in the employee's personnel file with the warning that a repeat offense will result in time off without pay; additional retraining is provided.

Fourth violation: The workforce member is suspended for three days without pay.

Fifth violation: The workforce member's employment is terminated.

Your policies and procedures also must indicate that the practice reserves the right to skip steps, repeat steps, or impose other sanctions, as it deems appropriate. It also may set time constraints, such as applying particular sanctions for a third violation within a 12-month period.

No sanctions are to be imposed against workforce members whose reason for conduct is in good faith and in accordance with HIPAA Privacy Rule provisions; for example:

- A whistleblower reporting to a government agency
- A workforce member crime victim reporting to a law enforcement official

Step 1H: Mitigation

Standard	Code of Federal Regulations	Privacy Management
Mitigation	45 CFR 164.530(f)	Administrative requirements

What to Do:

Mitigate, to the extent practicable, any harmful effect that is known to the covered entity of a use or disclosure of PHI in violation of its policies and procedures or requirements of the Privacy Rule by the covered entity or its business associate.

How to Do It:

Praise the workforce member who brings a complaint to the privacy official because that gives the organization an opportunity to take action to resolve the complaint before it goes to a higher level.

To mitigate something is to make it less harsh, less painful, or less severe. The Privacy Rule does not specify what steps a practice must take to resolve or mitigate harm to a patient from a privacy breach, but the rule does require the practice to try to resolve a complaint if the patient believes it has caused harm.

The normal human reaction is to try to mend a breach before the complaint goes to a supervisory level, but the best answer is to go directly to your privacy official with any complaint.

If a patient files a complaint with your privacy official and has chosen you as the person to blame, don't say, "She's out of her mind. That didn't happen." And don't say, "I'm really tired of hearing his whining." Do say, "Let's talk about what happened. My view may be different from the individual's."

Once you've presented the patient's complaint to the privacy official, step out of the picture. The privacy official is usually the only employee who can make mitigation recommendations.

For the privacy official:

- Document your conversation with the individual making a complaint.
- Do not offer any immediate solutions, but do promise to look into the event. The Breach Notification Rule requires a 30-day response time. Consult Chapter 5 on how to respond to an electronic breach.
- Consult the practice leaders to determine resources required to mitigate the violation. Resources may include the cost of a professional or legal consultant's time, internal resources, costs to remediate the data breach, and the costs of civil and/or criminal penalties.
- In accordance with the *guidance* contained in the Breach Notification Rule of August 24, 2009,[15] consult with legal counsel about any public notice that is required to be posted, and ensure encryption of server connections, portable computers, and all mobile devices to National Institute of Standards and Technology (NIST) standards as specified in the *guidance*. Consult Chapter 5 for more guidance on breach notification.
- In the event of a breach of unsecured PHI, evaluate the breach and follow requirements of the Breach Notification Rule and your policies and procedures for mitigation of harm.

- Depending on the nature of the complaint, mitigation responses may include:
  - ☐ Offering an apology in writing
  - ☐ Retrieving the PHI from where it was sent, accompanied by a letter notifying the individual of corrective actions
  - ☐ Adopting policies and procedures to clarify a situation that was not addressed before this incident
  - ☐ Retraining workforce members
  - ☐ Sanctioning an employee
- Certain breaches, such as accessing a patient record of a public figure without authorization or selling health information to a news media, are subject to criminal penalties. In this case, OCR may defer the case to a state attorney general, who will then provide more immediate and direct communication.

Most privacy violations are not intentional, but they do need to be corrected. If the violation was intentional, mitigation procedures can get complicated.

CRITICAL POINT

Demonstrating genuine concern about a possible privacy breach and providing a timely response with a plan to mitigate any harm may disarm an individual's more potent complaints filed against your organization with the HHS Office for Civil Rights.

Step 1I: Refraining from Intimidating or Retaliatory Acts

Standard	Code of Federal Regulations	Privacy Management
Refraining from intimidating or retaliatory acts	45 CFR 164.530(g)	Administrative requirements

What to Do:

A covered entity may not intimidate, threaten, coerce, discriminate against, or take other retaliatory action against any individual who exercises his or her right to file a complaint either with the HHS Office for Civil Rights or with the privacy official.

How to Do It:

Train workforce members that any workforce member who retaliates against an individual filing a complaint will be subject to sanctions, retraining, or immediate termination of employment.

Step 1J: Waiver of Rights

Standard	Code of Federal Regulations	Privacy Management
Waiver of rights	45 CFR 164.530(h)	Administrative requirements

What to Do:

A covered entity may not require an individual to waive his or her rights under the Privacy Rule, Security Rule, or Breach Notification Rule as a condition for obtaining treatment, enrollment in a health plan, or eligibility for benefits.

How to Do It:

The privacy official will confirm that the practice does not require patients to sign waivers of any of the following rights as a condition of receiving treatment, payment, enrollment in a health plan, or eligibility for benefits:

- Their rights to file a complaint with the practice or with HHS
- Their rights under the Security Rule
- Their rights under the Privacy Rule
- Their rights under the Breach Notification Rule

The privacy official must train workforce members not to request any patient to sign a waiver as a condition for obtaining treatment, payment, enrollment in a health plan, or eligibility for benefits. Workforce members who make such a request will be subject to the practice's sanctions policy, up to and including termination of employment.

Step 1K: Establish Minimum Necessary Limits for Use and Disclosures of Protected Health Information

Standard	Code of Federal Regulations	Protected Health Information Special Permissions
Minimum necessary	45 CFR 164.502(b); 45 CFR 164.514(d)	Uses and disclosures of PHI; other requirements relating to uses and disclosures of PHI

What to Do:

A covered entity must develop and implement policies and procedures to reasonably limit uses and disclosures of PHI to the minimum amount necessary to complete a task. The HIPAA Omnibus Rule also imposes these requirements on business associates but leaves the definition of minimum necessary up to both parties.

As it applies to a use or disclosure, a covered entity may not use, disclose, or request the entire medical record for a particular purpose unless it can specifically justify why it needs the whole record.

How to Do It:

Identify roles of workforce members and the appropriate amount of PHI that will be made available to each of them. Make reasonable efforts to limit the access of workforce members to the appropriate amount of PHI.

Implement policies and procedures for routine disclosures (which may be standard protocols) that limit the PHI disclosed to the amount reasonably necessary to achieve the purpose of the disclosure.

HIPAA did not offer well-defined direction for the minimum necessary requirement, but the HITECH Act offers some clarification: The entity disclosing the PHI (as opposed to the person or organization requesting the PHI) must make a responsible determination of what is the minimum amount necessary.

Your standard business associate agreement may need to be customized for some business associates who will need access to more PHI than other business associates. Your business associate's minimum necessary policies must be consistent with the covered entity's, and cannot be less stringent.[16] Subcontractors of the business associate also must agree to the minimum necessary policy.

EHR software automatically limits medically necessary information according to roles within the organization. An administrator would have to override those permissions to change medically necessary uses and disclosures.

A practice might assign access to PHI for purposes such as those listed in Table 3.2.

TABLE 3.2

Minimum Necessary Access Assignments

To complete this form, add Xs in the boxes as needed to indicate the types of protected health information (PHI) for which the individuals in each role have access privileges. Similar access can be provided via an electronic health record (EHR) system's role-based access functionality.

Name	Billing	Clinical		Administrative Access	Scheduling
		Vitals	Full		
(Physician)					
(Physician)					
(Nurse Practitioner)					
(Nurse)					
(Medical Assistant)					
(Receptionist)					
(Lab Technician)					

STEP 2: IDENTIFY PERMISSIONS FOR USE AND DISCLOSURE OF PROTECTED HEALTH INFORMATION

Most laws allow you to do anything you want, unless there is a provision against it. HIPAA is just the opposite. You can use and disclose patient information, but you have to find a reason for each use or disclosure. The core of the Privacy Rule is that you must identify permissions, even those that come with special requirements to use or disclose patient information.

CRITICAL POINT

To use or disclose PHI, you must first identify the permission (or reason) for the use or disclosure.

Under certain circumstances, HIPAA may permit or require a covered entity to use or disclose PHI without an individual's authorization. Under other circumstances a valid authorization from the individual is required. If the HIPAA Privacy Rule does not specifically permit or require a use or disclosure, you must obtain written authorization from the patient.

Itemized steps here provide how-to guidance for obtaining valid authorizations and situations where a covered entity may use and disclose patient information without the individual's authorization.[17]

In Step 2, we discuss the following permitted disclosures:

- Required disclosures (see Figure 3.2)
  - To HHS
  - To the patient or personal representative
- Permissible disclosures (see Figure 3.3)
  - For treatment, payment, and health care operations
  - For another covered entity's treatment, payment, and health care operations
  - To family, friends, and disaster relief agencies
  - Incidental to a use or disclosure otherwise permitted or required
  - Uses and disclosures for which an authorization or opportunity to agree or object is not required
- Uses and disclosures of de-identified PHI
- Limited data set for purposes of research, public health, or health care operations

FIGURE 3.2

Required Disclosures

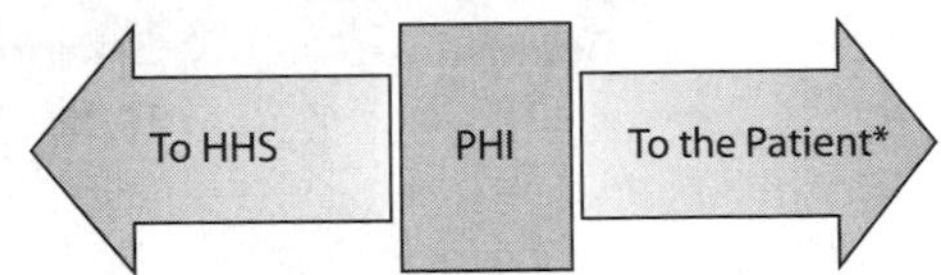

*Exceptions to patient disclosures are discussed in Step 6.

FIGURE 3.3

Permitted Disclosures

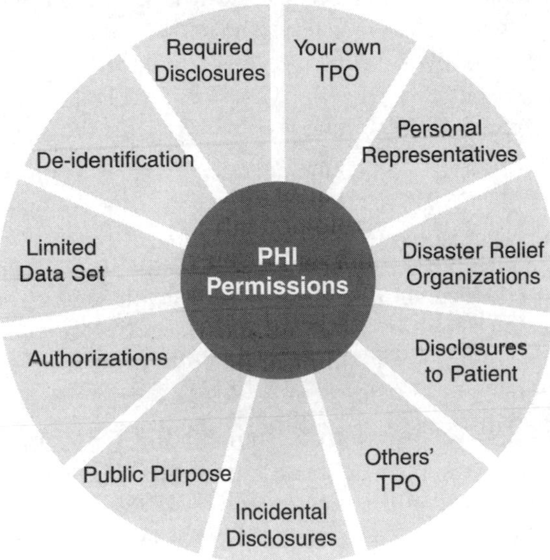

TPO indicates treatment, payment, and health care operations.
Reprinted with permission from Carolyn Hartley.

Step 2A: Required Disclosures

Standard	Code of Federal Regulations	Protected Health Information Permissions
Required disclosures	45 CFR 164.502(a)(2)	Uses and disclosures of protected health information: general rules

What to Do:

Unless a use or disclosure is required or permitted by the HIPAA Privacy Rule, as a covered entity, you must disclose PHI in only two situations:

- To individuals (or their personal representatives) specifically when they request access to, or an accounting of disclosures of, their PHI. However, there are circumstances where you would deny this.
- To a state attorney general, law enforcement officials, or local, state, or federal HHS officials when undertaking a compliance investigation or review or enforcement action.[18] In all situations, verify credentials.

How to Do It:

Your privacy official will determine whether a request for disclosure is required or permitted, if it requires special permission, and if an authorization is required.

Ensure that all workforce members from front office to clinic to back office are aware of the patient's right to request information. If your practice is engaged in quality reporting incentive programs such as the meaningful use incentive program, you have already experienced an increase in patient involvement. The Office of the National Coordinator for Health Information Technology (ONC) supports initiatives that educate consumers on accessing personal health information to better manage their care.

The Privacy Official's Response to a Request for PHI From a Patient:

First: If you do not know the person, obtain a photo ID. If this is a regular patient of the practice whom you recognize, then you are not required to obtain a photo ID.

Second: Ask what information is being requested. For example, is the request for a summary of a recent visit? Copies of radiographs or digital images? Payment history?

Third: Document the request in a log and in the patient's file.

Fourth: Provide requested information to the patient. If you are entitled to impose a fee in connection with the request, ask for payment, but first check to be sure you can impose a fee.[19]

The Privacy Official's Response to a Request for PHI From a Patient's Personal Representative:

First: Evaluate the relationship between the patient and personal representative, referring to the discussion of "personal representative" below, and examining and copying any applicable credentials or other documentation. Obtain a photo ID.

Second: Document the personal representative's request in the patient's record. If you provide the requested information, document your provision of the requested PHI and your basis for doing so. If you refuse to provide the requested information, document your refusal and your basis for refusing (eg, your reasonable belief that the personal representative did not provide necessary credentials and/or your belief that the personal representative might endanger the patient).

A personal representative[20] is legally responsible for the individual's care and general condition. A personal representative can be named in accordance with state or federal law. For example, the personal representative of a minor child is usually the child's parent or legal guardian.

In the case of a custody decree, the personal representative is the parent who can make health care decisions for the child under the decree. If you do not know the patient or parent, you should ask to see a copy of the divorce decree and a photo ID.

The personal representative may also present documentation including a health care power of attorney form. Make a copy of this document and include it in the patient's health record. Upon death of an individual, the executor or administrator of the deceased individual's estate is the personal representative for the deceased, and also is legally authorized by a court and/or state law to act on behalf of the deceased or the estate.

If you reasonably believe the personal representative might endanger the patient, such as in cases of domestic violence, abuse, or neglect, you can refuse to provide PHI. Be sure to document your decision. If you suspect the patient is a victim of abuse, neglect, or domestic violence, you may as a covered entity disclose PHI to appropriate government authorities regarding victims of abuse, neglect, or domestic violence.

Third: Document the request in a log and in the patient's file.

Fourth: Provide requested information to the personal representative. If you are entitled to impose a fee in connection with the request, ask for payment.

The Privacy Official's Response to a Request for PHI From an Agent of HHS or From a Law Enforcement Official:

First: Politely request to see the agent's or official's credentials, and inform the privacy official and the physician, who should determine whether the practice's attorney should be involved.

Second: Verify the agent's or official's credentials, and determine the nature of the inquiry. Consult with the practice's attorney to determine the practice's rights and obligations with respect to its response to the inquiry and the time frame for responding to the inquiry. Document all actions, times, and personnel involved that pertain to the inquiry and the practice's response.[21]

Step 2B: Permissible Disclosures: Treatment, Payment, and Health Care Operations

Standard	Code of Federal Regulations	Protected Health Information Permissions
Permissible disclosures: treatment, payment, and health care operations	45 CFR 164.506(c)	Uses and disclosures to carry out treatment, payment, or health care operations

What to Do:

A covered entity may use and disclose PHI for its own treatment, payment, and health care operations activities. A covered entity also may disclose PHI for the treatment activities of another health care provider, the payment activities of another covered entity or another health care provider, or the health care operations of another covered entity involving either quality or competency assurance activities or fraud and abuse detection and compliance activities, if both covered entities have or had a relationship with the individual and the PHI pertains to the relationship.

How to Do It:

In accordance with your NPP, you may use PHI for treatment, payment, and health care operations without obtaining authorization from the patient, except for cases where HIPAA authorization, state law, or other special requirements apply.

New *Patient Right:*

- The HIPAA Omnibus Rule added the right for an individual to request that his or her health information not be submitted to a health plan for purposes of payment or health care operations if the patient pays out of pocket and in full for the treatment. If the patient has paid in full and out of pocket for the services included in the restriction, you must comply with this restriction. The patient must complete a Request to Restrict Disclosure[22] form prior to making a decision to restrict the disclosure. In all cases, the privacy official shall determine whether to refuse or honor the request.

The privacy official is designated to be the contact person for questions, suggestions, or complaints relating to use or disclosure of PHI for the practice's treatment, payment, and health care operations.

Step 2C: Permissible Disclosures: Another Covered Entity's Treatment, Payment, and Health Care Operations

Standard	Code of Federal Regulations	Protected Health Information Permissions
Permissible disclosures: another covered entity's treatment, payment, or health care operations	45 CFR 164.506(c)	Uses and disclosures to carry out treatment, payment, or health care operations

What to Do:

A covered entity may disclose PHI for the treatment activities of any health care provider, the payment activities of another covered entity or health care provider, or the health care operations of another covered entity involving either quality or competency assurance activities or fraud and abuse detection and compliance activities, if both covered entities have or had a relationship with the individual and the PHI pertains to the relationship.

How to Do It:

Disclose PHI for treatment, payment, and health care operations of another health care provider if that request complies with the list below or is approved by the practice's privacy official.

Such a disclosure may be made for various reasons:

1. For treatment activities of another physician or health care provider
2. To another covered entity or health care provider for payment activities of the entity receiving the PHI
3. To another covered entity for its health care operations, as long as the other covered entity also has or had a relationship with the patient, the PHI pertains to that relationship, and the disclosure has one of the following purposes:
   (a) Quality assessment and improvement, including outcomes evaluation and developing clinical guidelines (but not primarily to obtain general knowledge)
   (b) Population-based activities related to improving health or reducing health care costs
   (c) Protocol development
   (d) Case management and care coordination
   (e) Contacting health care providers and patients with information about treatment alternatives
   (f) Functions not including treatment that are related to the purposes listed above
   (g) Performance evaluation, including reviewing the competence or qualifications of health care professionals
   (h) Evaluating practitioner or provider performance
   (i) Health plan performance
   (j) Conducting training programs in which health care students, trainees, or practitioners learn under supervision to practice or improve their skills
   (k) Training non-health care professionals
   (l) Accreditation, certification, licensing, or credentialing activities
   (m) Detecting health care fraud or abuse, or for compliance purposes if they are not listed above

Step 2D: Permissible Disclosures: Family, Friends, and Disaster Relief Agencies

Standard	Code of Federal Regulations	Protected Health Information Permissions
Permissible disclosures: family, friends, and disaster relief agencies	45 CFR 164.510	Use and disclosure requiring an opportunity for the individual to agree or to object

What to Do:

A covered entity may use or disclose PHI, provided that the individual is informed in advance of the use or disclosure and has the opportunity to agree to or prohibit or restrict the use or disclosure.

How to Do It:

In either verbal or written form, obtain the individual's agreement or objection to a use or disclosure requested by a friend, family member, or disaster relief agency.

CRITICAL POINT

Covered entities have frequently asked OCR about the rules for providing PHI to family, friends, and disaster relief agencies. OCR has prepared a document, Communicating with a Patient's Family, Friends, or Others Involved in the Patient's Care, which is available online[23] and is included in Appendix A. This document assists providers in determining what PHI can be shared with friends, family, or other caregivers in an emergency and other situations.

Disclose PHI to friends and family if:

- The patient is able to agree to the use or disclosure.
- The patient is incapacitated, and the disclosure is in his or her best interest, unless the disclosure has been previously prohibited by the patient.
- The patient is present and has the capacity to make decisions as to whether to share PHI with friends, family members, or disaster relief agencies.

If in your professional opinion, such as in cases of abuse, neglect, or domestic violence, you believe the disclosure is not in the patient's best interest, do not disclose PHI to friends or family members.

Possible disclosures include the following:

- An emergency room doctor may discuss a patient's treatment in front of the patient's friend if the patient asks that the friend come into the treatment room.
- A doctor's office may discuss a patient's bill with the patient's adult daughter who is with the patient at the patient's medical appointment and has questions about the charges.
- A doctor may discuss the drugs a patient needs to take with the patient's health aide who has accompanied the patient to a medical appointment.
- A doctor may give information about a patient's mobility limitations to the patient's sister who is driving the patient home from the hospital.

You may use or disclose PHI to a public or private disaster relief agency for the purpose of helping such entity notify a patient's family member, personal representative, or another person responsible for the patient's care, of the individual's location, general condition, or death. (See Step 2A for disclosures to the personal representative of a deceased patient.) You should comply with the procedures discussed above regarding communicating with family members and friends if in your professional judgment you determine that doing so will not interfere with the ability to respond to the emergency circumstances.

Step 2E: Incidental Uses or Disclosures

Standard	Code of Federal Regulations	Protected Health Information Permissions
Permissible disclosures: incident to a use or disclosure otherwise permitted or required	45 CFR 164.502(a)(1)(iii)	Uses and disclosures of PHI: general rules

What to Do:

HHS has provided guidance on what can be called an incidental use or disclosure: it cannot be a by-product of an underlying use or disclosure that violates *reasonable* Privacy Rule safeguards. *Translation*: You cannot rename a privacy violation an incidental disclosure.

How to Do It:

Put in place appropriate administrative, technical, and physical safeguards (see Step 10) that protect against uses and disclosures not permitted by the Privacy Rule and that limit incidental uses or disclosures.[24,25] Ensure that your organization also can meet the Privacy Rule *minimum necessary* standards.[26]

- Speak quietly when discussing a patient's condition with the patient and with family members in a waiting room or other public areas.
- Avoid using patients' names in public hallways and elevators.
- Post signs in the facility to remind workforce members to protect patient confidentiality.
- During the transition to an electronic workflow, store records in locked file cabinets until your system is nearly paperless.
- Do not share passwords.
- Turn computer monitors away to avoid public viewing access.
- Enforce sanctions against workforce members who do not keep voices low when discussing protected health information in public areas.

Step 2F: Other Uses or Disclosures for Which Authorization Is Not Required

Standard	Code of Federal Regulations	Protected Health Information Permissions
Other uses or disclosures for which authorization is not required	45 CFR 164.512; 45 CFR 164.512(b)	Uses and disclosure for which an authorization or opportunity to agree or object is not required

What to Do:

The HIPAA Privacy Rule provides details on specific circumstances in which a covered entity may be permitted to use or disclose PHI without the individual's authorization, including certain situations that involve:

- Public health activities, including requests for immunization records where state or local law requires the school to have such information prior to admitting the student. This is a new provision of the HIPAA Omnibus Rule.
- Victims of abuse, neglect, or domestic violence
- Health oversight activities
- Judicial and administrative proceedings
- Law enforcement purposes
- Decedents
- Organ and tissue donation
- Research
- Averting a serious threat to health or safety
- Specialized government functions (such as military and veterans, national security and intelligence, and correctional institutions)
- Workers' compensation

How to Do It:

Each of the permitted uses and disclosures involves detailed requirements that must be met prior to use or disclosure. In most cases, you should consult an attorney as necessary prior to using or disclosing PHI under these circumstances to be sure the requirements have been met.

Covered entities submitting immunization records to schools must document the request or agreement from the parent, guardian, or other person acting in loco parentis for the individual or if the individual is an adult or emancipated minor. Therefore, while written authorization is not required to share immunization records with schools, the practice must still document the request and what was provided. An individual, parent, or guardian can request immunization records be shared with the school by phone, written request, or e-mail. If by phone, make a notation in the patient's record. The school's request is not sufficient. The individual, parent, or guardian must agree to this public health disclosure.

Step 2G: Uses and Disclosures of De-identified Protected Health Information

Standard	Code of Federal Regulations	Protected Health Information Permissions
Uses and disclosures of de-identified PHI	45 CFR 164.502(d)(2); 45 CFR 164.514(a)-(c)	Uses and disclosures of PHI: general rules; other requirements relating to uses and disclosures of PHI

What to Do:

There are no restrictions on the use or disclosure of de-identified health information.

How to Do It:

De-identified health information is not PHI and therefore does not require an authorization for use or disclosure.

Follow one of the following two processes to de-identify health information:

1. Work with a credentialed statistician to de-identify the information.
2. Remove the following identifiers of the individual, the individual's relatives, household members, and employers:
   (a) Names
   (b) All geographic subdivisions smaller than a state, including street address, city, county, precinct, zip code, and their equivalent geocodes, except for the initial three digits of a zip code if, according to the current publicly available data from the Bureau of Census:
      i. The geographic unit formed by combining all zip codes with the same three initial digits contains more than 20,000 people; and
      ii. The initial three digits of a zip code for all such geographic units containing 20,000 or fewer people is changed to 000;
   (c) All elements of dates (except year) directly related to the individual, including birth date, admission date, discharge date, date of death; and all ages over 89 and all elements of dates (including year) indicative of such age, except that such ages and elements may be aggregated into a single category of age 90 or older
   (d) Telephone numbers
   (e) Fax numbers
   (f) E-mail addresses
   (g) Social Security numbers
   (h) Medical record numbers
   (i) Health plan beneficiary numbers
   (j) Account numbers
   (k) Certificate/license numbers
   (l) Vehicle identifiers and serial numbers, including license plate numbers
   (m) Device identifiers and serial numbers
   (n) Web universal resource locators (URLs)
   (o) Internet protocol (IP) address numbers
   (p) Biometric identifiers, including fingerprints and voice prints
   (q) Full-face photographic images and any comparable images
   (r) Any other unique identifying number, characteristic, or code, except as permitted for re-identification purposes provided certain conditions are met

If you develop a code or other means of re-identifying the information, you cannot derive the code using information about the individual.

The code must not be otherwise capable of being translated so as to identify the individual.

Do not disclose the code or the mechanism for re-identification for any other purpose.

Step 2H: Limited Data Set for Purposes of Research, Public Health, or Health Care Operations

Standard	Code of Federal Regulations	Protected Health Information Permissions
Limited data set for purposes of research, public health, or health care operations	45 CFR 164.514(e)	Other requirements relating to uses and disclosures of PHI

What to Do:

If your organization enters into a data use agreement with the recipient of a limited data set[27] as required by HIPAA, you may only use or disclose the limited data set for purposes of research, public health, or health care operations (as defined by HIPAA) if you remove the identifiers specified in this step. A limited data set is considered "unsecured" PHI under the January 25, 2013 Breach Notification Rule.

How to Do It:

If you participate in research, public health reporting (other than those disclosures required by law), or health care operations (as defined by HIPAA), your privacy official, in consultation with the practice's attorney, must either draft or review the data use agreement that safeguards PHI. Require any limited data set recipient to sign the appropriate data use agreement.

To meet the requirements of a limited data set, remove the following 16 identifiers from PHI:

1. Names
2. Postal address information, other than town or city, state, and zip code
3. Telephone numbers
4. Fax numbers
5. E-mail addresses
6. Social security numbers
7. Medical record numbers
8. Health plan beneficiary numbers
9. Account numbers
10. Certificate/license numbers
11. Vehicle identifiers and serial numbers, including license plate numbers
12. Device identifiers and serial numbers
13. Web universal resource locators (URLs)
14. Internet protocol (IP) address numbers
15. Biometric identifiers, including fingerprints and voice prints
16. Full-face photographic images and any comparable images

STEP 3: IDENTIFY USES AND DISCLOSURES THAT REQUIRE AUTHORIZATIONS

An authorization is written permission to disclose PHI to another person or entity. The authorization must be written in plain language so that the individual understands what is being disclosed and to whom.

Step 3A: Uses and Disclosures That Require Authorizations

Standard	Code of Federal Regulations	Protected Health Information Permissions
Authorizations	45 CFR 164.508	Uses and disclosures for which an authorization is required

What to Do:

If the use or disclosure is not permitted or required (Steps 1 through 2G), a covered entity must obtain a written "valid authorization" from the patient.[28] What constitutes a valid authorization?

- It must be in plain language.
- It must contain certain core elements and required statements:
  - ☐ A description of the protected health information to be used or disclosed
  - ☐ The name of the person authorized to make the use or disclosure[29]
  - ☐ The name of person(s) to whom the requested use or disclosure may be made
  - ☐ The purpose for the use or disclosure (if the patient has requested a use or disclosure, the privacy official may write "at the request of the individual")
  - ☐ An expiration date or expiration event
- It must be signed and dated by the patient.
- You must make a copy of the authorization for the patient.

How to Do It:

Your privacy official will determine uses and disclosures that require authorization. These may include the following:

- Requesting patients to sign up for and participate in using a patient portal
- Providing PHI for a long-term care application
- Providing PHI to a health benefits plan
- Using photos of patients as an example of treatment provided, such as before-and-after photos for plastic surgery, weight loss, or skin treatments. Photos of body sections that do not include the face are not de-identified and require authorization.
- See the sample authorization form in Appendix A.

New in the HIPAA Omnibus Rule:

Schools that are required to obtain immunization records before admitting students are not required to obtain an authorization prior to requesting immunization records; however, the parents must agree to the disclosure either orally (over the phone), via e-mail, or in writing. We discuss this in Step 2F and also in this chapter's section on patient rights.

Providers and business associates are required to obtain authorizations for subsidized communications that market a health-related product or service if the provider receives financial remuneration for the referral.[30]

Figure 3.4 provides an at-a-glance look at disclosures of PHI that require an authorization.

FIGURE 3.4

Special Requirements for Disclosing Protected Health Information (PHI)

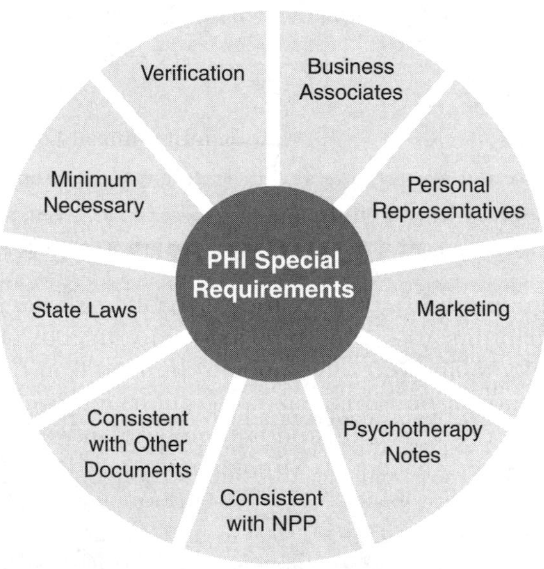
Nine Special Requirements
PHI Special Requirements
Verification
Business Associates
Personal Representatives
Marketing
Psychotherapy Notes
Consistent with NPP
Consistent with Other Documents
State Laws
Minimum Necessary

NPP indicates notice of privacy practices.
Reprinted with permission from Carolyn Hartley.

Authorizations Overview

Practices that participate in federal or state quality incentive programs are keenly aware of patient engagement initiatives. Individuals must sign an authorization form allowing the practice to download PHI onto a patient portal that most likely interfaces with the practice's EHR or practice management system. The company providing the patient portal is a business associate. The patient is not a covered entity, but it is a good practice to inform individuals of their privacy responsibilities if they print or download information from the portal onto their own devices.

An authorization cannot be combined with another document. "Compounded authorizations" are prohibited.

With certain exceptions, a covered entity may not place conditions on the individual for treatment, payment, enrollment in a health plan, or eligibility for benefits on the provision of an authorization (this is referred to as a *conditional authorization*). Consult an attorney before placing any conditions on an authorization.

The patient may revoke the authorization at any time, provided the revocation is in writing. However, an authorization cannot be revoked if the practice has already taken action, relying on information provided in the authorization.

Use the workflow in Figure 3.5 to obtain an individual's authorization prior to using or disclosing PHI when the use or disclosure requires the individual's permission. Authorizations may be completed in person or via fax.

An authorization is defective and not valid if any of the following is true:

- It has expired.
- It has not been filled out completely.
- The practice is aware that the authorization has been revoked.
- It is an impermissible *compound authorization*.
- It is an impermissible *conditional authorization*.
- The practice knows that material information in the authorization is false.

FIGURE 3.5

Authorization Workflow

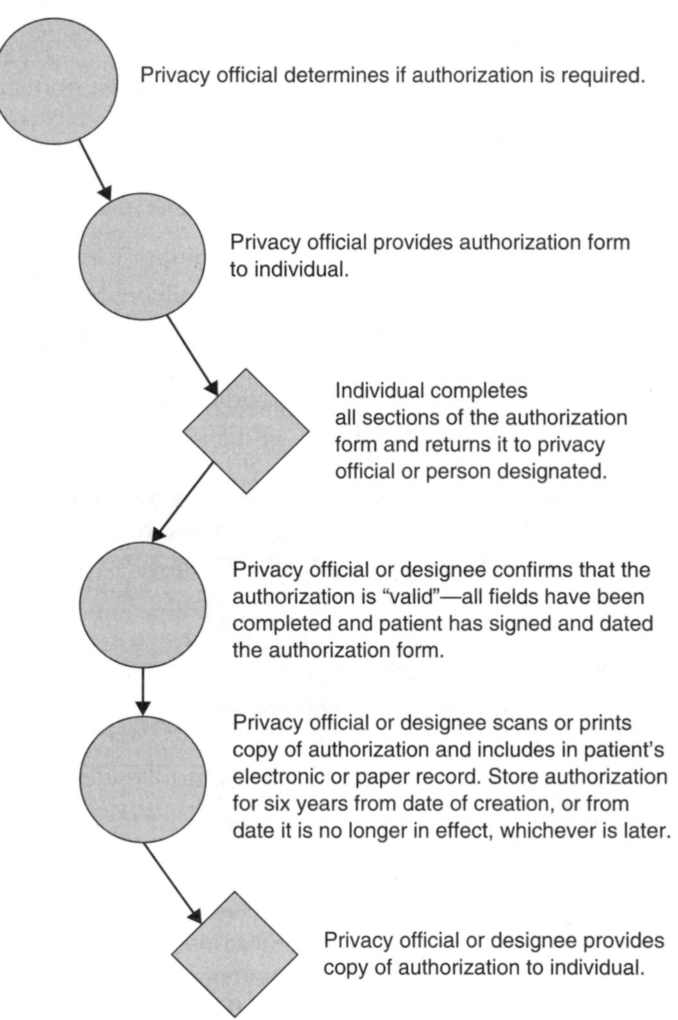

Privacy official determines if authorization is required.
Privacy official provides authorization form
to individual.
Individual completes
all sections of the authorization
form and returns it to privacy
official or person designated.
Privacy official or designee confirms that the
authorization is "valid"—all fields have been
completed and patient has signed and dated
the authorization form.
Privacy official or designee scans or prints
copy of authorization and includes in patient's
electronic or paper record. Store authorization
for six years from date of creation, or from
date it is no longer in effect, whichever is later.
Privacy official or designee provides
copy of authorization to individual.

CRITICAL POINT
If the use or disclosure is not for one of the following procedures, it will require an authorization.

Uses or disclosures not requiring authorization are as follows:

- Treatment, payment, or health care operations, which may include:
  - Quality assurance and quality reporting
  - Credentialing and licensing verification
  - Practitioner and provider evaluations
  - Insurance contracting and underwriting
  - Audits
  - Legal services
  - Compliance programs
  - Business planning and development
  - Management and general administration
- Requests by the patient or his or her personal representative. (See reasons to deny requests in Step 6.)
- Uses or disclosures required by HIPAA, including uses or disclosures required by HHS for compliance audit or complaint investigation purposes. (See Step 2.)

Step 3B: Psychotherapy Notes

Standard	Code of Federal Regulations	Protected Health Information Permissions
Psychotherapy notes	45 CFR 164.508(a)(2)	Uses and disclosures for which an authorization is required

What to Do:

Psychotherapy notes receive special protection under the HIPAA Privacy Rule. A medical practice may not use or disclose psychotherapy notes for any purpose, including most treatment, payment, or health care operations, without a written authorization signed by the patient. However, there are exceptions.

How to Do It:

Obtain an authorization from the individual prior to releasing any psychotherapy notes.

Authorizations are not necessary for the following purposes:

- The originator of the notes wants to review them.
- The medical practice can use or disclose psychotherapy notes to defend itself in a legal action or other proceedings brought on by the patient.
- HHS wants to review them, or a law requires the use or disclosure.
- You need to avert a serious threat to health or safety.

Consult an attorney if you have questions about the release of psychotherapy notes.

"*Psychotherapy notes* excludes medication prescription and monitoring, counseling session start and stop times, the modalities and frequencies of treatment furnished, results of clinical tests, and any summary of the following items: Diagnosis, functional status, the treatment plan, symptoms, prognosis, and progress to date."[31]

A white paper, *HIPAA for Behavioral Health in an Electronic Environment*, written by Carolyn P. Hartley for Sigmund Software and published by the Vendome Group, is included in Appendix A (reprinted with permission from Sigmund Software).

STEP 4: IDENTIFY PERSONAL IDENTITY AUTHENTICATION ISSUES

Standard	Code of Federal Regulations	Protected Health Information Special Permission
Verification requirements	45 CFR 164.514(h)(2)	Other requirements relating to uses and disclosures of PHI

What to Do:

Verify the identity of a person requesting PHI. If you do not know the person making the request, request documentation that verifies who he or she is.

How to Do It:

Providers pride themselves in knowing patients and families, including details about their children, grandchildren, pets, and other relevant connections. However, there may be times when you do not recognize someone who comes into the practice.

Before releasing any PHI to an individual or personal representative, ask for verification documents if you don't know the individual or if you aren't sure of the patient's name, and/or verify the identity and authority of that person using the following processes.

For New Patients:

- Upon entering the practice, each new patient is required to provide at least two forms of ID, with one being a photo ID.
- Verify that the name on a credit card is the same as the name on the photo ID.
- Make an electronic copy of the photo ID and scan it into the patient's chart. If you are still using paper records, attach the photocopy to the inside of the patient's chart.
- Using a digital or other electronic camera interfaced to the EHR, take a photo of the patient and upload it into the patient's electronic chart.
- Return both cards to the individual.

For Existing Patients Who Request PHI:

- Determine whether verification is needed (do we know this person?). If the patient is already in the EHR system, or if you can access a photo of the patient, you can ask if the patient's demographic information (address, phone number, preferred communication method) is still current.
- If you do not know the person, follow the if-then procedures in Table 3.3.

TABLE 3.3

If-Then Verification Procedures If You Do Not Know the Individual

IF	THEN
It's the patient in the practice or clinic.	Request a photo ID and one other form of ID, such as a credit card. You may also request an address or date of birth for verification.
It's the patient, but on the phone.	Ask the individual to provide details that would help identify the patient. This may include last name, date of birth, address, or approximate date last seen in your practice.
It's a friend or family member.	Request a photo ID; require signature from the person requesting PHI. When identity has been verified, see Step 2D regarding disclosures to friends or family members.
It's a personal representative.	If a personal representative accompanies the individual, exercise professional judgment to verify that this person is acting on behalf of the individual, and verify his or her identity. If you are unsure of the representative, request a copy of the power of attorney or other document, such as a document establishing legal guardianship, and request a photo ID. When identity has been verified, see Step 2A regarding disclosures to personal representatives.
It's a public official.	Contact the privacy official. Request to see the identification badge or other official credentials. If the request is in writing, review the appropriate government letterhead, insignia, address, and credentials. When identity has been verified, see Step 2F: Other Uses or Disclosures for Which Authorization Is Not Required, for more information regarding permissible disclosures to public officials.
It's a member of law enforcement.	Ask for credentials, including badge number. If you doubt the credentials, call the local police and ask if the person is a legitimate law enforcement officer. Then ask what specific details the law enforcement officer wishes to access. Write down the badge number, and provide only the details requested. Document what you provided.

When to Decline to Recognize Identity and Authority

If, in your professional opinion, you have followed verification procedures and you doubt the requester's credentials, politely tell the requester that you are unable to release the PHI. Document your decision in the verification log. If the person persists, he or she may request a meeting with the privacy official for the practice.

Require all persons receiving PHI to acknowledge receiving it by signing a verification of identity form.[32] This form will be scanned and saved in the patient's electronic record or copied and placed in the patient's paper chart.

STEP 5: UPDATE YOUR HIPAA PRIVACY SAFEGUARDS

Standard	Code of Federal Regulations	Privacy Management
Safeguards	45 CFR 164.530(c)	Administrative Requirements relating to uses and disclosures of PHI

What to Do:

A covered entity must have in place administrative, technical, and physical safeguards to protect the privacy of PHI. These safeguards must reasonably safeguard PHI from any intentional or unintentional use or disclosure that is in violation of the Privacy Rule.

To meet meaningful use Stage 1 core measures, you must complete an annual risk assessment and attest that you have completed this assessment. If questioned in a compliance audit, complaint, or breach investigation, you will be required to produce your risk assessment, verification of the date it was completed, and evidence that you are putting in place measures to mitigate your identified risks. This evidence may include policies and procedures, training, or revised workflows to mitigate risks.

Although the risk assessment also is a requirement of the Security Rule (discussed in Chapter 4), many of the safeguards in the HIPAA Privacy Rule cross-reference requirements in the Security Rule. These cross-references include the following:

Privacy Rule	Security Rule
Minimum necessary; authentication	Access control
Access permissions	Audit controls
Who can change PHI?	Integrity controls
Use and disclosure for treatment, payment, and health care operations	Transmission security
Workstation and device privacy	Workstation and device security

How to Do It:

Create, train workforce members on, and implement policies and procedures, including sanctions, that safeguard PHI in oral, hard-copy (paper and other physical documentation such as X rays), and electronic formats.[33]

Tables 3.4, 3.5, and 3.6 provide examples of administrative, physical, and technical safeguards for your practice.

The HIPAA Privacy Rule contains security provisions (often called the "mini-security rule"). The following tables provide safeguards addressed in the Privacy Rule.

TABLE 3.4

Sample Administrative Safeguards

Privacy Rule Safeguards	Required Actions
Sign-in sheets	Have patients sign in using last name and time of arrival only.
Communications	Avoid unnecessary disclosures of PHI by monitoring voice levels. Conduct dictation and telephone conversations in private areas.
Telephone messages	Telephone messages and appointment reminders may be left on answering machines and voice mail systems unless the patient has requested that he or she be contacted by alternative means, or you suspect abuse or neglect.
Faxes	Only the PHI that is necessary will be faxed. Use a cover sheet that includes a confidentiality notice.
Mail	Mailed PHI will be concealed and sent via first-class mail to the patient's primary address or the patient's alternative address.
Copies	Copies of records containing PHI will be stamped "Copy" in a color other than black.

TABLE 3.5

Sample Physical Safeguards

Privacy Rule Safeguards	Required Actions
Facility access controls	Outline procedures that allow facility access and support data restoration in a disaster or emergency. Control access daily.
Facility security plan	Outline procedures that safeguard the facility and the equipment inside from unauthorized physical access, tampering, and theft.
Access control and validation	Outline procedures that control and validate an individual's access to facilities based on the individual's role or function.
Maintenance records	Document repairs and modifications to the facility that may have an impact on security, such as changes in walls, hardware, doors, and locks.
Workstation use	Determine the functions to be performed at each workstation in the facility, the manner in which these functions are performed, and the physical attributes of the surroundings.
Workstation security	Outline physical safeguards for all workstations in the facility that allow access to PHI, and restrict access to authorized users.
Device and media controls	For media disposal, use software that completely sanitizes the magnetic area of the media that stores the PHI, such that it cannot be retrieved. Treat media to be reused in the same way as media intended for disposal. Outline procedures for documenting movements of either hardware or electronic media containing PHI.
Patients and visitors	Visitors and patients will be appropriately monitored during their visits at the practice. Patients will not be allowed to access other patients' records or other PHI.

TABLE 3.6

Sample Technical Safeguards

Privacy Rule Safeguards	Required Actions
Computer controls	Determine types of information that should be made available to workforce members. EHR access is typically role based, but the system administrator, with written justification, may modify access privileges.
Emergency access	Develop emergency operations procedures to follow in the event of, and during, a disaster or emergency. At least two individuals should be designated to have responsibility for emergency access to PHI.
Data integrity controls	Put security mechanisms in place and keep them in in working order to ensure transmission or receipt of PHI is completed securely.
Audit controls	Review system configurations and mechanisms for tracking access to and use of networks, workstations, and information. Be sure your EHR vendor trains the system administrator how to manage audit controls, as some vendors have not done so.
Encryption	Encrypt data that could be accessed on a portable or mobile device, desktop computer, server, or Internet connection by an unauthorized user.
Data authentication	Review system configuration and conduct audits to ensure data can only be created or modified by authorized users.

STEP 6: UPDATE NEW PATIENT RIGHTS, INCLUDING RIGHTS PROVIDED IN THE HITECH ACT

The HITECH Act added patient rights that will change your policies and procedures. Because these changes will affect your NPP, you will need to update it.

Steps 6A through 6G provide an overview of those changes and highlight updates to patient rights.

Step 6A: Right to Access Protected Health Information

Standard	Code of Federal Regulations	Patient Rights
Individuals' access to PHI	45 CFR 164.524	Access a copy of PHI

What to Do:

Unless a covered entity has grounds to deny an individual access, an individual has a right to access, inspect, and obtain a copy of the PHI about the individual in a designated record set for as long as the PHI is maintained in the designated record set. Right to access does not include:

- Psychotherapy notes
- Information compiled in reasonable anticipation of, or for use in, a civil, criminal, or administrative action or proceeding

- PHI maintained by a covered entity that is either (a) exempt from the Clinical Laboratory Improvements Amendments of 1988 (CLIA) or (b) subject to CLIA, to the extent that the provision of access to the individual would be prohibited by law

How to Do It:

According to your internal policies and procedures, a patient's request to access PHI should be directed to the privacy official or a person designated to act in the privacy official's absence, such as the security official if that role is held by a different individual.

Verify the patient's identity. If you know the patient, you are not required to obtain verification documentation. If you do not know the patient, ask for at least two forms of identification, with one being a photo ID. If the photo ID and second piece of identification do not match, the request must be denied. In most cases, your practice can honor the patient's request for access to PHI.

Ask the patient to complete the Patient Request to Access Protected Health Information form.[34] In completing this form, ask the patient to define the information requested, such as:

- Status of accounts payable
- Lab, imaging, or pathology results from last patient visit
- A record of a child's immunization dates

The HIPAA Privacy Rule allows the privacy official 30 days to respond to the request.

You may charge a reasonable cost-based fee as permitted by HIPAA, unless a more stringent state law applies. Fees may include:

- Charges for hard copies:
  - ☐ Copying, including the cost of supplies for the labor of copying the requested information
  - ☐ Postage, when the individual has requested the copy or a summary or explanation (see below) to be mailed
- A charge for preparing the summary or explanation, but only if both of the following are true:
  - ☐ The individual has agreed in advance to such a summary or explanation.
  - ☐ The individual has agreed in advance to the fees for preparing the summary or explanation.
- A fee for providing an individual with an electronic copy (or an electronic summary or explanation of ePHI). The fee may not be greater than the labor costs in responding to the request for the electronic copy (or summary or explanation).

Paper-based Process:

Record the request in a Request to Access PHI log.

Place a copy of the Patient Request for Access to PHI form in the patient's file.

Provide the requested PHI via US Postal Service.

Electronic Health Record Process:

Electronically scan the request into the patient's electronic chart.

Ask the patient to sign up for the practice's patient portal.

Use the practice's authorization form to ensure both the patient and practice understand their responsibilities to safeguard electronic PHI.

Provide the requested PHI into the patient's portal, or send a hard copy via US Postal Service. You may send the PHI electronically only if the patient has signed an authorization to provide information electronically.

If you are using EHR software, individuals also may request that PHI be provided to them in an electronic format, such as on a USB drive, a CD, or a SIM card, or to a secure patient portal. While it is wise to advise the patient to safeguard the patient-owned USB drive, security of the USB drive or other patient-owned media is the responsibility of the patient.

Establish protocols on what you will and will not download from your electronic patient record to a patient's electronic personal health record. Note that in such instances, state laws that are more stringent than HIPAA also may apply. For example, some states limit a minor's access to PHI.

Reasons to Deny Access:

- You determine the individual making the request is not the patient.
- You do not hold information requested in a designated record set.
- In your professional judgment, the patient's access is reasonably likely to endanger the life or physical safety of the individual or another person.
- The PHI makes reference to another person (unless the other person is a health care provider), and in your professional judgment, the access requested is reasonably likely to cause substantial harm to that other person.
- The request is made by a personal representative, and in your professional judgment, the personal representative is reasonably likely to cause substantial harm to the individual or another person.

In some cases, the individual may request that your denial be reviewed.[35] Unreviewable grounds for denial include the following:

- The covered entity does not hold the requested information in its designated record set.
- The information was compiled in reasonable anticipation of or for use in a civil, criminal, or administrative action or proceeding.
- Information was obtained from someone other than your clinicians under a promise of confidentiality, and access would reveal the source of the information.

Denial Procedures:

If your practice denies the request, put the reason for denial in a plain-language letter to the patient. The letter must include:

- A plain-language reason for the denial. If the denial is based on reviewable grounds, the denial must state that the individual may request a review of the denial and describe how the individual may exercise the review right.[36]
- A description of how the individual may complain to the practice (including the name or title and telephone number of the contact person or office that you have designated to receive complaints)[37] or to HHS.

If your practice does not maintain the PHI but knows where it is located, inform the patient where to redirect his or her request for access.

Document your decision to deny access to the patient's record, and keep a denial-of-access log. Consult a health law attorney if the individual requests a review of your denial and you are uncertain how to proceed.

Figure 3.6 outlines the access and denial decision paths for your practice.

FIGURE 3.6

Access and Denial Decision Paths

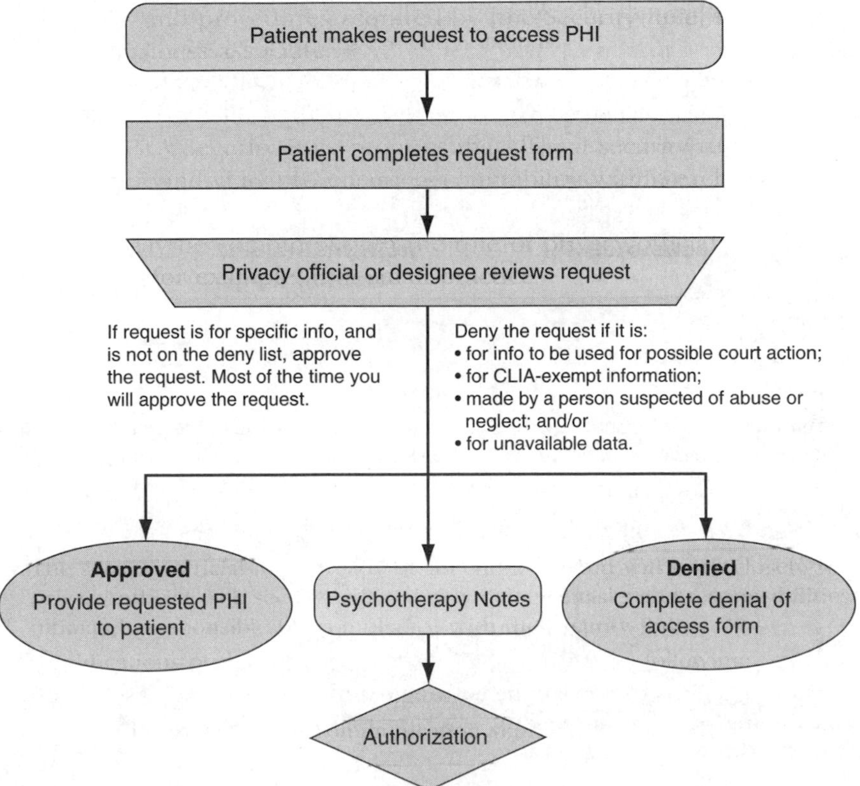

CLIA indicates Clinical Laboratory Improvement Amendments of 1988.

Step 6B: Patient's Right to Request an Amendment to Content in Patient Record

Standard	Code of Federal Regulations	Patient Rights
Request to amend	45 CFR 164.526	Amendment of PHI

What to Do:

You must allow an individual to request an amendment to content included in the patient's record. You may deny the individual's request to make the amendment, but if you agree with the request, then you must amend the record.

How to Do It:

In your NPP, you have stated that an individual may request in writing that you amend information in the individual's medical record if that information is incorrect.

Ask the patient to provide the amendment request in writing. If you agree to the amendment, you must amend the PHI in your designated record set(s). If you deny the request, notify the individual in writing why you are denying the request.

Complete the amendment within 60 days of receipt. You are entitled to one 30-day extension if you explain the delay to the individual in writing.[38]

Maintain documentation of each amendment request,[39] including a log of amendment requests.[40]

Reasons to Deny a Request for an Amendment

You may deny a request for an amendment if the information or record that is the subject of the request

- Is accurate and complete;
- Would not be available for access by the individual;[41]
- Was not created by the practice (unless the individual provides a reasonable basis to believe the originator is no longer available); or
- Is not part of the designated record set.[42]

If your practice grants a request to amend the patient's PHI, complete the following:

1. Inform the patient of your decision.
2. Identify the affected records and make the amendment.
3. Inform parties whom the patient identifies as requiring the newly amended information.
4. Make reasonable efforts to provide the amendment to identified and designated individuals in the amendment request (including your business associates).

Step 6C: Accounting of Disclosures

Standard	Code of Federal Regulations	Patient Rights
Accounting of disclosures	45 CFR 164.528	Accounting of disclosures of PHI

What to Do:

An individual has a right to receive an accounting of the disclosures of PHI made by a covered entity in the six years prior to the date in which the accounting is requested with certain exceptions. This accounting of disclosures does not include those for treatment, payment, and health care operations.

New: If your practice is using an EHR system, the individual also may now request an electronic accounting of disclosures. An EHR system's capability to do this is still an optional certification criterion for the meaningful use Stage 2 incentive program. An audit request to your system administrator should help you obtain an electronic accounting of disclosures. The rule did not shorten the time frame of 30 days to complete an accounting of disclosures to the patient. Covered entities may request an additional 30 days and also may charge a reasonable fee to produce the report.

Consult your EHR software company to determine when it will be able to provide an electronic accounting-of-disclosures function. Apply a statement of concern if the EHR vendor says it is not obligated to accommodate an accounting of disclosures. This generally is an indication that the EHR vendor is facing development challenges.

How to Do It:

Take all requests for an accounting of disclosures to the privacy official or person designated by the privacy official. Ask the patient to put the request for an accounting of disclosures in writing using the Request for Accounting of Disclosures form provided in Appendix A. You have 60 days from the date of receipt of the request to provide an accounting, with a one-time 30-day extension if you provide the individual with a written statement of the reasons for the delay and the date on which you will provide the accounting of disclosures.[43]

Use the Accounting of Disclosures Log provided in Appendix A. Maintain documentation of content provided in each disclosure, and the title of the person or office responsible for receiving and processing requests for an accounting, for six years from the date of its creation, or the date when it was last in effect, whichever is later.

You must provide the first accounting to the patient in any 12-month period without charge, but you may charge a reasonable cost-based fee for subsequent requests within the 12-month period if

- you have informed the patient in advance of the cost, and
- you have provided the patient with an opportunity to withdraw or modify the request to avoid or reduce the fee.

An individual has the right to request an accounting of disclosures made up to six years prior to the date of request, but not prior to April 14, 2003.

Guidance for Electronic Accounting of Disclosures

If a covered entity uses an EHR system, an individual has the right to receive an accounting of disclosures that the covered entity made for treatment, payment, and health care operations during the three years prior to the date of the request. The effective date of this requirement depends on when the EHR system was adopted. An entity that adopted EHRs before January 1, 2009, had to comply on January 1, 2011. A practice that adopted EHRs on or after January 1, 2009, must comply by January 1, 2014. HHS may extend that date.

For a discussion with your EHR software vendor, ask about forthcoming updates and functionalities that will allow you to generate an accounting of the following:

- Disclosures of PHI to individuals
- Disclosures made incident to a disclosure otherwise permitted or required under HIPAA privacy regulations
- Disclosures that were authorized by the individual[44]
- Appropriate disclosures to family and friends (see Step 2D)
- Certain disclosures for national security or intelligence[45] or to correctional institutions or law enforcement officials[46]
- Disclosures of information as part of a limited data set (see Step 2H)

The accounting of disclosures must include the following information regarding disclosures made by a practice or by one of the business associates during the applicable time period:

- Date of disclosure
- Name of the entity or person who received the information and, if known, the address of the entity or person
- A brief description of the PHI disclosed
- A brief statement of the purpose of the disclosure, or if applicable, a copy of the written request for disclosure[47]

Under certain circumstances, the practice may be required to suspend a patient's right to receive an accounting of his or her disclosures made to health oversight agencies or law enforcement officials.[48]

Step 6D: Confidential Communications Requirements

Standard	Code of Federal Regulations	Patient Rights
Confidential communications requirements	45 CFR 164.522 (b)	Request privacy protection for PHI

What to Do:

A covered entity must permit individuals to request and must accommodate reasonable requests by individuals to receive communications of PHI from the covered entity by alternative means or at alternative locations. For example, an individual may request to be contacted on a mobile phone rather than the home phone for any calls from the provider's office, including appointment reminder calls, test results, or other communications. You may set conditions for alternative communications to ensure that an address for billing purposes is included in your records.

How to Do It:

Require a new patient, upon signing in, to complete a Confidential Communications Information Sheet, which indicates that you may communicate with him or her at a specific telephone number or address if the alternative means or location is different from the primary address.

When making appointments for existing patients, ask if contact information has changed in the last year.

Step 6E: Right of an Individual to Request Restriction of Uses and Disclosures

Standard	Code of Federal Regulations	Patient Rights
Right of an individual to request restriction of uses and disclosure	45 CFR 164.522(a)	Request privacy protection for PHI

What to Do:

A covered entity must permit an individual to request that the covered entity restrict (1) uses or disclosures of PHI about the individual for treatment, payment, or health care operations[49] and (2) permitted disclosures involving the individual's care and notification purposes.[50]

As a covered entity, you are not required to agree to a restriction, but if you agree to the restriction, you must comply, except for the following reasons:

- ***Emergency Treatment:*** If the individual who requested the restriction needs emergency treatment and the restricted PHI is needed for such treatment, you may use the restricted information or may disclose the information to a health care provider to provide emergency treatment. The covered entity must request that the emergency care provider not further use or disclose the information.
- ***HHS Investigation:*** A covered entity is required to disclose PHI when required by HHS in connection with an investigation or to determine compliance with HIPAA privacy regulations.
- ***Permitted Uses and Disclosures:*** An agreement to restrict disclosure is not effective to prevent uses or disclosures for which an authorization or opportunity to agree or object is not required.[51]

New: As of the HIPAA Omnibus Rule compliance date, September 23, 2013, a covered entity must comply with an individual's request to restrict the disclosure of his or her PHI to a health plan for payment or health care operations (as defined by HIPAA), if the PHI pertains solely to a health care item or service for which the health care provider has been paid out of pocket in full.[52]

This restriction may adjust reimbursement workflows. For example, if a patient receives two or more services in one visit, pays for one of the services in full out of pocket, and requests that you not disclose information about the second service, you must determine how best to appropriately maintain the PHI in relation to the procedures to comply with the request.

Other than the out-of-pocket payment-in-full provision, the covered entity is not required to agree to a requested restriction. In general, most covered entities agree to restrictions only when exceptional circumstances exist and when they can reasonably accommodate them.

The privacy official should determine whether or not to agree to the request.

How to Do It:

Document the decision if you agree to a restriction request. You may use and disclose PHI for treatment, payment, and health care operations, except as noted in the out-of-pocket payment-in-full provision, and as required or permitted by HIPAA for emergency treatment, HHS investigation, and/or permitted uses and disclosures.

A restriction may be terminated if

- The patient agrees to or requests the termination in writing; or
- The patient orally agrees to the termination, and the oral agreement is documented.
- Inform the individual that you are terminating the restriction agreement. The termination applies only to PHI created or received after you have informed the patient that the restriction has been terminated.

Step 6F: Right to File a Complaint

Standard	Code of Federal Regulations	Privacy Management
Complaints	45 CFR 164,530(a)(ii); 45 CFR 164.520(b)(1)(vi); 45 CFR 164.530(d); 45 CFR 164.530(g)	Notice of Privacy Practices for PHI; administrative requirements

Since April 14, 2003, when HIPAA Privacy Rule became enforceable, complaints filed with OCR (see Table 3.7) have grown from 3743 in 2003 to a total of 80,836 as of April 2013. Of these, 91%, or 73,676, have been resolved.

TABLE 3.7

Top Five Issues in Investigated Cases Closed With Corrective Action[a]

1. Impermissible uses and disclosures of protected health information (PHI)
2. Lack of safeguards of PHI
3. Lack of patient access to PHI
4. Uses or disclosures of more than the minimum necessary PHI
5. Lack of administrative safeguards of electronic PHI

[a] Data accessed on June 17, 2013, from the Office for Civil Rights (OCR). "Enforcement Highlights." http://www.hhs.gov/ocr/privacy/hipaa/enforcement/highlights/index.html.

What to Do:

Designate the contact person or office responsible for receiving complaints and for providing further information about the NPP. To accommodate complaints, provide a process to receive and mitigate complaints.

Include a statement in your NPP that individuals may complain to the practice's privacy official and HHS if they believe their privacy rights have been violated. Provide a brief description of how the individual may file a complaint with the privacy official and a statement that the individual will not be retaliated against for filing a complaint.

The Privacy Rule and Breach Notification Rule require that a process be put in place to receive complaints. A covered entity may not intimidate or take retaliatory action against an individual for filing a complaint.

The Breach Notification Rule requires extensive communications for an electronic breach of PHI. Consult Chapter 5 for more information on this rule.

How to Do It:

Train all workforce members on the contents of the NPP and the procedure to enter the time, date, and a brief description of the complaint into a log.[53]

The privacy official's next steps include the following:

- Listen to the individual's complaint, and then ask the individual to document the details of the complaint to make sure that the practice has an understanding of the nature of the complaint and a record of the complaint.
- Make inquiries into the nature of the complaint to determine what has occurred and whether it constitutes a HIPAA privacy breach and/or a violation of the practice's policies and procedures.
- Put a response in writing to the complainant, either describing how the practice will address and resolve the complaint or explaining why the practice's action did not violate any policies or procedures and/or constitute a breach of PHI.
- Remind the individual that *at no time* will the practice retaliate against an individual for filing a privacy complaint.

Step 6G: Know About GINA

The HIPAA Omnibus Rule includes modifications related to the Genetic Information Nondiscrimination Act of 2008 (GINA),[54] a rule that applies to health plans and not to health care providers. The rule prohibits most health plans, including health maintenance organizations (HMOs) and issuers of Medicare supplemental policies, from using or disclosing genetic information for underwriting purposes. Health plans, therefore, must revise their NPPs to reflect this provision.[55]

The rule is important to health care providers who use genetic tests to confirm a diagnosis "as long as the diagnosis is not based solely or principally on the result of the genetic test."[56] An interpretation provided in the HIPAA Omnibus Rule reads as follows:

> If a neurologist sees a patient with uncontrolled movements, a loss of intellectual faculties, and emotional disturbances, and the neurologist suspects the presence of Huntington's disease, the neurologist may confirm the diagnosis with a genetic test. While genetic information is used as part of the diagnosis, the genetic information is not the sole or principal basis for the diagnosis, and, therefore, the Huntington's disease would be considered a manifested disease of the patient.[57]

We include information about GINA in the event a health plan's underwriting department requests genetic information about a patient's family. The physician may disclose the information, but the health plan may not use genetic information for underwriting purposes.

For more information about GINA, consult the National Human Genome Research Institute at http://www.genome.gov.

STEP 7: UPDATE BUSINESS ASSOCIATE CONTRACTS

Standard	Code of Federal Regulations	Protected Health Information Special Permissions
Disclosures to business associates	45 CFR 164.502(e); 45 CFR 164.504(e)	Uses and disclosures of PHI: general rules

CRITICAL POINT

Business associates have been under OCR's jurisdiction for purposes of the Breach Notification Rule since September 23, 2009, the effective date of the interim final rule. OCR will begin enforcing BA compliance with the Security Rule and certain portions of the Privacy Rule beginning on Sept. 23, 2013. Covered entities should be aware that business associate contractors that they hire as health information technology vendors, and business associate subcontractors that business associate contractors may hire as project managers or consultants working with or on behalf of a covered entity's PHI, are subject to the new Omnibus Security and certain Privacy Rule modifications on September 23, 2013.

What to Do:

A covered entity may disclose PHI to a business associate, and may allow a business associate to create or receive PHI on its behalf, if the covered entity obtains satisfactory assurance that the business associate will appropriately safeguard the information.

According to the HIPAA Omnibus Rule, covered entities and business associates must create new business associate agreements or amend existing agreements to incorporate relevant obligations for each party to the agreement.[58]

The HIPAA Omnibus Rule includes parallel provisions in §164.502(e) that allow a business associate to disclose PHI to a subcontractor acting on behalf of the business associate, but the covered entity is not required to obtain a business associate agreement from the subcontractor. Rather, the business associate contractor executes a business associate agreement with its subcontractors. Each is under the jurisdiction of OCR for purposes of Security and Privacy Rule enforcement. Business associates and covered entities have until September 23, 2014, to phase in amended contracts.[59]

In a business associate agreement, a covered entity and its business associates provide satisfactory assurances that PHI will be secure and that each develops and implements policies and procedures to safeguard PHI.

A covered entity may contractually hire a business associate to complete a task covered by the Privacy Rule, but the covered entity is still required to ensure the task is complete. For example, a practice hires an outside source to develop a revised NPP, distribute it, and post it on the practice's Web site. Yet the NPP does not get updated and is not posted on the Web site. The covered entity is still responsible for this activity, even though the business associate did not comply with the contractual obligations.

A covered entity is not in compliance with the business associate agreement standard if it knows of a pattern of activity or a practice of the business associate that constitutes a material breach or violation of the business associate's obligation under the contract, unless the covered entity takes reasonable steps to cure the breach or end the violation, as applicable. If such steps are unsuccessful, the covered entity must terminate the contract, if feasible, or if termination is not feasible, report the problem to HHS. This obligation works both ways: a business associate must report a violation or breach by the covered entity that the covered entity has not taken reasonable steps to end or cure, as applicable.

How to Do It:

The privacy official will work with the practice's attorney to identify business associates and other covered entities acting in business associate roles, and to develop an updated business associate agreement for the practice. Develop a policy stating that no member of the workforce is permitted to disclose PHI to a business associate unless the practice has an updated, executed agreement with that business associate.

The privacy official ensures that new business associate agreements incorporating privacy and security provisions of the HITECH Act and the HIPAA Omnibus Rule are in place with each of the practice's business associates.

Any business associate requesting access to PHI must first consult the privacy official.

The privacy official must train the workforce members to report any pattern of activity or practice of a business associate that constitutes a material breach or violation of the business associate's obligation under the agreement.

If a covered entity discovers such a pattern of activity or practice, it is the privacy official's duty to take reasonable steps to cure the breach or end the violation, as applicable. If corrective steps are unsuccessful, the practice may terminate the contract, if feasible, or if termination is not feasible, report the problem to HHS.

STEP 8: REVISE AND PROTECT FUNDRAISING AND MARKETING ACTIVITIES

Standard	Code of Federal Regulations	Protected Health Information Special Permissions
Disclosures to business associates	45 CFR 164.502(e); 45 CFR 164.504(e)	Uses and disclosures of PHI: general rules

What to Do:

New: Providing PHI for marketing purposes may only be completed after obtaining a "valid authorization" in connection with a marketing communication. This applies irrespective of whether the communication is made by your practice or by another entity. The marketing authorization must also contain additional provisions. This determination is a complex matter with many provisions and exceptions, and it becomes even more complicated as the HITECH Act takes effect. HIPAA, as amended by the HITECH Act, regulates the types of authorization that are required, which include the following situations:

- A covered entity uses PHI (such as patients' names and addresses, and/or information about their health conditions) to make a marketing communication about the covered entity's own products and services.
- A covered entity uses PHI to make a marketing communication in exchange for payment from an outside entity.
- A covered entity discloses PHI so that a business associate can make a marketing communication.
- A covered entity exchanges PHI for payment or other remuneration so that another entity can send a marketing communication.

How to Do It:

A covered entity may not use or disclose PHI for communication about a product or service that encourages the recipient of the communication to purchase the product or service unless the covered entity has obtained a certain form of "valid authorization"[60] from the individual.

An authorization is not required when communication occurs face to face with an individual or when communication is in the form of a promotional gift of nominal value.

Examples of marketing activities that require authorization include but are not limited to the following:

- A company that wants to send a marketing communication to all your patients with diabetes offers to give you direct or indirect remuneration or payment in exchange for these patients' names and addresses. You must obtain prior valid authorization from these patients. The authorization must state that remuneration is involved. As of 2011, the authorization is required to specify if the company receiving the data can further exchange it for remuneration.
- A company offers to pay you to send a communication to all your patients encouraging them to purchase one of the manufacturer's products. You will require authorization before sending such communications, and the communication must state that remuneration is involved.

Examples of communications that do not require authorizations include but are not limited to the following:

- You send out a notice to your patients that your office is relocating.
- You announce the arrival of a new physician or nurse practitioner.
- You recommend case management or care coordination for the individual, or recommend alternative treatments, therapies, health care providers, or settings of care to the individual, and you do not receive direct or indirect payment for making such communication.
- A pharmacy sends out a refill reminder for a medication that you prescribed for a patient.
- A pharmaceutical company offers to pay you to send a marketing communication to some of your patients, and the communication describes only a drug or biologic that is currently being prescribed for the recipients of the communication, and any payment that you receive in exchange for making the communication is reasonable in amount.

STEP 9: TRAIN YOUR STAFF ON NEW ISSUES AND PROVIDE REFRESHERS ON PRIVACY POLICIES AND PROCEDURES

The most dynamic privacy training sessions occurred in April 2003 when the Privacy Rule became enforceable. Informal training in most practices has continued as a reactive measure, primarily as issues come up.

In February 2009, when President Obama signed the American Recovery and Reinvestment Act, allocating billions of dollars to reimburse health care providers for adopting EHRs, the privacy safeguards and enforcement penalties escalated dramatically. Consumers needed additional confidence that taxpayer dollars would be used to benefit health information exchange and improved coordination of care, and that their PHI would be used and exchanged securely.

More information is provided about the Enforcement Rule in Chapters 1 and 5, but in a nutshell, it includes the following:

- Compliance is no longer voluntary but is driven by well-funded compliance officers hired to conduct random privacy and security audits.
- State attorneys general are authorized to conduct independent investigations into privacy and security breaches. On January 13, 2010, the state of Connecticut filed a historic lawsuit against Health Net for failing to secure patient medical records and financial information involving 446 000 Connecticut enrollees and to promptly notify customers endangered by the security breach.[61]
- The Secretary of HHS delegated OCR as the enforcement agency for HIPAA Administrative Simplification security and privacy matters, effective July 27, 2009.
- The Breach Notification Rule obligates covered entities to provide an expanded notice of incidents, using specific language, to "prominent media outlets," including HHS, if more than 500 residents in one state are affected by a breach. The privacy official, in collaboration with the security official, is required to notify patients of breaches of security that involve their medical information. Guidance on how to manage a breach is provided in Chapters 1 and 5. Because of the complexity of the Breach Notification Rule, physicians are strongly encouraged to create a breach notification plan that also includes consultation with legal counsel.
- A comprehensive document from the AMA, "What You Need to Know About the New HIPAA Breach Notification Rule," is included in Appendix C. Before building your training program, read the guidance in Appendix C and send a copy to your health law attorney. For training purposes, include at a minimum the following:
    - An overview of the Breach Notification Rule, including penalties
    - What the practice must do to inform patients of a security breach and the projected costs and reputation outcomes of those communications (specific guidance is provided in detail in Appendix C)
    - Policies and procedures about encrypting portable and mobile devices, and sanctions imposed against violators of that policy
    - Possible devices to track the location of portable, mobile, and stationary devices, including paper records, and measures to disengage access to medical information in the event a device is lost
- Covered entities must report to HHS within 60 days each discovered breach affecting 500 or more individuals, and annually provide HHS a log of all smaller reaches in the preceding calendar year.
- Covered entities, business associates, employers, and individuals may be subject to criminal liabilities if they use or disclose PHI without valid authorization.

In light of these additional enforcement approaches, let's take a look at the HIPAA Privacy Rule training requirements.

HIPAA Privacy Rule Training Requirements

- Workforce members include employees, volunteers, and trainees and may also include other persons whose conduct is under the direct control of the entity (whether or not they are paid by the entity).[62]
- A covered entity must train all workforce members on its privacy policies and procedures, as necessary and appropriate, for them to carry out their functions. New workforce members must be trained within a reasonable amount of time after they have been hired. Anytime a workforce member is promoted or changes his or her job position, you must provide privacy training according to the new job responsibilities.[63]
- A covered entity must have and must apply appropriate sanctions against workforce members who violate its privacy policies and procedures or the Privacy Rule.[64]

HITECH and HIPAA Training: Time to Double Down

by Edward Shay, Partner, Post, and Schell

As the healthcare industry continues to digest profound HITECH changes to HIPAA Privacy and Security rules, two observations already are apparent and indisputable for covered entities and their business associates. First, time and resources spent on a workforce that is well trained on the Privacy and Security rules will be an investment of exponential value. Second, enforcement of those same rules will make negligent and uncorrected errors very costly. A well-trained workforce makes fewer mistakes, and identifies and fixes those that it makes. A workforce that violates the rules because it does not know them or does not care to know them makes an inviting target for HITECH's new enforcement initiatives. The lesson seems clear: train on HITECH and re-train on existing HIPAA rules—or pay some new and onerous penalties for workforce mistakes.

Here are three hard truths about the HITECH amendments. First, after HITECH, penalties for each violation of HIPAA can now exceed civil penalties for violating the anti-kickback statute. Second, HITECH mandates much more enforcement by HHS, including compliance audits, and allows enforcement by state Attorneys General. Third, under the recently adopted breach notification rules, covered entities are required to submit annually logs of protected health information (PHI) breaches to the Secretary of HHS. Because by definition each of those reported breaches involves a violation of the Privacy Rule, covered entities also will be informing the Secretary of their Privacy Rule violations. You won't have to worry about possible whistleblowers; you are the whistleblower.

One major piece of good news in HITECH is that Congress provided that unless a violation is caused by willful neglect, penalties for the violation may be avoided by taking corrective action within 30 days. This is where training comes in, and where training pays off. A vigorous training program enables the workforce of a covered entity to identify violations quickly because the workforce knows what are proper PHI uses and disclosures and what are not. For example, if workforce members do not understand the concept of minimum necessary, they will not know that sending an entire medical record to a third party payer is highly likely to violate the Privacy Rule. If workforce members know what the minimum necessary disclosure is, they will either avoid an improper disclosure or move to correct it within the thirty-day corrective action grace period.

As with so many other areas of HIPAA, HITECH introduces many new concepts. New regulations have been published on unsecured breaches and more regulations are now here on privacy, security, and enforcement. Making these rules comprehensible to your workforce members (including management) and applicable to your environment requires training—and some re-training on the existing HIPAA Privacy and Security rules and how they all fit together.

This article was posted as a blog entry on HIPAA.com and is reprinted with permission.

Quick Training Tips

- Training keeps your workforce from making costly mistakes.
- Proof of attendance, such as signing a training attendance roster, verifies that the practice provided training in the event of an incident or breach.
- Don't let the fear of breaches drive your training program. Fear usually results in confused thinking and knee-jerk responses.
- Use a combination of media resources for training, including on-site sessions, group discussions, online training resources, and e-mail reminders.
- Training must be provided to the extent that is necessary for each employee to carry out his or her work functions.

No single training medium works all the time and/or for all employees, but privacy should always be the top priority. Determine how extensive your training should be by dividing your staff into three categories (see Table 3.8).

TABLE 3.8

Training by Job Category

Patient Contact Category	Amount of Training Needed
Employees with direct patient contact: physicians, nurses, office manager, privacy official	Extensive training, with regular updates and reminders throughout the year
Employees with some patient contact: receptionist, billing and insurance clerks, medical-records staff, lab technicians, volunteers, coders	Awareness training, with regular updates and reminders throughout the year
Employees with little or no patient contact: maintenance and housekeeping staff	Awareness training, with reminders or posters where employees can and will see them

Training Topics

A good training program, whether you develop it yourself or use an outside resource, should include the following topics:

- **Part I: HIPAA awareness (30 minutes to 1 hour)**
  - ☐ Overview of the HIPAA Privacy Rule and Breach Notification Rule
  - ☐ The practice's approach to protecting patient privacy
  - ☐ New and expanded patient rights, including a refresher on previous rights, and a definition of how the practice will honor those rights
  - ☐ The role of the privacy official
  - ☐ How the practice enforces the Privacy Rule and the Breach Notification Rule
  - ☐ Any updates that may be required
- **Part II: The practice's HIPAA policies and procedures (2 hours)**
  - ☐ Key terms
  - ☐ Permissions for use and disclosure of PHI
  - ☐ Special requirements for use and disclosure of PHI
  - ☐ Patient rights
  - ☐ Privacy management
- **Part III: Year-round training (15 to 30 minutes, once a month)**
  - ☐ Include training exercises and contingency scenarios as part of monthly staff meetings.
  - ☐ See Appendix B for a comprehensive training program, including month-by-month topics for discussion and an action approach to changing behavior, which can be very helpful as you build a privacy program in your medical practice.
  - ☐ **As part of each training session, you should also do the following:**
    - Test for understanding and keep records of each person's test.
    - Have employees sign an attendance register and maintain records and date(s) of attendance.
    - Ask employees and volunteers to sign a confidentiality agreement at the end of the HIPAA training.
    - Review confidentiality provisions with employees as part of the training, at least once a year.

STEP 10: IMPLEMENT YOUR PLAN AND EVALUATE YOUR COMPLIANCE STATUS

No office can avoid all privacy violations, but you must show good faith that you are trying to make the office violation free.

What to Do:

Safeguard your valued relationships with patients by implementing the new requirements of the Privacy Rule and Breach Notification Rule. It may save your practice significant embarrassment in the public media, as well as save the trust you've earned with patients.

How to Do It:

- Reinvigorate your privacy official, and show up for privacy training yourself. The privacy official's job has escalated, and the practice leaders must show support by participating in privacy training, which also is required under the Privacy Rule.
- Evaluate the privacy official's workload, especially if your privacy official is also your security official. Should some of this work be delegated or reassigned?
- Remind all clinicians that safeguards for incidental disclosures include keeping voices low when talking about patients in public areas.
- Using NIST standards (discussed in Chapter 4) to encrypt portable devices that contain or are used to access PHI.
- Implement sanctions! You must demonstrate through the HIPAA documentation requirements that you are following your policies and procedures. Failure to document compliance is tantamount to noncompliance.
- Communicate with everyone on staff about how they are doing.
- Tell your patients how you are managing patient privacy. Keep in mind that your patients and your staff have different approaches to privacy, but both desire the same outcome. Physicians and their workforce members have always believed that they practice confidentiality. Patients may believe what they read, hear, or see in the media, particularly stories about celebrities having their medical records looked at by unauthorized individuals, or the loss of a laptop with tens of thousands of sensitive financial or medical records that are not encrypted for security. If patients are informed about how you protect their PHI, they will trust and believe you. If they see that you are taking measures to protect their PHI, they will have more faith and believe you as well. Nothing can derail your privacy goals faster than revelation of a privacy or security breach in a 30-second sound bite on the evening news. Trustful patients make for good customer satisfaction, which also strengthens your foundation for successful HIPAA privacy procedures and the stability of your practice as a business.
- Evaluate your training status. Do you have new workforce members? Have current employees taken on new responsibilities that require retraining? Have your policies and procedures or HIPAA rules changed?
- Build new policies and procedures to accommodate updates to the Privacy Rule and Breach Notification Rule. Retrain the workforce on updated rules and changes.
- Conduct a monthly privacy check. Are you using your new documentation procedures? Are patients signing valid authorizations? Are you honoring patient requests that you have agreed to?

WHAT'S NEXT?

In the transition to the use of EHRs, security measures have become more prominent and have gained increasing momentum. Chapter 4 presents HIPAA security requirements effective since 2005 and updated in the HIPAA Omnibus Rule, and includes encryption implementation specifications.

ENDNOTES

1. Department of Health and Human Services, Office of the Secretary, "45 CFR Parts 160 and 164: Modifications to the HIPAA Privacy, Security, Enforcement, and Breach Notification Rules Under the Health Information Technology for Economic and Clinical Health Act and the Genetic Information Nondiscrimination Act; Other Modifications to the HIPAA Rules; Final Rule," Federal Register, v. 78, n. 17, January 25, 2013, pp. 5566-5702. Citations to this document hereafter are in the standard reference format of 78 Federal Register <page(s)> (eg, 78 Federal Register 5566). This document is available at http://www.gpo.gov/fdsys/pkg/FR-2013-01-25/pdf/2013-01073.pdf.
2. For information on how to participate in CMS incentive programs, go to http://www.CMS.gov/EHRIncentiveprograms.
3. 78 Federal Register 5625.
4. OCR's audit protocol is provided at http://www.hhs.gov/ocr/privacy/hipaa/enforcement/audit/protocol.html.
5. Meaningful use is the abbreviated term for the Medicare and Medicaid Programs EHR Incentive Programs, which define how eligible professionals and eligible hospitals can earn incentive funds by demonstrating that they are meaningful users of certified health information technology.
6. Department of Labor, "Civil Rights Center; Enforcement of Title VI of the Civil Rights Act of 1964; Policy Guidance to Federal Financial Assistance Recipients Regarding the Title VI Prohibition Against National Origin Discrimination Affecting Limited English Proficient Persons; Notice," Federal Register, v. 68, n. 103, May 29, 2003, pp. 32289-32305.
7. 78 Federal Register 5566, "Summary of Major Provisions."
8. 78 Federal Register 5617; 45 CFR 164.512(b)(1).
9. "Workforce means employees, volunteers, trainees, and other persons whose conduct, in the performance of work for a covered entity, is under the direct control of such entity, whether or not they are paid by the covered entity." 45 CFR 160.103.
10. See Chapter 4 for a discussion of business associate compliance with the Security Rule.
11. Consult Appendix B for a month-to-month sample training calendar.
12. 78 Federal Register 5634.
13. See Appendix A for a sample Workforce Training Session Attendee List.
14. American Health Information Management Assocation (AHIMA). "Sanction Guidelines for Privacy and Security Violations." J AHIMA. 2011;82(10):66-71. http://library.ahima.org/xpedio/groups/public/documents/ahima/bok1_049281.hcsp?dDocName=bok1_049281. Accessed May 15, 2013.
15. "Guidance Specifying the Technologies and Methodologies That Render Protected Health Information Unusable, Unreadable, or Indecipherable to Unauthorized Individuals," published in the *Federal Register* on August 24, 2009, as part of the interim final rule on breach notification. Department of Health and Human Services, "Breach Notification for Unsecured Protected Health Information; Interim Final Rule," *Federal Register*, v. 74, n. 162, pp. 42741-42743. Citations to this document hereafter are in the standard reference format of 74 Federal Register <page(s)> (eg, 74 Federal Register 42741).

16. 78 Federal Register 5599; 45 CFR 164.504(e).
17. 45 CFR 164.502(a)(1).
18. OCR provides guidance on the compliance and enforcement process for the Privacy Rule and Security Rule at http://www.hhs.gov/ocr/privacy/hipaa/enforcement/process/index.html.
19. A covered entity may impose a reasonable, cost-based fee when an individual requests a copy of his or her protected health information or agrees to a summary or explanation of such information, provided the fee includes ***only*** the cost of (1) copying (including the cost of supplies for and labor of copying the protected health information requested by the individual); (2) postage (when the individual has requested that the copy, or summary or explanation, be mailed); and (3) preparing an explanation or summary of the protected health information, if the individual has agreed in advance to the preparation of a summary or explanation and to any fees imposed by the covered entity for such summary or explanation. 45 CFR 164.524(c)(4).
20. See the OCR Web site for more details on personal representatives: http://www.hhs.gov/ocr/privacy/hipaa/understanding/consumers/personalreps.html.
21. Requests from law enforcement officials are treated in numerous sections of the HIPAA regulations. It is likely to be necessary to consult legal counsel in connection with matters that involve law enforcement officials.
22. 45 CFR 164.512(a), 164.512(b)(1)(ii), and 164.512(c).
23. For the OCR document "Communicating with a Patient's Family, Friends, or Others Involved in the Patient's Care," refer to Appendix A or http://www.hhs.gov/ocr/privacy/hipaa/understanding/coveredentities/provider_ffg.pdf.
24. See the OCR document *Incidental Uses and Disclosures,* which is available at http://www.hhs.gov/ocr/privacy/hipaa/understanding/coveredentities/incidentalusesanddisclosures.html.
25. See 45 CFR 164.530(c).
26. 45 CFR 164.502(b); 45 CFR 164.514(d).
27. De-identified PHI removes 18 direct identifiers. A limited data set removes 16 identifiers, permitting only elements of dates, such as dates of birth, and town or city, state, and zip code to remain in the limited data set.
28. See Appendix A for a sample Authorization form.
29. Be sure to request and verify positive identification of the individual requesting the authorization, especially if that individual is not known to your practice.
30. 78 Federal Register 5595.
31. 45 CFR 164.501.
32. See Appendix A for a sample Verification of Identity form.
33. The HIPAA Security Rule covers the administrative, physical, and technical safeguard implementation specifications for electronic PHI. The security safeguards are discussed in Chapter 4.
34. A sample Patient Request to Access Protected Health Information form is provided in Appendix A.
35. See 45 CFR 164.524(a)(2) for the full list of unreviewable grounds for denial, which also include certain provisions relating to psychotherapy notes, the Clinical

Laboratory Improvement Amendments of 1988 (42 USC 263a), inmates of correctional institutions, research, and the Privacy Act (5 USC 552a).

36. In general, if an individual requests a review, the covered entity must designate a licensed health care professional who was not directly involved in the denial to review the decision and must promptly refer the request for review to such professional. The professional must determine, within a reasonable period of time, whether or not to deny access. The covered entity must promptly provide written notice to the individual of the determination and must take any action required to carry out the determination. Reviewable grounds for denying access are listed at 45 CFR 164.524(a)(3). The procedures for responding to a review of a denial of access are found in 45 CFR 164.524(a)(4) and 164.524(d)(4).
37. See Step 6F: Right to File a Complaint for further discussion of complaints.
38. 45 CFR 164.526(b)(2)(ii).
39. See Appendix A for a sample Patient Request for Amendment of Patient's Protected Health Information form.
40. See Appendix A for a sample Amendment Request Log.
41. See Step 6A: Right to Access Protected Health Information, in this chapter, or 45 CFR 164.524 for more information about when information is available for access by the individual.
42. A *designated record set* generally includes medical records, billing records, health plan enrollment, payment, claims adjudication, and case management records, or other records that are used to make decisions about individuals. For purposes of defining a *designated record set*, the word record includes any item, collection, or grouping of information that includes PHI that is maintained, collected, used, or disseminated by or for the practice. For the complete definition, see 45 CFR 164.501 or the Glossary.
43. 45 CFR 164.528(c)(1)(ii).
44. 45 CFR 164.508.
45. 45 CFR 164.512(k)(2).
46. 45 CFR 164.512(k)(5).
47. A copy of the written request for disclosure may be provided instead of a brief statement of the purpose of the disclosure if the disclosure was made to HHS in connection with an investigation or determination of HIPAA Privacy Rule compliance under 45 CFR 164.528(b)(2)(iv) and 45 CFR 164.502(a)(2)(ii) or if the disclosure was required by law; for public health activities; about victims of abuse, neglect, or domestic violence; for health oversight activities; for judicial and administrative proceedings; for law enforcement purposes; about decedents; for organ or tissue donation purposes; for research purposes; to avert a serious threat to health or safety; for specialized government functions (such as military and veterans activities, and government programs providing public benefits); or for workers compensation purposes (see 45 CFR 164.512).
48. 45 CFR 164.528(a)(2).
49. See Step 2B: Permissible Disclosures: Treatment, Payment, and Health Care Operations.
50. See Step 2C: Permissible Disclosures: Another Covered Entity's Treatment, Payment, and Health Care Operations.

51. See 45 CFR 164.512, which covers certain uses and disclosures required by law and certain uses and disclosures pertaining to public health activities; victims of abuse, neglect, or domestic violence; health oversight activities; judicial and administrative proceedings; law enforcement purposes; decedents; organ or tissue donation; research purposes; serious threats to health or safety; specialized government functions; and workers' compensation.
52. 45 CFR 164.522(a)(1)(vi)(B).
53. See Appendix A for a sample Complaint Log.
54. 45 CFR 164.520(b)(1)(iii)(D), 164.502(a)(5)(i).
55. §105 of Title I adds to §1180 of the Social Security Act to require HHS to revise the HIPAA privacy regulations to clarify that genetic information is health information under the rule and prohibits the use of genetic information for underwriting purposes.
56. 78 Federal Register 5664.
57. Ibid.
58. See 42 USC 17931 (security obligations) and 42 USC 17934 (privacy obligations).
59. 78 Federal Register 5677.
60. 45 CFR 164.508.
61. "Attorney General Sues Health Net for Massive Security Breach Involving Private Medical Records and Financial Information on 446,000 Enrollees." Press release on the Connecticut Attorney General's Office Web site. http://www.ct.gov/ag/cwp/view.asp?A=2341&Q=453918. Published January 13, 2010. Accessed May 8, 2013.
62. 45 CFR 160.103.
63. 45 CFR 164.530(b).
64. 45 CFR 164.530(e).

chapter 4

HIPAA Security: Tougher, but with Safe Harbors

The purpose of this chapter is to provide you with a basic understanding of the HIPAA Administrative Simplification Security Rule that was published in the *Federal Register* on February 20, 2003,[1] and required compliance by covered entities on April 21, 2005,[2] and with the HITECH Act Security Rule modifications published in the *Federal Register* on January 25, 2013,[3] which required compliance by covered entities *and* business associates by September 23, 2013.

What You Will Learn in This Chapter

- The basic structure of the Security Rule and how it was modified in 2013
- The basic foundation of the Security Rule
- How the Security Rule relates to the Privacy Rule and to the Breach Notification Rule
- Why the Security Rule is technologically neutral and scalable
- How the Security Rule is designed to provide scalability and flexibility
- How to conduct a risk analysis
- What the difference is between *required* and *addressable* implementation specifications that underpin the security standards, and how to manage those concepts when implementing the Security Rule
- Why reasonable and appropriate actions provide the framework for the Security Rule, irrespective of size, complexity, or environment in which the covered entity or business associate operates
- What the characteristics of the administrative, physical, and technical security safeguards are
- Why cost is a consideration in exercising responsibility to comply with the Security Rule, but "cost is not meant to free covered entities from this responsibility"[4]

Key Terms

- Addressable
- Administrative safeguards
- Availability
- Breach
- Business associate
- Confidentiality
- Covered entity
- Electronic media
- Electronic protected health information (ePHI)
- Encryption
- Guidance
- Implementation specification
- Integrity
- Person
- Physical safeguards
- Protected health information (PHI)
- Required
- Security incident
- Subcontractor
- Technical safeguards
- Unsecured protected health information

ABOUT HIPAA'S SECURITY RULE

The Security Rule became effective April 21, 2003, and required compliance no later than April 21, 2005, for most covered entities: health plans, health care clearinghouses, and health care providers who transmit any health information in electronic form in connection with a standard transaction.[5]

The Privacy Rule, which required compliance by covered entities by April 14, 2003,[6] also required that administrative, technical, and physical safeguards of protected health information (PHI) in oral, hard copy, and electronic forms be in effect as of that date.[7] As a result, the Privacy Rule accelerated the need for implementation of security provisions, and the final Security Rule provided guidance for the appropriate security safeguards required under the Privacy Rule.

Unlike the Privacy Rule, which applies to PHI in oral, hard copy, and electronic form, the Security Rule applies only to *electronic* protected health information (ePHI). Both rules cover protected health information *in use* (creation, retrieval, revision, and deletion), *at rest* (database), and *in motion* (transmission).

The Privacy Rule defines authorized and required uses and disclosures of PHI and the rights patients have with respect to it. The Security Rule defines safeguards for such information. Three key properties[8] are the foundation of privacy and security working together:

- ***Confidentiality*** is the property that PHI is "not made available or disclosed to unauthorized persons or processes."
- ***Integrity*** is the property that PHI "has not been altered or destroyed in an unauthorized manner."
- ***Availability*** is the property that PHI "is accessible and useable upon demand by an authorized person."

These properties, and other security attributes, are embodied in three types of security standards: administrative safeguards, physical safeguards, and technical safeguards.

Within the administrative, physical, and technical safeguard categories are standards and implementation specifications that are examined in detail in this chapter. Covered entities have been required to comply with the Security Rule standards and implementation specifications since April 21, 2005, and business associates will have to comply "in the same manner as these requirements apply to covered entities" by September 23, 2013.[9] Compliance is designed to provide "a floor of protection of all electronic protected health information" but takes into consideration that covered entities and business associates are of different sizes and complexities, and, thus, are likely to require different means to achieve protection of such information. As a result, the Security Rule is considered "technologically neutral."[10]

CRITICAL POINT

HIPAA's Security Rule is technologically neutral. The Security Rule does not tell your organization what technology choices (inputs) to make, just what protections (outputs) to achieve.

The foundation of the Security Rule is that security protections must be "reasonable and appropriate,"[11] as assessed in a required risk analysis and study of risk-management measures. The Security Rule is designed to be "scalable and flexible."[12] As a result, a small physician practice will have a different array of security protections than a large practice, clinic, or hospital, with the selection of security protections determined by the risk analysis. Many of these protections will be reflected and documented in written policies and procedures that your organization must keep current. Documentation may be in hard copy or electronic form and must be retained for six years from the date of creation or the date last in effect, whichever is later. Your organization also must similarly document "actions, activities, and assessments"[13] related to its Security Rule policies and procedures. Both types of documentation must be made available to your organization's workforce[14] members who are responsible for or affected by the Security Rule.

CRITICAL POINT

Your organization must document its Security Rule policies, procedures, actions, activities, and assessments, and retain such documentation in hard copy or electronic form for six years from its date of creation or the date last in effect, whichever is later.

There are five parts of the Security General Rules:

- General requirements
- Flexibility of approach
- Standards
- Implementation specifications
- Maintenance

General Requirements

There are four general requirements:

- Ensure the confidentiality, integrity, and availability of all electronic protected health information the covered entity [or business associate] creates, receives, maintains, or transmits.
- Protect against any reasonably anticipated threats or hazards to the security or integrity of such information.
- Protect against any reasonably anticipated uses or disclosures of such information that are not permitted or required under [the Privacy of Individually Identifiable Health Information standards].
- Ensure compliance with [the Security Rule] by its workforce.[15]

These requirements serve as the foundation for the administrative, physical, and technical safeguards.

Flexibility of Approach

The general requirements provide for flexibility of approach in complying with the Security Rule. Because of the importance of a flexible approach in providing a foundation for the scalability of administrative, physical, and technical safeguards, the two parts of this rule are reproduced here:

1. Covered entities and business associates may use any security measures that allow the covered entity to reasonably and appropriately implement the standards and implementation specifications as specified in [the Security Standards for the Protection of Electronic Protected Health Information].
2. In deciding which security measures to use, a covered entity or business associate must take into account the following factors:
   (i) The size, complexity, and capabilities of the covered entity or business associate
   (ii) The covered entity's or the business associate's technical infrastructure, hardware, and software security capabilities
   (iii) The costs of security measures
   (iv) The probability and criticality of potential risks to electronic protected health information[16]

CRITICAL POINT
To determine what are reasonable and appropriate security measures for your organization, you must take the four factors listed above into account in your risk analysis.

Standards

This part of the general rules requires that covered entities and business associates comply with the security standards with respect to all ePHI.

> Before the HITECH Act, the Security Rule did not directly apply to business associates of covered entities. However, section 13401 of the HITECH Act provides that the Security Rule's administrative, physical, and technical safeguards requirements . . . , as well as the Rule's policies and procedures and documentation requirements . . . , apply to business associates in the same manner as these requirements apply to covered entities, and that business associates are civilly and criminally liable for violations of these provisions.[17]

Business associates, as well as covered entities, must comply with the HITECH Act modifications to the Security Rule by September 23, 2013.

Implementation Specifications

There are two types of implementation specifications, *required* and *addressable*, and each implementation specification is so designated. If an implementation specification is designated *required*, a covered entity or business associate must implement the specification. The term *addressable* is more complicated and gives the covered entity options. These options are outcomes of the risk analysis that the practice conducts. When analyzing a particular addressable implementation specification for a standard, the organization must determine "whether each implementation specification is a *reasonable and appropriate* safeguard in its environment, when analyzed with reference to the likely contribution to protecting the entity's or business associate's electronic protected health information."[18] For example, in a large physician practice, you likely would conduct a detailed background investigation of a person seeking employment (clearance implementation specification). In a solo practice with only the physician's spouse as the "workforce," such a clearance procedure likely would not be considered reasonable or appropriate.

In this and other addressable implementation specifications, the covered entity or business associate must balance the safeguard specification with the degree of risk mitigation the specification affords, taking into consideration its analysis of risk, strategy for risk mitigation, security protections already in place, and cost of implementation. If the covered entity or business associate determines that the implementation specification is a reasonable and appropriate safeguard, it must implement the specification.

If your organization determines that the implementation specification is not reasonable and appropriate, you have two options, and for each of them you must document why the implementation specification is not reasonable and appropriate. First, you must document why it is not reasonable and appropriate and implement one or more alternative equivalent measures, or a combination of such measures, if reasonable and appropriate. Second, if you can otherwise document that the standard can be met, you may choose to implement neither the implementation specification nor the alternative equivalent measure(s). In either circumstance, written documentation of the decision is critical.

Maintenance

This part of the general rules requires that covered entities and business associates review their security measures periodically, make modifications as necessary to ensure that they continue to provide "reasonable and appropriate protection of electronic protected health information,"[19] and update documentation accordingly.

SECURITY STANDARDS AND IMPLEMENTATION SPECIFICATIONS

Table 4.1 outlines the 18 administrative, physical, and technical safeguard standards of the Security Rule, which are defined as follows.

- Nine administrative safeguard standards are "administrative actions, and policies and procedures, to manage the selection, development, implementation, and maintenance of security measures to protect electronic protected health information and to manage the conduct of the covered entity's or business associate's workforce in relation to the protection of that information."[20]
- Four physical safeguard standards are "physical measures, policies, and procedures to protect a covered entity's or business associate's electronic information systems and related buildings and equipment, from natural and environmental hazards, and unauthorized intrusion."[21]
- Five technical safeguard standards are "the technology and the policy and procedures for its use that protect electronic protected health information and control access to it."[22]

There are 36 defined implementation specifications for the safeguard standards, which can be either *required* or *addressable*. Six standards do not have defined implementation specifications, and for these standards, the language of the standard explains what is *required* to be implemented.

TABLE 4.1

Security Safeguard Standards and Implementation Specifications

Standard	Code of Federal Regulations (CFR) Section	Implementation Specifications	Required (R) or Addressable (A)
Administrative Safeguards[23]			
Security management process	164.308(a)(1)	A. Risk analysis	R
		B. Risk management	R
		C. Sanction policy	R
		D. Information system activity review	R
Assigned security responsibility	164.308(a)(2)		R
Workforce security	164.308(a)(3)	A. Authorization and/or supervision	A
		B. Workforce clearance procedure	A
		C. Termination procedures	A
Information access management	164.308(a)(4)	A. Isolating health care clearing-house functions	R
		B. Access authorization	A
		C. Access establishment and modification	A
Security awareness and training	164.308(a)(5)	A. Security reminders	A
		B. Protection from malicious software	A
		C. Log-in monitoring	A
		D. Password management	A
Security incident procedures	164.308(a)(6)	Response and reporting	R
Contingency plan	164.308(a)(7)	A. Data backup plan	R
		B. Disaster recovery plan	R
		C. Emergency mode operation plan	R
		D. Testing and revision procedures	A
		E. Applications and data criticality analysis	A
Evaluation	164.308(a)(8)		R
Business associate contracts and other arrangements	164.308(b)(1)	Written contract or other arrangement	R

Continued

TABLE 4.1 (continued)

Security Safeguard Standards and Implementation Specifications

Standard	Code of Federal Regulations (CFR) Section	Implementation Specifications	Required (R) or Addressable (A)
Physical Safeguards[24]			
Facility access controls	164.310(a)(1)	i. Contingency operations	A
		ii. Facility security plan	A
		iii. Access control and validation procedures	A
		iv. Maintenance records	A
Workstation use	164.310(b)		R
Workstation security	164.310(c)		R
Device and media controls	164.310(d)(1)	i. Disposal	R
		ii. Media re-use	R
		iii. Accountability	A
		iv. Data backup and storage	A
Technical Safeguards[25]			
Access control	164.312(a)(1)	i. Unique user identification	R
		ii. Emergency access procedure	R
		iii. Automatic log-off	A
		iv. Encryption and decryption	A
Audit controls	164.312(b)		R
Integrity	164.312(c)(1)	Mechanism to authenticate electronic protected health information	A
Person or entity authentication	164.312(d)		R
Transmission security	164.312(e)(1)	i. Integrity controls	A
		ii. Encryption	A

In the sections that follow, we outline the administrative, physical, and technical standards and implementation specifications. For each standard, we identify the implementation specifications and references. References include the following:

- Relevant location in Title 45 (Public Welfare), Subtitle A (Department of Health and Human Services), Subchapter C (Administrative Data Standards and Related Requirements), Part 164 (Security and Privacy), Subpart C (Security Standards for the Protection of Electronic Protected Health Information), of the Code of Federal Regulations (CFR)[26]
- The National Institute of Standards and Technology (NIST) document *An Introductory Resource Guide for Implementing the Health Insurance*

Portability and Accountability Act (HIPAA) Security Rule, Special Publication (SP) 800-66, Revision 1, October 2008[27]

- Each Security Rule standard and implementation specification as it appears in 45 CFR 164.308, 164.310, and 164.312, or as modified by the January 25, 2013, HITECH Act modifications to the Security Rule. Applicable modifications to the language of the administrative standards and implementation specifications are discussed in this chapter; there were no modifications to the language of the physical or technical safeguards. The introductory text for administrative, physical, and technical safeguards was modified to include business associates: "A covered entity or business associate must, in accordance with §164.306 . . . "[28]
- Throughout the remainder of this chapter, when we use the terms *practice* and *organization*, unless otherwise specified, think in terms of a business context broader than that of just a medical practice, applying to organizations that must implement standards and implementation specifications to achieve compliance with the HITECH Act modifications of the HIPAA Security Rule, namely, covered entities, business associates, and subcontractors required to safeguard ePHI that is created, received, maintained, or transmitted.[29]
- As you examine the administrative, physical, and technical standards and implementation specifications, you may find it useful to examine two recent online resources that elaborate on provisions you may wish to consider as you design and implement your safeguard policies and procedures.
  - The first, published by NIST, is the *Security Content Automation Protocol (SCAP) HIPAA Security Rule Toolkit*, which is available at http://scap.nist.gov/hipaa and was last updated on November 2, 2012 (as of this writing in February 2013). This resource lists questions you may address, broken down by HIPAA security standard and implementation specification, and provides references for those questions to other NIST publications.
  - The second was published by the HHS Office for Civil Rights (OCR)—the HIPAA/HITECH Act enforcement arm for privacy, security, and breach notification—and lists, as of this writing, 169 audit inquiries an auditor would select from to determine a covered entity's or business associate's compliance with HIPAA/HITECH Act rules, processes, controls, and policies and procedures. The audit protocol was released on June 26, 2012, and is available at http://www.hhs.gov/ocr/privacy/hipaa/enforcement/audit/protocol.html. Be sure to check this site for updates that reflect modifications of HIPAA/HITECH Act enabling regulations that were published in the *Federal Register* on January 25, 2013.

Security Management Process

Standard	Implementation Specifications	References
Security management process	A. Risk analysis (R)	45 CFR 164.308(a)(1)(i)
	B. Risk management (R)	NIST SP 800-66, pp. 17-19
	C. Sanction policy (R)	68 Federal Register 8377
	D. Information system activity review (R)	78 Federal Register 5694

What the Standard Requires

The standard requires that a covered entity or business associate "[i]mplement policies and procedures to prevent, detect, contain, and correct security violations."[30] This standard and the four required implementation specifications "form the foundation upon which an entity's necessary security activities are built."[31]

- In essence, a covered entity or business associate is to evaluate and manage its security risks, establish sanctions as a disincentive for or deterrent to noncompliant behavior, and periodically review its security controls. Covered entities and business associates "have the flexibility to implement the standard in a manner consistent with numerous factors, including such things as, but not limited to, their size, degree of risk, and environment."[32]
- A covered entity or business associate can find guidance for implementing these specifications from the NIST Computer Security Resource Center.[33]

CRITICAL POINT

"Your first priority is to develop a way to quantify and evaluate risk. You need to know what you are protecting and how much it's worth before you can decide how to protect it."[34]

Risk Analysis

Standard	Implementation Specification	Reference
Security management process	A. Risk analysis (R)	164.308(a)(1)(ii)(A)

What to Do:

Conduct an accurate and thorough assessment of the potential risks and vulnerabilities to the confidentiality, integrity, and availability of ePHI held by the covered entity or business associate.

How to Do It:

- Consult the NIST publication *Guide for Conducting Risk Assessments.*[35]
- There are nine steps to conduct during a risk analysis:
  1. Define the scope of the risk analysis pertaining to your practice's electronic systems that contain ePHI.
  2. Identify and compile relevant information.
  3. Identify realistic threats.
  4. Identify potential vulnerabilities.
  5. Assess current security controls in your practice.
  6. Determine the likelihood and impact of a threat exercising a vulnerability that would affect your electronic systems containing ePHI.
  7. Determine levels of risk to your practice's electronic systems that contain ePHI.
  8. Recommend security controls to mitigate such risk levels.
  9. Document the risk assessment findings.

CRITICAL POINT

Be sure to include in your risk analysis portable and mobile electronic devices and media along with stationary electronic networks, systems, applications, and workstations.

CRITICAL POINT

Your organization's risk analysis is the foundation of your risk mitigation strategy and the source of guidance for implementing administrative, physical, and technical safeguards to protect electronic systems that contain ePHI.

Risk Management

Standard	Implementation Specification	Reference
Security management process	B. Risk management (R)	164.308(a)(1)(ii)(B)

What to Do:

Implement security measures sufficient to reduce risks and vulnerabilities to a reasonable and appropriate level to comply with the general requirements of the Security Rule.[36]

How to Do It:

The threat-management outcomes of the risk analysis that you conduct will provide the foundation for your organization's policies and procedures. Your organization is unique, so you must evaluate your threats and vulnerabilities to be able to implement an effective security strategy to safeguard your electronic systems that contain ePHI.

Sanction Policy

Standard	Implementation Specification	Reference
Security management process	C. Sanction policy (R)	164.308(a)(1)(ii)(C)

What to Do:

Apply appropriate sanctions against workforce members who fail to comply with the security policies and procedures of the covered entity or business associate.

How to Do It:

Your organization must determine appropriate internal penalties for violations of your practice's security policies and procedures by the practice workforce. Such penalties should be an incentive to comply with your practice's policies and procedures and should deter noncompliant actions (for example, posting passwords on computer terminals or desktops). Your sanction policies and procedures will be an outcome of your practice's risk analysis and should be related to the practice's determination of harm pertaining to a particular security incident.

Information System Activity Review

Standard	Implementation Specification	Reference
Security management process	D. Information system activity review (R)	164.308(a)(1)(ii)(D)

What to Do:

Implement procedures to regularly review records of information system activity, such as audit logs, access reports, and security incident tracking reports.

How to Do It:

Ask your practice-management system vendor for help in setting up system audit logs, access reports, and security incident tracking reports. As part of your security-management process, identify all reporting requirements and establish procedures for compiling requisite information, creating log entries, safeguarding the documentation, and maintaining the documentation for "6 years from the date of its creation or the date when it last was in effect, whichever is later."[37]

Assigned Security Responsibility

Standard	Implementation Specification	References
Assigned security responsibility		45 CFR 164.308(a)(2) NIST SP 800-66, p. 20 68 Federal Register 8377 78 Federal Register 5694

What the Standard Requires

The standard requires that a covered entity or business associate "[i]dentify the security official who is responsible for the development and implementation of the policies and procedures required by [the Security Rule] for the covered entity or business associate."[38]

The implementation specification is contained in the language of the standard and, thus, is required.

The HIPAA Security Rule requires that "[f]inal security responsibility must rest with one individual to ensure accountability within each covered entity"[39] for the security of the electronic systems that contain ePHI. The role of security official may be combined with the role of privacy official if reasonable and appropriate, for example, in a small practice.

Security Official Job Description

The Security Official

The security official will have overall responsibility in the practice for compliance with the Security Rule generally and, in particular, for implementing policies and procedures that ensure the confidentiality, integrity, and availability of the practice's electronic protected health information.

The security official may already be an employee and will work closely with the privacy official. The security official may delegate tasks and responsibilities but is ultimately responsible for compliance with the Security Rule.

Qualifications of the security official should include the following:

- Knowledgeable about technological and business applications in the practice
- Good oral and written communication skills with the ability to discuss technical terms in plain language
- Ability to compile, update, and maintain documentation of policies, procedures, actions, and assessments pertaining to implementation specifications of the security standards
- Good people management skills inside the practice and with business associates such as electronic system vendors
- Ability to enforce security policies, procedures, and sanctions in the practice
- Ability to lead risk analysis processes and training programs in the practice

Critical Functions

The security official is responsible for the following activities:

- Prepare and manage the budget allocated to the practice's security program and be responsible for protecting the practice's information system assets, including an up-to-date record of inventory of hardware and software
- Develop and implement security policies, procedures, and guidelines to direct and carry out the objectives of the practice's security program; research and recommend new security measures for the practice; and monitor and test the practice's security program for effectiveness

Continued

Security Official Job Description (continued)

- Ensure that the following policies and procedures are in place: security policies and procedures, baseline security safeguards, security risk management, security administration, security of the computer network, security of servers, security of personal computers, physical security, disaster recovery plan, and security awareness training
- Maintain documentation regarding levels of access granted to each information system user in the practice, and review these levels of access periodically and when the status of a workforce member changes, controlling access as appropriate
- Investigate, respond to, and remedy security incidents
- Supervise personnel of vendors or business associates who perform technical system maintenance activities in the practice, and provide and document that such personnel have security awareness training, as appropriate
- Document and maintain system access authorization records, which will be signed by personnel of vendors or business associates who perform technical system maintenance activities in the practice

Workforce Security

Standard	Implementation Specifications	References
Workforce security	A. Authorization and/or supervision (A) B. Workforce clearance procedure (A) C. Termination procedures (A)	45 CFR 164.308(a)(3)(i) NIST SP 800-66, pp. 21-22 68 Federal Register 8377 78 Federal Register 5694

What the Standard Requires

The standard requires that a covered entity or business associate "[i]mplement policies and procedures to ensure that all members of its workforce have appropriate access to electronic protected health information, as provided under [the Information Access Management standard], and to prevent those workforce members who do not have access under [the Information Access Management standard] from obtaining access to electronic protected health information."[40]

This standard requires your practice to control access to ePHI in the practice. Simply put, you must have controls in place to allow appropriate access to ePHI for workforce members to perform their job responsibilities and to preclude such access for workforce members who do not need such information to conduct their job responsibilities. The requirement to preclude access to ePHI also includes workforce members whose job responsibilities may have changed to no longer require such information and those who have left the practice or have been terminated from employment.

The three implementation specifications for this standard illustrate the concept of addressability (as opposed to requirement), especially with regard to risk analyses pertaining to small physician practices. For example, in designing a clearance procedure, the "need for and extent of a screening process is normally based on an assessment of the risk, cost, benefit, and feasibility as well as other protective measures in place. . . . For example, a personal clearance may not be reasonable or appropriate for a small provider whose only assistant is his or her spouse."[41] Similarly, with regard to termination procedures, "in certain circumstances . . . in a solo physician practice whose staff consists only of the physician's spouse, formal procedures may not be necessary."[42] Finally, "the purpose of termination procedure documentation is to ensure that termination procedures include security-unique actions to be followed, for example, revoking passwords and retrieving keys when a termination occurs."[43] Certainly, the procedures in the solo practice example above would be different from those in a multiphysician practice with a large workforce. In each case, however, given that the implementation specifications are addressable, it is required that the policies and procedures to comply with the standard be documented in writing.

Authorization and/or Supervision

Standard	Implementation Specification	Reference
Workforce security	A. Authorization and/or supervision (A)	164.308(a)(3)(ii)(A)

What to Do:

Implement procedures for the authorization[44] and/or supervision of workforce members who work with ePHI or in locations where it might be accessed.

How to Do It:

As part of your practice's risk analysis, determine which workforce members have a need for access to ePHI as part of their job responsibilities. Describe such needs, corresponding authorization, and supervision responsibilities in job descriptions. Ensure that each member of the workforce understands those responsibilities.

Workforce Clearance Procedure

Standard	Implementation Specification	Reference
Workforce security	B. Workforce clearance procedure (A)	164.308(a)(3)(ii)(B)

What to Do:

Implement procedures to determine that the access of a workforce member to ePHI is appropriate.

How to Do It:

Clearance will be an outcome of the risk analysis and an elaboration of the authorization contained in job descriptions. As part of the risk analysis, the practice should consider criteria for a background check for each workforce member candidate.

Termination Procedures

Standard	Implementation Specification	Reference
Workforce security	C. Termination procedures (A)	164.308(a)(3)(ii)(C)

What to Do:

Implement procedures for terminating access to ePHI when the employment of, or other arrangement with, a workforce member ends or as required by determinations made as specified in the Workforce Clearance implementation specification of this standard.

How to Do It:

The January 25, 2013, addition of "or other arrangement with" to the implementation specification recognizes that "not all workforce members are employees (eg, some may be volunteers) of a covered entity or business associate."[45] Establish an exit-interview format in which passwords are invalidated, terminated workforce members are informed that any authorizations are denied, federal penalties for unauthorized access to ePHI in the practice are outlined, and the terminated employee acknowledges in writing the receipt and understanding of the information conveyed in the exit interview.

Information Access Management

Standard	Implementation Specifications	References
Information access management	A. Isolating health care clearinghouse functions (R) B. Access authorization (A) C. Access establishment and modification (A)	45 CFR 164.308(a)(4)(i) NIST SP 800-66, pp. 23-24 68 Federal Register 8377 78 Federal Register 5694

What the Standard Requires

The standard requires that a covered entity or business associate "[i]mplement policies and procedures for authorizing access to electronic protected health information that are consistent with the applicable requirements of [the HIPAA Privacy Rule]."[46]

This standard is analogous to other HIPAA administrative simplification standards in the Privacy Rule that restrict access to PHI to authorized users. It requires that your practice have a management system in place to authorize workforce members to have access to ePHI through a "workstation, transaction, program, process, or other mechanism."[47] Today, another mechanism could be a mobile device such as a smart phone, a technology that was in its infancy when the HIPAA Security Rule was promulgated.

Isolating Health Care Clearinghouse Functions

Standard	Implementation Specifications	Reference
Information access management	A. Isolating health care clearinghouse functions (R)	164.308(a)(4)(ii)(A)

What to Do:

If a health care clearinghouse is part of a larger organization, the clearinghouse must implement policies and procedures that protect the ePHI of the clearinghouse from unauthorized access by the larger organization.

How to Do It:

A practice will not have to address this implementation specification directly, but the practice needs to know about it if the practice engages a health care clearinghouse as a business associate. Health care clearinghouses function almost entirely as business associates with respect to the PHI they maintain and process,[48] but as HIPAA-defined covered entities, they were required to comply with the HIPAA Security Rule prior to the HITECH Act, so they should be able to provide "satisfactory assurances"[49] of that compliance under the business associate agreement.[50]

Access Authorization

Standard	Implementation Specifications	Reference
Information access management	B. Access authorization (A)	164.308(a)(4)(ii)(B)

What to Do:

Implement policies and procedures for granting access to ePHI, for example, through access to a workstation, transaction, program, process, or other mechanism.

How to Do It:

Determine through the risk analysis which workforce members have a need for access to ePHI. Include the need for such access in job responsibilities incorporated into job descriptions. Ask for help from your business associate electronic systems vendors about system capacities for setting access controls, and address such capacities as part of your practice's risk analysis. In addition, determine which business associates need access to your electronic systems containing ePHI, and consider the implications of such access authorization in your risk analysis.[51] Your practice's privacy and security officials should jointly develop policies and procedures related to access that are consistent with the access authorization provisions of the Privacy Rule and the Security Rule.

Access Establishment and Modification

Standard	Implementation Specification	Reference
Information access management	C. Access establishment and modification (A)	164.308(a)(4)(ii)(C)

What to Do:

Implement policies and procedures that, based upon the covered entity's or the business associate's access authorization policies, establish, document, review, and modify a user's right of access to a workstation, transaction, program, or process.

How to Do It:

Establish procedures for periodically reviewing and modifying access based on a change in an authorized workforce member's modified job responsibilities. Document and maintain access authorization records according to the HIPAA documentation standard. Such records should include changes in authorization due to modification of job responsibilities relating to grants of access, levels of access, times of access, and place(s) or system(s) of access, as applicable.

CRITICAL POINT

The addressable *Access Authorization* and *Access Establishment and Modification* implementation specifications recognize the existence of alternatives in complying with the Information Access Management standard that may be based on a practice's size and degree of electronic system automation.

Security Awareness and Training

Standard	Implementation Specifications	References
Security awareness and training	A. Security reminders (A) B. Protection from malicious software (A) C. Log-in monitoring (A) D. Password management (A)	45 CFR 164.308(a)(5)(1) NIST SP 800-66, pp. 25-26 68 Federal Register 8377

What the Standard Requires

The standard requires that a covered entity or business associate "[i]mplement a security awareness and training program for all members of its workforce (including management)."[52]

Training is an ongoing internal process for safeguarding PHI from unauthorized use or disclosure as business policies and procedures evolve and regulatory standards are initiated or modified.

Furthermore, the training standard requires that workforce members, including management, demonstrate awareness and understanding on an ongoing basis and that covered entities and business associates document that their workforce members have been trained. As examples, the first implementation specification of the Security Awareness and Training standard of the Security Rule is "Security reminders"; this addressable specification requires that the covered entity or business associate implement "[p]eriodic security updates."[53] One part of the implementation specification for the Privacy Rule's training standard states that a "covered entity must provide training . . . [t]o each member of covered entity's workforce whose functions are affected by a material change in the policies or procedures required by [the Privacy Rule], within a reasonable period of time after the material change becomes effective."[54]

Whether it is Privacy Rule, Security Rule, or Breach Notification Rule training, each member of the workforce, including the management of the practice, must participate in training. It is important that training be coordinated across each of the rules as they are interrelated. It also is important that each member of the workforce receive the same training so that workforce members reinforce one another in safeguarding PHI in the practice in any form: oral, hard copy, or electronic.

Your practice must make your business associates aware of your security policies and procedures. As of the HITECH Act compliance date of September 23, 2013, business associates must comply with the Security Rule and so must have their own security awareness and training programs in place. It would be prudent business practice to determine how your practice's business associates are training their workforce members to safeguard your ePHI.

Because your practice generates revenue on a transactional basis during the business day, it may be costly and inconvenient to take time away from patients to conduct training. Your practice may wish to consider online training programs that your workforce members can take outside of the business day at their convenience, such as in the evening or on weekends.[55] Be sure to document your training programs, including the time, curriculum, and results for each workforce member.

Each of the four implementation specifications within this standard is addressable. Even though the implementation specifications are addressable, "[s]ecurity awareness training is a critical activity, regardless of an organization's size."[56] Although training is required, its content and method are addressable. That the implementation specifications are addressable reflects several considerations discussed in the preamble to the Security Rule, namely, that training is "[d]ependent upon an entity's configuration and security risks" and is "[a]n on-going, evolving process as an entity's security needs and procedures change."[57]

Each person with access to ePHI must be knowledgeable about and understand the appropriate security measures to reduce the risk of improper access, use, and disclosure. Awareness is the first goal of training. Awareness is not a one-time outcome for the workforce, but rather a continuing responsibility as technology changes, as new technology is introduced into the practice,[58] and as policies and procedures change in response to modifications of the HIPAA standards.[59] These modifications occurred with the HITECH Act and were promulgated on January 25, 2013, with a compliance date of September 23, 2013. The practice is not responsible for providing training to anyone outside of its workforce, but the practice is responsible for ensuring that its business associates are aware of the practice's security policies and procedures and the requirement that business associates inform the covered entity of any discovered breaches of ePHI for which they are responsible. This level of awareness of policies and procedures also should be imparted to representatives of business associates who may be at your practice facility or facilities for a limited period of time, such as vendors, maintenance personnel, and others. Such representatives can be made aware of the covered entity's safeguard policies and procedures by giving them pamphlets or copies of the safeguards for which compliance is required.

NIST highlights the importance of awareness and training programs:

> Awareness programs set the stage for training by changing organizational attitudes to realize the importance of security and the adverse consequences of its failure. The purpose of training is to teach people the skills that will enable them to perform their jobs more effectively.[60]

This quotation highlights two important attributes of a successful awareness and training program: a change in corporate culture is required, and the payoff can be greater workforce productivity. When the practice's workforce pulls together to conduct a risk analysis, each member has a stake in the inputs and in the security safeguards. Management plays an important role in effecting change and in realizing the risk mitigation payoff. Quite simply, the intersecting roles of management and the workforce in ensuring security of PHI are reflected in the language of the standard.

CRITICAL POINT

All members of your practice workforce, including management, are required to participate in security awareness and training. When the practice workforce pulls together to conduct a risk analysis, each member has a stake in the inputs and in the security safeguards, and the practice can effect change and realize risk mitigation payoffs.

Security Reminders

Standard	Implementation Specification	Reference
Security awareness and training	A. Security reminders (A)	164.308(a)(5)(ii)(A)

What to Do:

Implement periodic security reminders.

How to Do It:

Post security reminders in work areas, and periodically broadcast security reminders via e-mail to workforce members. At meetings of workforce members, be sure to include at least one security safeguard topic on the agenda.

Protection From Malicious Software

Standard	Implementation Specification	Reference
Security awareness and training	B. Protection from malicious software (A)	164.308(a)(5)(ii)(B)

What to Do:

Implement procedures for guarding against, detecting, and reporting malicious software.

How to Do It:

Discuss technologies for guarding against, detecting, and reporting malicious software with your systems vendor(s). Install commercially available virus detection and firewall software programs on all of the practice's electronic devices and media. Apply sanctions to any workforce member who does not comply with the practice's procedures relating to safeguarding ePHI from malicious software.

Log-in Monitoring

Standard	Implementation Specification	Reference
Security awareness and training	C. Log-in monitoring (A)	164.308(a)(5)(ii)(C)

What to Do:

Implement procedures for monitoring log-in attempts and reporting discrepancies.

How to Do It:

Discuss with your practice-management software vendor how to monitor and track log-in attempts and report discrepancies. Check the documentation of your operating system to determine its capability for tracking authorized log-ins and unauthorized log-in attempts. Either implement the operating system's capability or acquire and activate a viable commercial software program for doing so. Maintain log-in activity reports according to the HIPAA documentation standard.

Password Management

Standard	Implementation Specification	Reference
Security awareness and training	D. Password management (A)	164.308(a)(5)(ii)(D)

What to Do:

Implement procedures for creating, changing, and safeguarding passwords.

How to Do It:

Develop a policy and corresponding procedures for password management. The practice's designated system administrator and security official should be the only persons with access to passwords of other workforce members.[61] Passwords should be changed periodically based on threat exposures (eg, every 30, 60, or 90 days, with timing an output of the practice's risk analysis). Implement and carry out sanctions for any workforce member who posts a password on a workstation terminal or desktop, or who shares a password with other workforce members.

Security Incident Procedures

Standard	Implementation Specification	References
Security incident procedures	Response and reporting (R)	45 CFR 164.308(a)(6)(i) NIST SP 800-66, pp. 27-28 68 Federal Register 8377 78 Federal Register 5694

What the Standard Requires

The standard requires that a covered entity or business associate "[i]mplement policies and procedures to address security incidents."[62]

A security incident is defined as "the attempted or successful unauthorized access, use, disclosure, modification, or destruction of information or interference with system operations in an information system."[63] Your practice must consider the wide variety of risks that this definition encompasses as you assess threats and vulnerabilities in your risk analysis.

The HITECH Act, discussed in Chapter 1, provided for breach notification, the requirement of which was embodied in an interim final rule published in the *Federal Register* on August 24, 2009, and modified in a final rule published in the *Federal Register* on January 25, 2013. If your practice fails to encrypt ePHI in your practice database(s) (data at rest) or in your transactions (data in motion), and there is a breach of your ***unsecured*** ePHI, then your practice is subject to the response and reporting requirements of the Breach Notification Rule discussed in Chapter 1.

Response and Reporting

Standard	Implementation Specification	Reference
Security incident procedures	Response and reporting (R)	164.308(a)(6)(ii)

What to Do:

Identify and respond to suspected or known security incidents; mitigate, to the extent practicable, harmful effects of security incidents that are known to the covered entity or business associate; and document security incidents and their outcomes.

How to Do It:

Prior to enactment of the HITECH Act, this required implementation specification did not mandate reporting security incidents to outside authorities. The Security Rule indicated that such decisions should be based upon "business and legal considerations."[64] Then, as now, your practice had an obligation to respond and report, keeping track of your practice's actions, in writing, if your practice experienced a security incident. Your practice also was required to mitigate harms arising from the incident, put in place more effective safeguards to mitigate the risk of the incident occurring again, and update its risk analysis. With the HITECH Act came requirements for responding to a security breach of unsecured ePHI, discussed in Chapter 1. We recommend, here as elsewhere in this chapter, that your practice encrypt its ePHI in its databases (data at rest) and in its transactions (data in motion) in order to avoid the consequences of a security incident in which unsecured ePHI is impermissibly used by or disclosed to unauthorized individuals. With significantly increased civil penalties for a security violation that became effective with enactment of the HITECH Act on February 17, 2009, and with federal enforcement effective on February 22, 2010, for discovered breaches occurring on or after that date, the consequences of a security incident could be costly. Use the sample security incident report in Figure 4.1 and the sample security incident log in Figure 4.2 to document and maintain records of any security incidents that your practice experiences.

CRITICAL POINT

Your practice is required to respond to and mitigate any harmful effects of security incidents and to document and maintain a log of all security incidents.

FIGURE 4.1

Sample Security Incident Report

Description of Attempted or Actual Security Incident: ______________________

____

____

Date: __________ Time: __________ Location: ______________________

Who Discovered the Security Incident: ______________________

How the Security Incident Was Discovered: ______________________

____

____

Evidence of Incident: ______________________

____

____

Actions Taken to Minimize Damages to Practice's Systems and Electronic Data:

____

____

____

____

Policy and Procedural Changes Implemented to Avoid Recurrence: __________

____

____

____

Security Official Name ______________ Signature ________ Date ______________

FIGURE 4.2

Sample Security Incident Log

Date	Location	Description	Severity Level of Incident 1 ⟶ 5 Least Serious — Most Serious

Contingency Plan

Standard	Implementation Specifications	References
Contingency plan	A. Data backup plan (R) B. Disaster recovery plan (R) C. Emergency mode operation plan (R) D. Testing and revision procedures (A) E. Applications and data criticality analysis (A)	45 CFR 164.308(a)(7)(i) NIST SP 800-66, pp. 29-30 68 Federal Register 8377-8378

What the Standard Requires

The standard requires that a covered entity or business associate "[e]stablish (and implement as needed) policies and procedures for responding to an emergency or other occurrence (for example, fire, vandalism, system failure, and natural disaster) that damages systems that contain electronic protected health information."[65]

As your practice comes to rely increasingly on electronic systems to conduct business, it is vital to create, test, and update plans to respond to and recover from a contingency that impairs your ability to access electronic systems that contain ePHI. Those systems and the PHI therein are the lifeblood of your business as a medical practice. Part of your strategy for response and recovery is to develop data backup, disaster recovery, and emergency mode operation plans. Your practice needs to develop contingency plans around answers to these questions:

- How will the practice's patients be affected?
- What practice resources could be lost?
- What costs are associated with any loss?
- What efforts, costs, resources, and time would be required to achieve recovery?
- What would be the overall effect of the loss on the viability of the business as a medical practice?

This standard has five implementation specifications, with three required and two addressable.

Data Backup Plan

Standard	Implementation Specification	Reference
Contingency plan	A. Data backup plan (R)	164.308(a)(7)(ii)(A)

What to Do:

Establish and implement procedures to create and maintain retrievable exact copies of ePHI.

How to Do It:

Check with your practice-management software vendor to determine if your software accommodates backups with exact-copy capability. If your practice is small, you might consider using a daily tape, CD, DVD, or external hard drive backup and maintaining that electronic media off-site in a secure location.[66] If your practice is large, you might consider using a more complex procedure, such as a real-time, online, encrypted data stream or periodic batch download of duplicate data to a secure off-site location. Maintaining the integrity of your ePHI is paramount and, in fact, is a technical safeguard standard.

Disaster Recovery Plan

Standard	Implementation Specification	Reference
Contingency plan	B. Disaster recovery plan (R)	164.308(a)(7)(ii)(B)

What to Do:

Establish (and implement as needed) procedures to restore any loss of data.

How to Do It:

Disaster recovery planning will be an outgrowth of the identification of threats in the risk analysis. Your practice will need to determine outcomes of threats and the effect on the operations of the practice. Plan for the worst outcomes! Develop safeguards to mitigate those outcomes, and identify key workforce members in the practice to take responsibility for recovery should those outcomes become a reality. "The final rule calls for covered entities [and business associates] to consider how natural disasters could damage systems that contain electronic protected health information and develop policies and procedures for responding to such situations. We [HHS] consider this to be a reasonable precautionary step to take since in many cases the risk would be deemed to be low."[67]

With regard to preparing a disaster recovery plan, we recommend that your practice consult NIST Special Publication 800-34, *Contingency Planning Guide for Federal Information Systems*.[68]

Emergency Mode Operation Plan

Standard	Implementation Specification	Reference
Contingency plan	C. Emergency mode operation plan (R)	164.308(a)(7)(ii)(C)

What to Do:

Establish (and implement as needed) procedures to enable continuation of critical business processes for protection of the security of ePHI while operating in emergency mode.

How to Do It:

This plan will be a component of your disaster recovery plan. It is important to get input from each workforce member as to duties and workflow in order to establish a workable emergency mode operation plan. Use that information to prepare a workflow map of how your practice operates, which will prove useful in normal operations as well. Even when you are in an emergency mode, your practice must still safeguard ePHI. Develop a plan to securely access electronic systems (including servers and workstations) that contain an exact copy of your practice's current ePHI. Select and maintain an alternative site to perform the practice's data processing functions if a disaster seriously disrupts access and availability of ePHI at your practice facility. Ensure hardware and software compatibility at primary and backup sites. Provide backup power and communications in the event of an emergency. Appoint personnel to the emergency mode operations team. Train all personnel in the emergency mode operation plan, with emphasis on the circumstances under which a key workforce member initiates emergency mode operations and who may do so. Test the emergency mode operation plan and make modifications as necessary. Document all plans and actions, including test results, in writing, and maintain the documentation according to the HIPAA documentation standard.

CRITICAL POINT

Consider in your disaster recovery planning that loss of electricity in your practice curtails your access to electronic systems that contain ePHI, thereby triggering an emergency mode operation plan.

Testing and Revision Procedures

Standard	Implementation Specification	Reference
Contingency plan	D. Testing and revision procedures (A)	164.308(a)(7)(ii)(D)

What to Do:

Implement procedures for periodic testing and revision of contingency plans.

How to Do It:

After the disaster recovery plan is created, test the plan by creating a disaster scenario and going through the recovery steps in the plan. This test should be planned in advance and conducted at a time when the practice is not open for business, such as a weekend afternoon. Be sure to document the successful provisions of the plan, response times, and, most importantly, any failures that require correction. Make corrections to the plan as soon as possible, and make sure all workforce members know the new procedures and why they are being implemented. Test the plan at least annually, making sure that any deficiencies from the preceding test are evaluated to ensure that they have been corrected.

Applications and Data Criticality Analysis

Standard	Implementation Specification	Reference
Contingency plan	E. Applications and data criticality analysis (A)	164.308(a)(7)(ii)(E)

What to Do:

Assess the relative criticality of specific applications and data in support of other contingency plan components.

How to Do It:

Determine the applications and data that are most critical to the operation of your business as a medical practice. Prioritize decisions and actions, starting with answers to these questions that will inform your practice's risk analysis:

- What are the most important considerations in safeguarding the practice's electronic systems that contain ePHI?
- What are the practice's biggest security threats?
- What are the areas in which the practice is most vulnerable from a security perspective?
- What steps should be taken first, and in what order should they be taken, to recover critical business functions in the event of a contingency?

Remediation will be part of determining risk mitigation strategies. As your practice experiences growing use of electronic business processes, it is prudent to have in place the three required implementation specifications relating to contingencies: data backup, disaster recovery, and emergency mode operation plans.

CRITICAL POINT

"Contingency planning will be scalable based upon other factors, office configuration, and risk assessment."[69] Some scenarios that might invoke a disaster recovery and emergency mode operation plan for a covered entity would be just an inconvenience in other businesses. Electricity, for example, is critical to a covered entity such as a medical practice, whereas loss of electricity might just be an inconvenience to another type of business.

Evaluation

Standard	Implementation Specification	References
Evaluation		45 CFR 164.308(a)(8) NIST SP 800-66, pp. 31-32 68 Federal Register 8378 78 Federal Register 5694

What the Standard Requires

The standard requires that a covered entity or business associate "[p]erform a periodic technical and nontechnical evaluation, based initially upon the standards implemented under this rule and, subsequently, in response to environmental or operational changes affecting the security of electronic protected health information, that establishes the extent to which a covered entity's or business associate's security policies and procedures meet the requirements of [the HIPAA Security Rule]."[70]

The implementation specification is contained in the language of the standard and, thus, is required.

Your practice should design an evaluation format, establish an evaluation committee chaired by the security official and composed of workforce members, and set up a schedule for evaluating security systems, risk mitigation, and compliance with Security Rule safeguard standards. While your practice must perform periodic evaluations, you have the option of conducting the evaluations internally using your own workforce or using an external accreditation agency. The preamble to the Security Rule recognizes that cost may be a consideration for an external evaluation, especially for some entities such as small physician practices. Good sources of information and guidance pertaining to evaluation of standards under the Security Rule are the following:

- National Institute of Standards and Technology[71]
- URAC[72]
- Electronic Healthcare Network Accreditation Commission (EHNAC)[73]
- Workgroup for Electronic Data Interchange (WEDI)[74]

Your practice is required under the Security Rule to maintain acceptable levels of risk. If risks are not acceptable, your practice is required to effect changes in its policies and procedures to move to acceptable levels of risk. In an evaluation of the cost of attaining acceptable levels of risk, be sure to include consideration of the civil monetary penalties for violations of the Security Rule. Note that the HITECH Act significantly increased the penalties, with the maximum fine for repeated incidence of a single violation increasing 60-fold to $1.5 million per calendar year. Also, note that the 2011 cost per customer record for a breach in the health care industry was estimated by survey to be $240, which was based on a combination of "direct and indirect expenses."[75]

Business Associate Contracts and Other Arrangements

Standard	Implementation Specification	References
Business associate contracts and other arrangements	Written contract or other arrangement (R)	45 CFR 164.308(b)(1) and 45 CFR 164.308(b)(2) NIST SP 800-66, pp. 33-34 68 Federal Register 8378 78 Federal Register 5694

What the Standard Requires

The standard specifies the following:

> (b)(1) *Business associate contracts and other arrangements.* A covered entity may permit a business associate to create, receive, maintain, or transmit electronic protected health information on the covered entity's behalf only if the covered entity obtains satisfactory assurances, in accordance with [45 CFR] 164.314(a),[76] that the business associate will appropriately safeguard the information. A covered entity is not required to obtain such satisfactory assurances from a business associate that is a subcontractor.[77]
>
> (2) A business associate may permit a business associate that is a subcontractor to create, receive, maintain, or transmit electronic protected health information on its behalf only if the business associate obtains satisfactory assurances, in accordance with [45 CFR] 164.314(a),[78] that the subcontractor will appropriately safeguard the information.[79]

The HITECH Act statutorily established, and the modifications to the HIPAA rules by the January 25, 2013, final rule enable by regulation, that business associates are directly regulated by the federal government in a manner similar to that of covered entities.[80] This standard requires your practice to have appropriate written business associate agreements in place for any person[81] that creates, receives, maintains, or transmits ePHI on the covered entity's behalf in a contractor relationship. Under the HITECH Act, the relationship changed in four ways, discussed in Chapter 1. First, business associates are required to implement and comply with the Security Rule. Second, a business associate is required to report a discovered security incident or privacy breach to the covered entity and provide requisite information that will facilitate the covered entity's fulfillment of breach notification requirements. The reporting role of a business associate in a subcontractor capacity is discussed below. Third, with one exception, a business associate in any capacity is subject to the same penalties as a covered entity for violations of the Security Rule and Privacy Rule, as modified January 25, 2013, effective March 26, 2013, and with compliance required by September 23, 2013. The exception is breach notification; federal enforcement of covered entities and business associates commenced February 22, 2010, for breaches discovered on or after that date. Finally, business associate agreements had to incorporate specific security and privacy provisions.[82]

The January 25, 2013, final rule establishes a clear distinction between a business associate that is a contractor to a covered entity, and a business associate that engages one or more subcontractors that also are business associates. According to the final rule:

> A covered entity is not required to enter into a business associate agreement with a business associate that is a subcontractor; rather, this is the obligation of the business associate that has engaged the subcontractor to perform a function or service that involves the use or disclosure of protected health information.[83]

Regarding satisfactory assurances, the final rule states:

> [C]overed entities must ensure that they obtain satisfactory assurances required by the Rules from their business associates, and business associates must do the same

with regard to subcontractors, and so on, no matter how far "down the chain" the information flows. This ensures that individuals' health information remains protected by all parties that create, receive, maintain, or transmit the information in order for a covered entity to perform its health care functions. For example, a covered entity may contract with a business associate (contractor), the contractor may delegate to a subcontractor (subcontractor 1) one or more functions, services, or activities the business associate has agreed to perform for the covered entity that require access to protected health information, and the subcontractor may in turn delegate to another subcontractor (subcontractor 2) one or more functions, services, or activities it has agreed to perform for the contractor that require access to protected health information, and so on. Both the contractor and all of the subcontractors are business associates under the final rule to the extent they create, receive, maintain, or transmit protected health information.[84]

Written Contract or Other Arrangement

Standard	Implementation Specification	Reference
Business associate contracts and other arrangements	Written contract or other arrangement (R)	164.308(b)(3)

What to Do:

Document the satisfactory assurances required in paragraph (b)(1) or (b)(2) of the Business Associate Contracts and Other Arrangements standard through a written contract or other arrangement with the business associate that meets the applicable requirements of 45 CFR 164.314(a).

How to Do It:

The HITECH Act requires that covered entities amend their business associate agreements to reflect new requirements and changes in the relationship between a covered entity and its business associates. For information on how the final rule modified business associate agreement provisions, see OCR, "Business Associate Contracts: Sample Business Associate Agreement Provisions," which is available at http://www.hhs.gov/ocr/privacy/hipaa/understanding/coveredentities/contractprov.html.

PHYSICAL SAFEGUARD STANDARDS AND IMPLEMENTATION SPECIFICATIONS

"Physical safeguards are physical measures, policies, and procedures to protect a covered entity's or business associate's electronic information systems and related buildings and equipment, from natural and environmental hazards, and unauthorized intrusion."[85] They are designed to help you protect your investment in the facilities and electronic systems, devices, and media that contain ePHI. Covered entities have been required to comply with the Security Rule since April 21, 2005. The final Security Rule modifications published in the *Federal Register* on January 25, 2013, required business associates also to implement Security Rule standards and implementation specifications, but did not otherwise modify the language of the physical safeguard regulations. Physical safeguards are designed to help you protect your investment in the facilities and electronic systems, devices, and media that contain ePHI.

Facility Access Controls

Standard	Implementation Specifications	References
Facility access controls	i. Contingency operations (A) ii. Facility security plan (A) iii. Access control and validation procedures (A) iv. Maintenance records (A)	45 CFR 164.310(a)(1) NIST SP 800-66, pp. 35-36 68 Federal Register 8378

What the Standard Requires

The standard requires that a covered entity or business associate "[i]mplement policies and procedures to limit physical access to its electronic information systems and the facility or facilities in which they are housed, while ensuring that properly authorized access is allowed."[86]

This standard has four implementation specifications, each of which is addressable, which means that you may tailor your policies and procedures for controlling access to your practice's particular physical environment. The language of the implementation specifications is straightforward. Specifications will be determined based on a covered entity's risk analysis and other factors, such as the characteristics of the practice facility itself. Two clarifications are important with respect to this standard. First, the facility access controls standard applies to a covered entity or business associate's location or locations, and the facility includes "physical premises and the interior and exterior of a building(s)."[87] Please note that the term *facility* includes premises for workforce members who may be authorized to work with ePHI from their homes and covers *electronic systems, devices*, and *media* that may be used in a home environment or mobile capacity. Second, a covered entity "retains responsibility for considering facility security even where it shares space . . . with other organizations."[88]

Contingency Operations

Standard	Implementation Specification	Reference
Facility access controls	i. Contingency operations (A)	164.310(a)(2)(i)

What to Do:

Establish (and implement as needed) procedures that allow facility access in support of restoration of lost data under the disaster recovery plan and emergency mode operations plan in the event of an emergency.

How to Do It:

This implementation specification is related to the administrative safeguard contingency plan and outlines the procedures to be followed to restore ePHI in the event of an emergency situation, so compliance with this standard requires coordination of the procedures here with the disaster and emergency mode operation plans that are covered by that administrative safeguard standard. The procedures will be based on outcomes of your practice's risk analysis. Questions to address include the following examples:

- What are your procedures for recovery if your practice is damaged by fire?
- What are your procedures for recovery if your practice loses its electricity supply for a prolonged period of time, such as from a natural disaster?
- Where would your practice relocate in the event of a natural disaster?[89]

Remember, the critical outcome is reestablishing access to the practice's electronic systems that contain ePHI. Identify your software vendor(s) and key workforce members that will be responsible for achieving that outcome. Finally, have a procedure for keeping your patients informed of your progress in restoring practice operations.

Facility Security Plan

Standard	Implementation Specification	Reference
Facility access controls	ii. Facility security plan (A)	164.310(a)(2)(ii)

What to Do:

Implement policies and procedures to safeguard the facility and the equipment therein from unauthorized physical access, tampering, and theft.

How to Do It:

Develop procedures to protect your practice's facility and electronic systems, devices, and media from unauthorized physical access, tampering, and theft. Include policies regarding building exteriors, interiors, access, tampering, and theft. Also, include procedures for handling intrusions and deliberate impairment of systems, which may include computer systems and electricity serving your facility location. Develop access policies and implement procedures to safeguard your practice's facility and electronic systems, using locks, alarm systems, identification systems such as pass cards, anti-intrusion systems, and similar devices that are suitable for your practice as a business environment. See Figure 4.3 for a sample checklist of facility access controls.

CRITICAL POINT

During practice hours, the receptionist can play a key role in controlling access and ensuring that only authorized individuals have access to systems containing ePHI.

FIGURE 4.3

Sample Checklist of Facility Access Controls

- ☐ Who is authorized to have access to your electronic systems containing ePHI, what is their mode of access, and how is access controlled? What are your opening and closing procedures?
- ☐ Who maintains the layout and design of the facility? Who authorizes access to the facility?
- ☐ Who has control over locks and keys?
- ☐ What are the locking mechanisms for doors, gates, windows, and other access points?
- ☐ Do workforce members have access badges and cards, door keys, etc?
- ☐ Do you have sign-in and sign-out procedures?
- ☐ Do you have door and window locations and security devices for each?
- ☐ Are you in a flood zone? Are there fire or water hazards on the premises?
- ☐ Who is authorized to handle contingencies?
- ☐ Are there environmental controls (heating, ventilation, and air conditioning) for electronic systems?
- ☐ Do you have a plan for monitoring and periodically evaluating the facility security plan?

Access Control and Validation Procedures

Standard	Implementation Specification	Reference
Facility access controls	iii. Access control and validation procedures (A)	164.310(a)(2)(iii)

What to Do

Implement procedures to control and validate a person's access to facilities based on his or her role or function, including visitor control, and control of access to software programs for testing and revision.

How to Do It:

This implementation specification typically is based on job function and need. Your practice needs to implement procedures to control access to electronic systems that contain ePHI. In accordance with the minimum necessary requirement of the Privacy Rule, these Security Rule access procedures should cross-reference the Privacy Rule access controls to avoid conflicting policies. Your procedures should verify authorization for any workforce member or business associate to access electronic systems that contain ePHI. In addition, your practice should control access and movement within the practice. For business associates and any other nonpatient visitors to the practice, your practice should use Business Associate and Visitor sign-in and badge systems. Your practice should escort visitors in areas that contain access to ePHI, should there be a reason for them to be in such areas. The security official should be aware of and oversee business associates responsible for software testing and revision and should document all such activities as to time and result.

Maintenance Records

Standard	Implementation Specification	Reference
Facility access controls	iv. Maintenance records (A)	164.310(a)(2)(iv)

What to Do:

Implement policies and procedures to document repairs and modifications to the physical components of a facility that are related to security (for example, hardware, walls, doors, and locks).

How to Do It:

Create a log and description of repairs or modifications made to the facility's physical security components, including hardware, walls, doors, and locks. The log should document each repair in writing and be maintained according to the HIPAA documentation standard. Electronic documentation is permissible, but be sure to routinely back up the log after each new entry.

Workstation Use

Standard	Implementation Specification	References
Workstation use		45 CFR 164.310(b) NIST SP 800-66, p. 37 68 Federal Register 8378

What the Standard Requires

The standard requires that a covered entity or business associate "[i]mplement policies and procedures that specify the proper functions to be performed, the manner in which those functions are to be performed, and the physical attributes of the surroundings of a specific workstation or class of workstation that can access electronic protected health information."[90]

The implementation specification is contained in the language of the standard, and, thus, is required.

Note the definition of workstation in the Security Rule: "[A]n electronic computing device, for example, a laptop or desktop computer, or any other device that performs similar functions, and electronic media stored in its immediate environment."[91] Accordingly, this standard applies to workstations and electronic media that are stationary in the practice as well as those that may be portable or mobile and used outside the practice. An example of a policy and accompanying procedure pertaining to this standard would be that workforce members must log off before leaving a workstation unattended. Another example would be that a receptionist has to make sure that the workstation he or she uses to log patients into the practice for an encounter is shielded from the patients signing in. A third example would be that workstations used throughout the practice should not have screens visible to passersby, such as patients and visitors unauthorized to access ePHI. A final example would be that any workstation containing ePHI must not have Internet access over an open network and that any workforce members using an authorized portable or mobile device must have encryption that safeguards ePHI at rest and in motion.

Workstation Security

Standard	Implementation Specification	References
Workstation security		45 CFR 164.310(c) NIST SP 800-66, p. 38 68 Federal Register 8378

What the Standard Requires

The standard requires that a covered entity or business associate "[i]mplement physical safeguards for all workstations that access electronic protected health information, to restrict access to authorized users."[92]

The implementation specification is contained in the language of the standard and, thus, is required.

The compliance solution for this standard will be "dependent on the entity's risk analysis and risk management process."[93] All electronic systems and workstations in the practice that contain ePHI must have authentication[94] controls to allow access to authorized users while precluding access by unauthorized individuals. In addition to this safeguard, the practice must consider in its risk analysis the physical location and working environment in the practice for further safeguard possibilities. An example is shielding the screen of the receptionist's computer from the view of a patient signing in for an encounter, as mentioned in the discussion of the previous standard. Another example is having automatic log-off on all workstations; an automatic log-off would activate after a period of time determined as an outcome of the practice's risk analysis. Workstation security also pertains to portable and mobile devices used inside and outside the practice, all of which should be safeguarded through authentication and encryption controls.

Device and Media Controls

Standard	Implementation Specifications	References
Device and media controls	i. Disposal (R) ii. Media re-use (R) iii. Accountability (A) iv. Data backup and storage (A)	45 CFR 164.310(d)(1) NIST SP 800-66, p. 39 68 Federal Register 8378

What the Standard Requires

The standard requires that a covered entity or business associate "[i]mplement policies and procedures that govern the receipt and removal of hardware and electronic media that contain electronic protected health information into and out of a facility, and the movement of these items within the facility."[95]

This standard, which has two required implementation specifications and two addressable implementation specifications, requires your practice to establish policies and implement procedures to account for hardware and electronic media that contain ePHI. We discussed the August 24, 2009, *Guidance Specifying the Technologies and Methodologies That Render Protected Health Information Unusable, Unreadable, or Indecipherable to Unauthorized Individuals*[96] in Chapter 1, and the provisions of that *guidance* inform the discussion that follows on the implementation specifications. The *guidance* applies to the required implementation specifications for disposal and media re-use.

Disposal

Standard	Implementation Specification	Reference
Device and media controls	i. Disposal (R)	164.310(d)(2)(i)

What to Do:

Implement policies and procedures to address the final disposition of ePHI and/or the hardware or electronic media on which it is stored.

How to Do It:

We repeat here the relevant portion of the *guidance*:

> Protected health information (PHI) is rendered unusable, unreadable, or indecipherable to unauthorized individuals if one or more of the following applies: . . .
>
> (b) The media on which the PHI is stored or recorded have been destroyed in one of the following ways: . . .
>
> (ii) Electronic media have been cleared, purged, or destroyed consistent with NIST Special Publication 800-88, *Guidelines for Media Sanitation,*[97] such that the PHI cannot be retrieved.[98]

We recommend that your practice follow the *guidance* for disposal of hardware and electronic media. This guidance, which was published in updated form within the preamble to the interim final rule and made available on the HHS Web site,[99] specifies that only encryption and destruction, consistent with NIST guidelines, renders PHI unusable, unreadable, or indecipherable to unauthorized individuals such that notification is not required in the event of a breach of such information.[100] Consult your hardware and software vendors for help on interpreting the NIST *Guidelines for Media Sanitation*, referred to above.

Media Re-use

Standard	Implementation Specification	Reference
Device and media controls	ii. Media re-use (R)	164.310(d)(2)(ii)

What to Do:

Implement procedures for removal of ePHI from electronic media before the media are made available for re-use.

How to Do It:

How to handle media re-use will be an outcome of your practice's risk analysis. Since this implementation specification was promulgated, electronic media have become relatively inexpensive and are becoming more so with each passing year. Accordingly, in your risk analysis, your practice needs to compare the cost of replacing rather than re-using electronic media, with the latter including expected costs (based on risk) that you might incur should a breach occur from re-used electronic media. The expected costs should now include the costs of having to conduct breach notification. Given how inexpensive electronic media have become, we recommend ***not*** re-using electronic media, but rather destroying such media according to the procedure outlined in the preceding implementation specification (disposal).

Accountability

Standard	Implementation Specification	Reference
Device and media controls	iii. Accountability (A)	164.310(d)(2)(iii)

What to Do:

Maintain a record of the movements of hardware and electronic media and any person responsible therefor.

How to Do It:

Create and maintain an inventory and track movement of electronic systems, workstations, devices, and media within your practice. The inventory should include model and serial number, date purchased, place of purchase, warranty and/or maintenance contract (if applicable), location, workforce member responsible, and any movement from one location to another (if applicable). This implementation specification does not address audit trails within systems and/or software. Rather it requires a record of the actions of a person relative to the receipt and removal of hardware and/or software into and out of a facility that are traceable to that person. The impact of maintaining accountability on system resources and services will depend upon the complexity of the mechanism to establish accountability . . . such as receipt and removal restricted to specific persons, with logs kept.[101] Please keep in mind that this implementation specification is addressable: "[S]mall providers would be unlikely to be involved in large-scale moves of equipment that would require systematic tracking, unlike, for example, large health care providers or health plans."[102]

Data Backup and Storage

Standard	Implementation Specification	Reference
Device and media controls	iv. Data backup and storage (A)	164.310(d)(2)(iv)

What to Do:

Create a retrievable, exact copy of ePHI, when needed, before movement of equipment.

How to Do It:

Prior to moving any electronic systems, workstations, devices, or electronic media in the practice, make sure that you create an exact copy of ePHI contained therein. Maintain that copy in a separate file backed up in a secure off-site database environment. This copy must be readily retrievable in the event that hardware or electronic media are damaged in movement or if a disaster or other contingency affects the practice.

TECHNICAL SAFEGUARD STANDARDS AND IMPLEMENTATION SPECIFICATIONS

"Technical safeguards mean the technology and the policy and procedures for its use that protect electronic protected health information and control access to it."[103] Covered entities have had to comply with the Security Rule since April 2005, with small health plans having an additional year to do so. The final Security Rule modifications published in the *Federal Register* on January 25, 2013, required business associates also to implement Security Rule standards and implementation specifications, but did not otherwise change the language of the technical safeguards.

As security becomes even more important with the growing use of electronic health record (EHR)[104] systems and e-prescribing[105] by health care providers, you will find the policy and procedure information in this chapter useful as your practice checks on its own policies and procedures to ensure they are current.

Many of the technical safeguards may require information from your hardware or software vendor. Be sure to ask your vendor if you have any questions. Remember, you may use *reasonable* and *appropriate* measures to demonstrate compliance.

Access Control

Standard	Implementation Specifications	References
Access control	i. Unique user identification (R) ii. Emergency access procedure (R) iii. Automatic log-off (A) iv. Encryption and decryption (A)	45 CFR 164.312(a)(1) NIST SP 800-66, pp. 40-41 68 Federal Register 8378

What the Standard Requires

The standard requires that a covered entity or business associate "[i]mplement technical policies and procedures for electronic information systems that maintain electronic protected health information to allow access only to those persons or software programs that have been granted access rights as specified in [the administrative safeguard Information Access Management standard]."[106]

Unique User Identification

Standard	Implementation Specification	Reference
Access control	i. Unique user identification (R)	164.312(a)(2)(i)

What to Do:

Assign a unique name and/or number for identifying and tracking user identity.

How to Do It:

The security official should do the following:

- Assign unique user identification to each workforce member.
- Manage and track user identities, especially when new workforce members come on board and when current employees change jobs or names.
- Change passwords according to a timetable based on your risk analysis and policies and procedures. We recommend that passwords contain at least seven alphanumeric characters to make them difficult to decode or guess and that they be changed every 30, 60, or 90 days, depending on outcomes from your practice's risk analysis.

Emergency Access Procedure

Standard	Implementation Specification	Reference
Access control	ii. Emergency access procedure (R)	164.312(a)(2)(ii)

What to Do:

Establish (and implement as needed) procedures for obtaining necessary ePHI during an emergency.

How to Do It:

The security official should do the following:

- Determine types of situations that warrant immediate access to your practice's ePHI.
- Work with your practice's information technology (IT) vendors to establish emergency access procedures to accommodate various situations.[107]
- Coordinate your practice's emergency access procedures with your practice's administrative safeguard contingency plan and physical safeguard contingency operations procedures.
- Document procedures for emergency access, and train workforce members on their use.
- Develop strict alarm procedures, such as audit trails, to avoid abuse of emergency access, and hold users accountable for their actions.

Automatic Log-off

Standard	Implementation Specification	Reference
Access control	iii. Automatic log-off (A)	164.312(a)(2)(iii)

What to Do:

Implement electronic procedures that terminate an electronic session after a predetermined time of inactivity.

How to Do It:

The security official should do the following:

- Activate a password-protected screen saver that automatically prevents unauthorized users from viewing or accessing ePHI on unattended computer workstations
- Establish a timeout period before the log-off capability locks the computer workstation and makes information inaccessible.[108]
- Work with your practice's IT vendors to ensure that all workstations containing ePHI have activated log-off features in place.

Encryption and Decryption

Standard	Implementation Specification	Reference
Access control	iv. Encryption and decryption (A)	164.312(a)(2)(iv)

What to Do:

Implement a mechanism to encrypt and decrypt ePHI.

How to Do It:

This implementation specification focuses on encryption and decryption[109] of data at rest. The security official should ensure that all ePHI at rest in a database is encrypted.

On August 24, 2009, HHS published in the *Federal Register* an interim final rule, "*Breach Notification for Unsecured Protected Health Information.*"[110] Section 13402 of the HITECH Act, part of the American Recovery and Reinvestment Act of 2009 (ARRA) enacted February 17, 2009, required HHS to issue interim final regulations within 180 days to require covered entities under HIPAA and their business associates to provide notification in the case of breaches of unsecured PHI. HHS included in the August 24, 2009, interim final rule an update of guidance that it had earlier published in the *Federal Register* on April 27, 2009,[111] to conform with HITECH Act provisions, which explained the meaning of "unsecured protected health information." The August 24, 2009 guidance, entitled *Guidance Specifying the Technologies and Methodologies That Render Protected Health Information Unusable, Unreadable, or Indecipherable to Unauthorized Individuals,*[112] is reproduced here, with the content relevant to this implementation specification at (a) and (a)(i):

> Protected health information (PHI) is rendered unusable, unreadable, or indecipherable to unauthorized individuals if one or more of the following applies:
>
> (a) Electronic PHI has been encrypted as specified in the HIPAA Security Rule by "the use of an algorithmic process to transform data into a form in which there is a low probability of assigning meaning without use of a confidential process or key"[113] and such confidential process or key that might enable decryption has not been breached. To avoid a breach of the confidential process or key, these decryption tools should be stored on a device or at a location separate from the data they are used to encrypt or decrypt. The encryption processes identified below have been tested by the National Institute of Standards and Technology (NIST) and judged to meet this standard.
>
> (i) Valid encryption processes for data at rest are consistent with NIST Special Publication 800-111, *Guide to Storage Encryption Technologies for End User Devices.*[114]
>
> (ii) Valid encryption processes for data in motion are those which comply, as appropriate, with NIST Special Publications 800-52, *Guidelines for the Selection and Use of Transport Layer Security (TLS) Implementations*; 800-77, *Guide to IPsec VPNs*; or 800-113, *Guide to SSL VPNs*, or others which are Federal Information Processing Standards (FIPS) 140-2 validated.[115]
>
> (b) The media on which the PHI is stored or recorded has been destroyed in one of the following ways:
>
> (i) Paper, film, or other hard copy media have been shredded or destroyed such that the PHI cannot be read or otherwise cannot be reconstructed. Redaction is specifically excluded as a means of data destruction.
>
> (ii) Electronic media have been cleared, purged, or destroyed consistent with NIST Special Publication 800-88, *Guidelines for Media Sanitization,*[116] such that the PHI cannot be retrieved.

We highly recommend that your practice encrypt its ePHI according to the recommendations in this *guidance*, whether that information is *at rest* in a database, or *in motion* over a communications network as discussed in the sections on the transmission security standard and encryption implementation specification below. If your practice uses portable or mobile electronic devices outside the practice that could be misplaced, lost, or stolen, it is essential that you encrypt your data. In your risk analysis, be sure to compare the cost of encrypting your ePHI to make it *secure* with the potential costs to your practice of having *unsecured* ePHI accessible to unauthorized individuals, meeting breach notification requirements, and incurring federal fines.

Audit Controls

Standard	Implementation Specification	References
Audit controls		45 CFR 164.312(b) NIST SP 800-66, pp. 42-43 68 Federal Register 8378

What the Standard Requires

The standard requires that a covered entity or business associate "[i]mplement hardware, software, and/or procedural mechanisms that record and examine activity in information systems that contain or use electronic protected health information."[117]

The implementation specification is contained in the language of the standard and, thus, is required.

Audit controls allow your practice to monitor who is accessing information, when they access it, and what they do with it. Small and large practices are required to have audit controls in place to monitor activity on their electronic systems. They must also review audit control records to ensure all activity is appropriate. This requirement may include reviewing and monitoring log-ons and log-offs, file accesses, updates, edits, system activity, and security incidents. How your practice meets this requirement will be an outcome of your risk analysis.

How to Do It:

To implement this standard, the security official should do the following:

- Define the reason for the audit trail (eg, system troubleshooting, policy enforcement, security incident, etc).
- Determine whether workforce members are accessing information or performing tasks beyond the scope of their job responsibilities.
- Determine whether workforce members are sharing their user IDs. One measure of evidence that a user is sharing his or her ID is that the user is logged on to two or more computer workstations simultaneously.
- Determine if the user is logged on over a period of several days, which indicates that the user does not log off at the end of a work session.[118]
- Maintain and periodically review audit trails[119] or activity logs for critical application systems, including user-written applications.
- Follow up on suspicious entries, such as unauthorized accesses and attempts, and identify and resolve inappropriate activity.

The security official should also do the following:

- Determine if unauthorized users are looking at ePHI. Workforce members may be curious about friends, family members, coworkers, or celebrities. Without authorization, such curiosity may provide proof of a breach of confidentiality.
- Review Internet audit trails. If employees are bored, they may be logging onto inappropriate Web sites and exposing your practice to a potential breach if

unsecured ePHI is intercepted and accessed by an unauthorized individual. Check for evidence of streaming videos, audio files, or other non-business-related programs that slow your network.

- Determine if users are downloading executable files that make your practice liable for software licensing agreement violations.
- Measure the effect of auditing on system performance.

Integrity

Standard	Implementation Specification	References
Integrity	Mechanism to authenticate electronic protected health information (A)	45 CFR 164.312(c)(1) NIST SP 800-66, pp. 44-45 68 Federal Register 8378-8379

What the Standard Requires

The standard requires that a covered entity or business associate "[i]mplement policies and procedures to protect electronic protected health information from improper alteration or destruction."[120]

Integrity is "the property that data or information has not been altered or destroyed in an unauthorized manner."[121] Along with *confidentiality* and *availability*, integrity is one of the three key pillars of the security rule. It means in practice that the right person can access the right information at the right time and that the data are not altered or destroyed in any manner. Inaccurate data could result in harm to or even potential death of a patient.

Access controls and audit trails can keep individuals from breaching confidentiality, but data can become corrupt from several sources: data entry errors, hacking or tampering, mechanical errors in storage devices, transmission error, and poor data integration, such as downloading lab reports into an EHR or other database system. Software or programming bugs, computer viruses, and human error also can cause corruption. A practice must ensure that its ePHI has not been altered without its knowledge and approval.

Mechanism to Authenticate Electronic Protected Health Information

Standard	Implementation Specification	Reference
Integrity	Mechanism to authenticate electronic protected health information (A)	164.312(c)(2)

What to Do:

Implement electronic mechanisms to corroborate that ePHI has not been altered or destroyed in an unauthorized manner.

How to Do It:

The security official should do the following:

- Verify with the practice's IT vendors that the practice's electronic systems have mechanisms to detect unauthorized intrusion and data corruption and to verify data integrity.
- Ensure that the practice's electronic systems, applications, and databases are backed up regularly, with backups tested on a routine schedule.
- Use and review daily audit trails of intrusion detection systems to identify any system hacking attempts.

Person or Entity Authentication

Standard	Implementation Specification	References
Person or entity authentication		45 CFR 164.312(d) NIST SP 800-66, p. 46 68 Federal Register 8379

What the Standard Requires

The standard requires that a covered entity or business associate "[i]mplement procedures to verify that a person or entity seeking access to electronic protected health information is the one claimed."[122]

The implementation specification is contained in the language of the standard and, thus, is required.

This standard requires password management and audit trails that enable your practice to authenticate who is accessing, reading, altering, or transmitting ePHI. A person or entity authentication involves a mechanism such as a username/password query.

The security official should ensure that your practice's electronic systems certify that the user or entity seeking access to the practice's ePHI can provide verification of identity.[123]

Transmission Security

Standard	Implementation Specifications	References
Transmission security	i. Integrity controls (A) ii. Encryption (A)	45 CFR 164.312(e)(1) NIST SP 800-66, p. 47 68 Federal Register 8379

What the Standard Requires

The standard requires that a covered entity or business associate "[i]mplement technical security measures to guard against unauthorized access to electronic protected health information that is being transmitted over an electronic communications network."[124]

Your practice's local network may have no connectivity to any entity outside your practice, but in today's electronic environment this is increasingly rare. Your IT vendors likely have some connection to your network so that they can provide your practice with IT support. Because many practices also are considering going wireless or using mobile devices, such as multifunction personal digital assistants (PDAs) or smart phones, the use of a poorly designed local network or communications over open external networks can threaten your information system, especially if it compromises the availability and integrity of your data.

Today's systems are more secure, but older systems likely contain unused or unnecessary programs that leave your practice exposed to open networks. Ask your practice's IT vendor or an IT consultant to help your practice identify systems that can be replaced or updated to mitigate potential transmission threats.

Integrity Controls

Standard	Implementation Specification	Reference
Transmission security	i. Integrity controls (A)	164.312(e)(2)(i)

What to Do:

Implement security measures to ensure that electronically transmitted ePHI is not improperly modified without detection until it is disposed of.

How to Do It:

The security official should do the following:

- Assign a unique user ID to each workforce member authorized to log onto the practice's information systems, which ensures that entries by those users can be identified and tracked appropriately.
- Make sure that your audit trails track username/password entries so that your information system can track unauthorized changes to electronic records by the person making the changes.
- Apply appropriate sanctions to workforce members if changes to ePHI are made without authorization.

CRITICAL POINT

If someone changed the telephone numbers and addresses in your personal database without your permission, you would question whether the remainder of the information in the database was accurate. Ensuring data integrity means ensuring that ePHI has not been altered or destroyed without appropriate knowledge and approval.

Encryption

Standard	Implementation Specification	Reference
Transmission security	ii. Encryption (A)	164.312(e)(2)(ii)

What to Do:

Implement a mechanism to encrypt ePHI whenever encryption is deemed appropriate.

How to Do It:

This implementation specification focuses on encryption of data in motion. The security official should ensure that all ePHI in motion transmitted from the practice is encrypted. The encryption and decryption implementation specification of the technical safeguard standard on access controls (discussed earlier in this chapter) focuses on preventing a person or entity from deciphering ePHI should the person or entity gain entry to a *database* on an information system without authorization for access. This encryption implementation specification relates to the *movement* of ePHI in transmission over a network.

Encryption is appropriate if the practice is using open networks such as the Internet for transmission of ePHI. Because practices increasingly are using e-mail for communications between physician and patient, adopting EHR systems, and transmitting and receiving ePHI from labs and pharmacies, encryption is a must. Your IT vendor can assist the practice in making sure that all transmissions over open networks are encrypted.

Encryption also is a must for portable and mobile devices—PDAs, smart phones, notebook computers, and tablets—that may be mislaid, lost, or stolen. The practice's Notice of Privacy Practices should address the practice's policy and procedures regarding encryption of ePHI, especially as it relates to physician-to-patient and patient-to-physician e-mail communications.[125]

We recommend that you read carefully the resources listed at (a)(ii) of the guidance quoted above, in the section on the encryption and decryption implementation specification of the technical safeguard Access Control standard, and discuss the encryption options therein with your practice's IT vendor.

ENDNOTES

1. Department of Health and Human Services, Office of the Secretary, "45 CFR Parts 160, 162, and 164: Health Insurance Reform: Security Standards; Final Rule," *Federal Register*, v. 68, n. 34, February 20, 2003, pp. 8333-8381. Citations to this document hereafter are in the standard reference format of 68 *Federal Register* <page(s)> (eg, 68 *Federal Register* 8333). This document is available at http://www.gpo.gov/fdsys/pkg/FR-2003-02-20/pdf/FR-2003-02-20.pdf. Comprehensive information about the HIPAA Security Rule and helpful links also are available at http://www.hhs.gov/ocr/privacy/hipaa/administrative/securityrule/.
2. Small health plans had an additional year to comply by April 21, 2006 (68 *Federal Register* 8334).
3. Department of Health and Human Services, Office of the Secretary, "45 CFR Parts 160 and 164: Modifications to the HIPAA Privacy, Security, Enforcement, and Breach Notification Rules Under the Health Information Technology for Economic and Clinical Health Act and the Genetic Information Nondiscrimination Act; Other Modifications to the HIPAA Rules; Final Rule," *Federal Register*, v. 78, n. 17, January 25, 2013, pp. 5566-5702. Citations to this document hereafter are in the standard reference format of 78 *Federal Register* <page(s)> (eg, 78 *Federal Register* 5566). This document is available at http://www.gpo.gov/fdsys/pkg/FR-2013-01-25/pdf/2013-01073.pdf.
4. 68 *Federal Register* 8343.
5. 68 *Federal Register* 8334.
6. Small health plans had an additional year to comply.
7. 45 CFR 164.530(c)(1).
8. 45 CFR 164.304.
9. 78 *Federal Register* 5589.
10. "The standards do not allow organizations to make their own rules, only their own technology choices." 68 *Federal Register* 8343. As we shall see in the discussion of encryption in the section on technical safeguards later in this chapter, the one exception to technology neutrality is the specification of acceptable encryption technologies to secure ePHI in the August 24, 2009, *Guidance Specifying the Technologies and Methodologies That Render Protected Health Information Unusable, Unreadable, or Indecipherable to Unauthorized Individuals*, pp. 42742-42743 in Department of Health and Human Services, Office of the Secretary, "45 CFR Parts 160 and 164: Breach Notification for Unsecured Protected Health Information; Interim Final Rule," *Federal Register*, v. 74, n. 162, August 24, 2009, pp. 42740-42770. Citations to this document hereafter are in the standard reference format of 74 *Federal Register* <page(s)> (eg, 74 *Federal Register* 42740). This document is available at http://www.gpo.gov/fdsys/pkg/FR-2009-08-24/pdf/E9-20169.pdf. The guidance is also available at http://www.hhs.gov/ocr/privacy/hipaa/administrative/breachnotificationrule/brguidance.html.
11. 45 CFR 164.306(b)(1).
12. 45 CFR 164.306(b)(2).
13. 45 CFR 164.316(b)(1)(ii).
14. "*Workforce* means employees, volunteers, trainees, and other persons whose conduct, in the performance of the work for a covered entity or business associate, is

under the direct control of such covered entity or business associate, whether or not they are paid by the covered entity or business associate." 45 CFR 160.103.

15. 68 *Federal Register* 8376.
16. 68 *Federal Register* 8376-8377; 78 *Federal Register* 5693.
17. 78 *Federal Register* 5589. See Table 2, 78 *Federal Register* 5583. Also visit the Office for Civil Rights (OCR) Web site for examples of resolution agreements and civil money penalties at http://www.hhs.gov/ocr/privacy/hipaa/enforcement/examples/index.html.
18. 68 *Federal Register* 8377.
19. 45 CFR 164.306(e).
20. 78 *Federal Register* 5693. See 68 *Federal Register* 8346-8353 for discussion of administrative safeguards (45 CFR 164.308) in the preamble of the final Security Rule.
21. 78 *Federal Register* 5693. See 68 *Federal Register* 8353-8354 for discussion of physical safeguards (45 CFR 164.310) in the preamble of the final Security Rule.
22. 68 *Federal Register* 8376. See 68 *Federal Register* 8354-8358 for discussion of technical safeguards (45 CFR 164.312) in the preamble of the final Security Rule.
23. See 68 *Federal Register* 8346-8353 for discussion of administrative safeguards (45 CFR 164.308) in the preamble of the final Security Rule.
24. See 68 *Federal Register* 8353-8354 for discussion of physical safeguards (45 CFR 164.310) in the preamble of the final Security Rule.
25. See 68 *Federal Register* 8354-8358 for discussion of technical safeguards (45 CFR 164.312) in the preamble of the final Security Rule.
26. The most up-to-date CFR source is the electronic CFR, which is available at http://www.ecfr.gov.
27. National Institute of Standards and Technology (NIST). *An Introductory Resource Guide for Implementing the Health Insurance Portability and Accountability Act (HIPAA) Security Rule*. Special Publication (SP) 800-66, Revision 1, October 2008. http://csrc.nist.gov/publications/nistpubs/800-66-Rev1/SP-800-66-Revision1.pdf. Accessed February 14, 2013. Page references refer to key activities, sample questions, and a description of activities relevant to each standard. Check the NIST Web site periodically as this document likely will be revised to reflect the January 25, 2013, HITECH Act modifications to the HIPAA Security Rule.
28. 78 *Federal Register* 5694.
29. 78 *Federal Register* 5590-5591.
30. 45 CFR 164.308(a)(1)(i).
31. 68 *Federal Register* 8346.
32. Ibid.
33. See NIST, *Guide for Conducting Risk Assessments*, Special Publication (SP) 800-30 Revision 1, September 2012, which is available at http://csrc.nist.gov/publications/nistpubs/800-30-rev1/sp800_30_r1.pdf.
34. Al Berg, "6 Myths About Security Policies: Leave Your Preconceptions Behind and Write Policies That Work in the Real World," *Information Security*, October 2002, p. 49.

35. NIST. *Guide for Conducting Risk Assessments*. Special Publication (SP) 800-30, Revision 1, September 2012. http://csrc.nist.gov/publications/nistpubs/800-30-rev1/sp800_30_r1.pdf.
36. The general requirements were outlined earlier in this chapter.
37. 45 CFR 164.316(b)(2)(i).
38. 45 CFR 164.308(a)(2).
39. 68 *Federal Register* 8347.
40. 45 CFR 164.308(a)(3)(i).
41. 68 *Federal Register* 8348.
42. Ibid.
43. 68 *Federal Register* 8349.
44. Authorization means "access privileges granted to a user, program, or process or the act of granting those privileges." NIST, *Glossary of Key Information Security Terms*, NIST IR 7298, Revision 1, February 2011.
45. 78 *Federal Register* 5590.
46. 45 CFR 164.308(a)(4)(i).
47. 68 *Federal Register* 8377; 45 CFR 164.308(a)(4)(ii)(B).
48. 78 *Federal Register* 5676.
49. 45 CFR 164.308(b).
50. For additional information, see Office for Civil Rights (OCR), "Business Associate Contract: Sample Business Associate Agreement Provisions," which is available at http://www.hhs.gov/ocr/privacy/hipaa/understanding/coveredentities/contractprov.html, and was published contemporaneously with the modifications to the HIPAA rules on January 25, 2013.
51. For example, does a member of the workforce accompany authorized business associate representatives when they are performing system maintenance? Are such representatives given background checks by the covered entity? Are such representatives' actions with regard to the electronic systems audited or tracked, and are audit logs or tracking reports examined to ensure that such actions conform to your practice's policies and procedures?
52. 45 CFR 164.308(a)(5)(i).
53. Ibid.
54. 45 CFR 164.530(b)(2)(i); 45 CFR 164.530(b)(2)(i)(C).
55. The American Medical Association offers online HIPAA/HITECH Act privacy and security training at http://ama.hipaaschool.com.
56. 68 *Federal Register* 8350.
57. Ibid.
58. An example is the growing use of mobile technologies and portable computers in the medical practice. Such devices with ePHI therein are at a different risk level due to the potential for being mislaid, stolen, or lost if used outside of the practice than stationary workstations in the practice under physical safeguards. Retraining on the use of these devices is critical to avoid the consequences of a breach.
59. Training is a dynamic process. Although the comment in the preamble of the January 16, 2009, final rule pertaining to HIPAA electronic transaction standards

(discussed in Chapter 2) refers to "administrative transactions," it may be instructive in the context of training as well: "HHS does not recognize certification of any systems or software for purposes of HIPAA compliance" (Department of Health and Human Services, Office of the Secretary, "45 CFR Part 162: Health Insurance Reform; Modifications to the Health Insurance Portability and Accountability Act (HIPAA) Electronic Transaction Standards; Final Rule," *Federal Register*, v. 74, n. 11, January 16, 2009, p. 3310). The burden on a covered entity or business associate is to conduct and periodically review its risk assessment, implement policies and procedures to safeguard protected health information, conduct awareness training for all workforce members based on those policies and procedures, update that training if policies and procedures change or HIPAA privacy and security regulations are initiated or modified, and document in writing those activities. Certification, which relates only to a static point in time, is not a requirement in that process.

60. NIST. *Information Security Training Requirements: A Role- and Performance-Based Model*. NIST Special Publication 800-16 Revision 1 (Draft), March 2009, p. 36. http://csrc.nist.gov/publications/drafts/800-16-rev1/Draft-SP800-16-Rev1.pdf.
61. In the discussion of the administrative safeguard contingency plan standard, we recommend that the security official have a sealed envelope of passwords of key workforce members who would be responsible for disaster recovery, along with an emergency password for use in emergency mode operations.
62. 45 CFR 164.308(a)(6)(i).
63. 68 *Federal Register* 8376; 45 CFR 164.304.
64. 68 *Federal Register* 8350.
65. 45 CFR 164.308(a)(7)(i).
66. If you do so, be sure that you encrypt the electronic media to prevent a breach of unsecured ePHI should the electronic media be mislaid, lost, or stolen in transit to a secure location.
67. 68 *Federal Register* 8351.
68. NIST. *Contingency Planning Guide for Federal Information Systems*. Special Publication 800-34 Revision 1, May 2010. http://csrc.nist.gov/publications/nistpubs/800-34-rev1/sp800-34-rev1_errata-Nov11-2010.pdf. See Appendix I: Resources (2 pages) for a list of print and online resources related to contingency and disaster recovery planning.
69. 68 *Federal Register* 8351. Also, "[w]hen the Department of Health and Human Services' Office for Civil Rights will conduct audits of organizations' compliance with the HIPAA security rule, a comprehensive business continuity contingency plan is one of many pieces investigators will be looking for. . . . That means data back-up and disaster recovery plans are required." See J. Goedert, "OCR: We Want to See Contingency Plans," *HDM Breaking News*, May 13, 2010, http://www.healthdatamanagement.com/news/ocr-disaster-recovery-contingency-hipaa-security-40277-1.html. You can check out the OCR Audit Protocol Program at http://www.hhs.gov/ocr/privacy/hipaa/enforcement/audit/protocol.html.
70. 45 CFR 164.308(a)(8).
71. National Institute of Standards and Technology, Computer Security Resource Center. http://www.csrc.nist.gov.
72. URAC. http://www.urac.org.
73. Electronic Healthcare Network Accreditation Commission (EHNAC). http://www.ehnac.org.

74. Workgroup for Electronic Data Interchange (WEDI). http://www.wedi.org. WEDI is charged in the HIPAA legislation and enabling regulations as an adviser to the Secretary of HHS and to the National Committee on Vital and Health Statistics (NCVHS) on matters related to HIPAA administrative simplification.

75. "For purposes of this study, direct costs refer to the direct expense outlay to accomplish a given activity such as hiring a law firm or offering victims identity protection services. Indirect costs are related to the amount of time, effort and other organizational resources spent such as using existing employees to help in the data breach notification efforts or in the investigation of the incident." See Ponemon Institute, *2011 Cost of Data Breach Study: United States*, March 2012, p. 18, which is available at http://www.symantec.com/about/news/resources/press_kits/detail.jsp?pkid=ponemon-cost-of-a-data-breach-2011.

76. "Organizational requirements. (a)(1) *Standard: Business associate contracts or other arrangements.* The contract or other arrangement required by [the *Written contract or other arrangement* implementation specification] § 164.308(b)(3) must meet the requirements of paragraph (a)(2)(i), (a)(2)(ii), or (a)(2)(iii) of this section, as applicable. (2) *Implementation specifications* (Required). (i) *Business associate contracts.* The contract must provide that the business associate will—(A) Comply with the applicable requirements of [the Security Rule]; (B) In accordance with § 164.308(b)(2), ensure that any subcontractors that create, receive, maintain, or transmit electronic protected health information on behalf of the business associate agree to comply with the applicable requirements of [the Security Rule] by entering into a contract or other arrangement that complies with this section; and (C) Report to the covered entity any security incident of which it becomes aware, including breaches of unsecured protected health information as required by [the *Notification by a business associate* standard (164.410) of the Breach Notification Rule]. (ii) *Other arrangements.* The covered entity is in compliance with paragraph (a)(1) of this section if it has another arrangement in place that meets the requirements of [the Privacy Rule *Uses and Disclosures: Organizational requirements—Other arrangements* implementation specification (164.504(e)(3)]. (iii) *Business associate contracts with subcontractors.* The requirements of paragraphs (a)(2)(i) and (a)(2)(ii) of this section apply to the contract or other arrangement between a business associate and a subcontractor required by § 164.308(b)(3) in the same manner as such requirements apply to contracts or other arrangements between a covered entity and business associate." 45 CFR 164.314, at 78 *Federal Register* 5694.

77. "*Subcontractor* means a person to whom a business associate delegates a function, activity, or service, other than in the capacity of a member of the workforce of such business associate." 45 CFR 160.103, at 78 *Federal Register* 5689.

78. See note 76.

79. 78 *Federal Register* 5694.

80. It is important to note that business associates are *not* covered entities. Rather, the HITECH Act and enabling regulations require certain obligations of business associates in the same manner as they are required of covered entities. In contrast, there are examples of covered entities acting in a business associate role, such as a health care clearinghouse processing electronic transactions for a physician practice.

81. "*Person* means a natural person, trust or estate, partnership, corporation, professional association or corporation, or other entity, public or private." 45 CFR 160.103.

82. For information on how the Final Rule modified business associate agreement provisions, see the OCR Web site, published January 25, 2013, titled "Business Associate Contracts: Sample Business Associate Agreement Provisions," at http://www.hhs.gov/ocr/privacy/hipaa/understanding/coveredentities/contractprov.html.
83. 78 *Federal Register* 5590.
84. 78 *Federal Register* 5574.
85. 45 CFR 164.304, at 78 *Federal Register* 5693.
86. 45 CFR 164.310(a)(1).
87. 68 *Federal Register* 8354.
88. 68 *Federal Register* 8353.
89. A home office and electronic system that was not configured for compliance with the Security Rule and Privacy Rule prior to an emergency is not a suitable recovery environment. Consider instead a hot site, from which you could access an exact backup copy of your ePHI and be back in operation in an emergency situation.
90. 45 CFR 164.310(b).
91. 68 *Federal Register* 8376; 45 CFR 164.304.
92. 45 CFR 164.310(c).
93. 68 *Federal Register* 8354.
94. "*Authentication* means the corroboration that a person is the one claimed." 45 CFR 164.304.
95. 45 CFR 164.310(d)(1).
96. 74 *Federal Register* 42742-42743. The guidance is a part of the Breach Notification Interim Final Rule, published August 24, 2009, and is available at http://www.hhs.gov/ocr/privacy/hipaa/administrative/breachnotificationrule/brguidance.html.
97. The NIST document *Guidelines for Media Sanitation*, Special Publication 800-88, Revision 1 (Draft), September 2012, is available at http://csrc.nist.gov/publications/drafts/800-88-rev1/sp800_88_r1_draft.pdf.
98. See note 97.
99. See note 97.
100. 78 *Federal Register* 5647.
101. 68 *Federal Register* 8354.
102. Ibid.
103. 45 CFR 164.304.
104. See C. P. Hartley and E. D. Jones III, *EHR Implementation: A Step-by-Step Guide for the Medical Practice*, 2nd ed., Chicago, IL: American Medical Association, 2012.
105. Electronic prescribing (e-prescribing) was included in the Medicare Modernization Act (MMA) of 2003. The final rule pertaining to formulary and benefit transactions, medication history transactions, and fill status notifications was published in the *Federal Register* on April 7, 2008 (73 *Federal Register* 18917-18942).
106. 45 CFR 164.310(d)(1).
107. For example, you may wish to establish a special user password that allows full access to all ePHI and safeguard the use of that password by creating a special audit log when it is used.
108. Workstations in high-traffic areas should have a timeout of 2 to 3 minutes. Those in protected areas with limited access, such as a laboratory or an isolated office,

may have a longer timeout period, eg, 10 minutes. A log-off requires the user to reenter a password to gain access to data.

109. *Encryption* converts a message in a file or document from a readable format to an unreadable format. *Decryption* does the reverse: it allows an encrypted, or unreadable, message to be converted into a readable format.

110. 74 *Federal Register* 42740. The definition of unsecured PHI at 45 CFR 164.402 was modified in the final rule published January 25, 2013, to read: "Unsecured protected health information means protected health information that is not rendered unusable, unreadable, or indecipherable to unauthorized persons through the use of a technology or methodology specified by the Secretary in the guidance issued under section 13402(h)(2) of Public Law 111-5." 78 *Federal Register* 5695.

111. Department of Health and Human Services, Office of the Secretary, "45 CFR Parts 160 and 164: Guidance Specifying the Technologies and Methodologies That Render Protected Health Information Unusable, Unreadable, or Indecipherable to Unauthorized Individuals for Purposes of the Breach Notification Requirements Under Section 13402 of Title XIII (Health Information Technology for Economic and Clinical Health Act) of the American Recovery and Reinvestment Act of 2009; Request for Information," *Federal Register*, v. 74, n. 79, April 27, 2009, pp. 19006-19010.

112. 74 *Federal Register* 42742-42743.

113. 45 CFR 164.304, definition of "encryption."

114. Available at http://csrc.nist.gov; NIST Roadmap plans include the development of security guidelines for enterprise-level storage devices and such guidelines will be considered in updates to this guidance, when available.

115. Available at http://csrc.nist.gov.

116. Available at http://csrc.nist.gov.

117. 45 CFR 164.312(b).

118. This may not be an issue if your practice has automatic log-off capabilities in place and in force.

119. Failure to regularly review audit trails may mean that a security incident goes undetected for a period of time, which may be construed as willful neglect, which is defined as "conscious, intentional failure or reckless indifference to the obligation to comply with the administrative simplification provision violated." 45 CFR 160.401.

120. 45 CFR 164.312(c)(1).

121. 45 CFR 164.304.

122. 45 CFR 164.312(d).

123. Proof of identity can be authenticated in one of several ways:
    - Something you know (eg, user ID, mother's maiden name, personal ID number such as a national provider identifier, or password)
    - Something you have (eg, smart card, token, swipe card, or badge)
    - Something you are (eg, biometric such as finger image, voice scan, or iris or retina scan)

    See NIST, *Electronic Authentication Guideline*, Special Publication 800-63-1, December 2011, which is available at http://csrc.nist.gov/publications/nistpubs/800-63-1/SP-800-63-1.pdf.

124. 45 CFR 164.312(e)(1).

125. It is a good idea for physician practices to use a secure e-mail server for communicating with patients that is separate from the database server containing ePHI. Once a patient authorizes in writing electronic communications, the practice should issue the patient a username/password for access to the secure e-mail server and a decryption key for reading encrypted files from that server. If the patient requests ePHI from the practice, an encrypted file can be placed on the e-mail server and a message can be sent to the patient to log onto the e-mail server to retrieve the file. Even with encryption, this is the appropriate procedure to follow because the physician is a covered entity with obligations for safeguarding ePHI even though the patient is not subject to those obligations.

chapter 5

HIPAA Communications: Patient Engagement and Social Networking

Oral, written, and electronic communications often say more about how your practice safeguards protected health information (PHI) than your written HIPAA policies and procedures do. When patients and their families visit the practice, they don't ask to see your policies. Instead, they receive a snapshot in time that gives insight into how you safeguard PHI. Your approach to communicating privacy and security using standardized talking points informs patients and visitors that privacy and security are part of your culture and not just a set of rules.

In this chapter, we focus on communication strategies to support how you implement privacy and security regulations, and in doing so, we reference the HIPAA standards discussed in detail in Chapters 3 and 4. Talking points provided here are for demonstration purposes only; your practice's talking points should be coordinated with your HIPAA policies and procedures, your Notice of Privacy Practices, and the recommendations of your privacy and security officials.

What You Will Learn in This Chapter

- What patients want to know about HIPAA
- The value of a communications plan in small and large practices
- The relationship of e-mail, electronic health record (EHR) messaging, and text messaging to patient communications
- Crisis communication management for audits, breaches, and patient complaints
- An overview of social networking, and why it makes good sense for your practice
- Communications and HIPAA training

Key Terms

- Protected health information (PHI)
- Incidental use and disclosure
- Social media
- Social networking

WHAT PATIENTS WANT TO KNOW ABOUT HIPAA

During most patient visits, patients just want to know how soon they will feel better. Inside the exam room, the physician and clinical staff build a level of intimacy and trust enabling the patient to discuss important details about their care, family life, and overall management of a health problem.

Patients also want to make sure their health information is kept in strict confidence. Physician practices tend to be skeptical when a patient's request for confidentiality seems excessive, but there likely is a reason why a patient may seem overprotective about his or her privacy. For example:

- A patient needs an HIV test and wants to pay out of pocket for the test so that the payer doesn't get involved; nor does the patient want the results to get in the hands of the payer.
- A teenager is experimenting with drugs and calls your office for help.
- A man tests positive for hepatitis C and is afraid he will lose his job.
- One of the practice's employees becomes a patient in the practice and wants only those fellow clinical staff involved in the patient's care to access the medical chart.

There are thousands of examples, many of which you have already heard. Patients want to know what you are doing to protect their privacy. They are unlikely to ask whether you lock the doors at night, but no patient wants health details overhead by others. They don't want to hear their PHI has been breached, nor do they want medical records faxed to the wrong location. They likely have already read or seen a story on TV about a doctor or hospital employee losing a laptop, raising the level of computer security awareness.

We, the authors, have been tracking consumer stories and ongoing privacy violations for more than 10 years, so we've heard some pretty outrageous stories. We've learned that privacy ranks highest among consumers' concerns surrounding the transition from paper medical charts to EHR software. The presence of patient portals, electronic gateways that allow patients and physicians to communicate electronically, adds a new dimension to the privacy landscape: the developers of patient portals and personal health records are considered business associates and must comply with the HIPAA Security Rule and Breach Notification Rule.

In this chapter, we provide sample talking points and emphasize the importance of a communications plan to effectively share information with your core audiences. Let's start with some initial talking points you may have already adopted when communicating with patients about HIPAA. Table 5.1 provides a list of patients' frequently asked questions and suggested responses you will want to customize for your practice.

TABLE 5.1

Patients' Frequently Asked Questions

Patient's Question	Possible Response
Can I get a copy of my medical record?	You sure can. Please complete this form (Access Medical Chart) and let us know what you'd like to see.
Please send my medical chart to this specialist.	Referral process: As part of our referral, we will electronically send the provider details about this visit. (In the event the specialist is outside the health system network, the patient may need to pick up X rays, CT [computed tomography] scans, or MRI [magnetic resonance imaging] results and hand deliver them to the specialist.)
Who in this office has seen my medical chart?	That is a question for our privacy official. Would you like to speak with her (him)?
When you moved my records into the computer, several things were entered incorrectly. Can you fix this? And how will I know when it's been corrected?	Did you speak with the doctor about making changes? If not, I can have you talk to our privacy official.
We are moving to another city. Can you give me a copy of my medical chart?	Yes, I can. Please provide additional instructions as there are several ways for us to manage this. 1. We can send your medical chart directly to your new doctor. 2. If you want access to your chart, please fill out this form and let me know what you'd like to have copied. 3. You can sign onto our patient portal, and I will download content from your medical chart into your account.
I just read this Privacy Notice, and I do not want my name on any fund-raiser list.	You would only receive marketing materials from us if you agreed in writing to receive it.
I demand to know why my son/daughter was here.	We follow state and federal laws that dictate when we can release patient information about a minor. Would you like to speak with our privacy official?
Why did you give information about me to the police?	Would you like to speak with our privacy official? (Agents representing the US Department of Health and Human Services [HHS], members of law enforcement, and agents representing the US Department of Transportation are generally exempt from HIPAA if they present legitimate credentials and are engaged in an official investigation seeking medical evidence to effectively investigate a case. The National District Attorneys Association provides additional guidance on HIPAA and law enforcement,[1] and also cross-references all guidance back to the HIPAA Privacy Rule and Security Rule.)
I didn't like the way that billing clerk was talking about me on the phone. Everyone around could hear what she said. I'm going to file a complaint.	You have a right to do that. We hope we can solve the problem before you leave. Would you like to speak with our privacy official?

Privacy complaints such as the one in the last item of Table 5.1 are a part of the health care process. No one likes to receive a complaint, but a compliance training program can help you minimize those complaints. Because of the final rule published in the *Federal Register* on January 25, 2013, referred to as the HIPAA Omnibus Rule,[2] you will need to expand your communications and training program to include new requirements.

IMPLEMENTING AN INTERNAL AND EXTERNAL COMMUNICATIONS PLAN

Whether written into a strategic document, or left open for discussion, your practice has a HIPAA communications plan. In any communication plan, you have internal and external audiences. Internal audiences include your workforce members and board members, whereas external audiences include your patients, referral partners such as hospitals and health care professionals, public health agencies, state and federal departments of health and human services, law enforcement, billing and collections companies, pharmaceutical companies, and business associates.

Updating and managing your HIPAA policies and procedures is a continuous communications and training activity that involves adapting your practice's culture (behavior and actions) to help you meet new HIPAA patient rights discussed in Chapters 3 and 4. The first step in understanding and applying HIPAA is to recognize that it is a lengthy statute filled with standards (what to do) and implementation specifications (how to do it) on how to confidentially manage the patient encounter. General guidelines on how to manage culture and behavioral change are not included in the HIPAA regulations. HIPAA interpretation is an activity that involves interaction among covered entities, business associates, regulators, attorneys, and the courts, but applying HIPAA principles to your practice involves setting policies and then presenting those policies via a communications and training program.

CRITICAL POINT

Talking about patient privacy for a few hours once a year will meet the training requirement, but it won't change anyone's actions unless there is a cohesive training and communication plan with consequences for those who do not adhere to it.

Follow this six-step plan to implement your communications process to standardize the key messages you present to your patients and to the public.

Step 1: Refer to your security risk analysis as a starting point for your communications plan. Get department heads or appointees engaged as risk managers.

- Consider the exposures you documented during the previous year and analyze which ones could be managed better or differently this year.

- Ask staff to point out where privacy issues have occurred in the past. This is not a finger-pointing exercise but an opportunity to identify where exposures are most likely to occur so that you can better manage them moving forward.

Step 2: Identify the core audiences most likely to recognize whether you are communicating your HIPAA policies, and know what they want. Manage your audiences' communications expectations. You can do this by knowing where you might face potential risks and understanding each audience's concerns about HIPAA. Table 5.2 provides an overview of these audiences and what your communications messages mean to them.

TABLE 5.2

Core Audiences and What They Want

Audience	What They Want
Patient	Be treated with respect and confidentiality, and get better.
Family, friends, and personal representatives	Ensure the patient receives respect and is treated with confidentiality; may also serve as the patient's advocate.
Referring physicians	Confidently refer patients to you.
Business associates	Continue to do business with you. (You must ensure they meet HIPAA security and breach notification requirements, effective September 23, 2013.)
Office for Civil Rights	Ensure you have implemented your privacy and security policies and procedures, including training on those policies.
Internal workforce members	Ensure they meet the patient's needs in a trustful and respectful manner.
Public health agencies	Obtain data that will help improve population health.

Step 3: Evaluate your front-office, clinic, and back-office workflows to determine where your privacy and security messages may be put to the test.

- By evaluating the privacy complaints most frequently reported to the Office for Civil Rights (OCR), you can then evaluate where they are most likely to occur. Table 5.3 provides the most frequently investigated privacy issues reported to OCR since 2003.
- Evaluate where these incidents are likely to occur inside your practice, using the examples in Table 5.3 as a starting point.

TABLE 5.3

OCR's Most Frequently Reported Privacy Issues[3]

Compliance Issue	Where in Your Practice These Issues Could Occur[4]
Impermissible uses and disclosures of protected health information (PHI)	Leaving telephone messages with the patient's daughter detailing the patient's medical condition and treatment Providing x-ray results of a sports figure's injury to the media
Lack of safeguards of PHI	Discussing HIV treatment with a patient in the waiting room
Lack of patient access to PHI	Not allowing patient access to the medical record Charging an impermissible records-review fee upon a patient's request to access a copy of the medical record
Uses or disclosures of more than the minimum necessary PHI	Payer sending a patient's entire medical chart to disability insurance without authorization
Lack of administrative safeguards of electronic PHI	Patient in exam room overhearing collections discussion and then recounting the conversation to the person in default of payment

Step 4: Develop levels of accountability.

- The Privacy Rule, Security Rule, and Breach Notification Rule require your practice to identify a contact person to serve as the privacy or security official and manage patient complaints. If your original appointee is no longer with the practice, appoint and train a new one.
- Train a backup privacy and security team that would be able to respond should the privacy official not be available when an incident occurs. Often, practices name risk managers to be part of the risk management team and serve as immediate points of contact if there is an event or question. Ultimately, the privacy official is the party to whom workforce members look for guidance and leadership.

Step 5: Create a no-blame work environment.

The Institute of Medicine's report *To Err Is Human: Building a Safer Health System* fundamentally changed how the health care system assigns blame by shifting from blaming individuals to analyzing processes.[5] "No blame" was initially directed to redesign health care processes, but privacy and security also have benefited, especially as workforce members collaborate to identify a problem and fix it. For example, a physician's laptop was stolen, exposing the practice to a significant amount of work to manage the breach. To counter the problem not just for one but for all physicians in the practice, the EHR system administrator altered network and EHR settings so that PHI could be accessed only through a secure local area network (LAN) and could no longer be downloaded onto a local device.

Step 6: Conquer the fear of conflict, whether it may be with patients, coworkers, or other external audiences.

- Assign risk managers to be the "go-to person" in the event of a question. Risk managers may be department specific or, if you have multiple locations, may be geographically based.
- Provide one-on-one additional training for workforce members who are likely to let an incident go unresolved rather than report the incident.
- Ask reticent workforce members to serve on a HIPAA committee.
- Train all workforce members on new or modified HIPAA requirements.
- Acknowledge the potential for mistakes.
  - No practice will be HIPAA compliant all of the time. People will unintentionally and inadvertently say the wrong thing at the wrong time, or access the wrong patient's chart. Mistakes can be fixed before they become major incidents. If you discover you've made a mistake, tell your privacy official right away so the practice can begin to look for a solution. Mistakes that remain unresolved become incidents. Incidents cost time and money and can damage your credibility, reputation, and business.
  - If someone in your office makes the same mistake several times and doesn't show signs of understanding the privacy or security policy, the employee may need retraining or disciplinary action, such as time off without pay, depending on how your office has structured sanctions in your policies and procedures.
  - If you are unsure of what to do in the event of a mistake, go to the regulations for clarification or call your attorney for legal advice.
- Give your staff fallback talking points. For example, a patient, sales representative, or family member exhibits aggressive behavior and is challenging a HIPAA policy. One fallback talking point could be: "Would you like to speak to our privacy official?"

YOUR HIPAA COMMUNICATIONS PLAN

In Robin Cohn's book, *The PR Crisis Bible*, he writes, "Learn by the mistakes of others—you can't live long enough to make them all yourself."[6] A HIPAA communications plan is a management tool and a change agent that must be continuously in effect and easily understood by all workforce members.

Communications templates and approaches vary, but all include the content found in Table 5.4. If you have been named to your practice's leadership communications team, this section is for you. Your communications plan, at a minimum, should include how to address the following HIPAA requirements, all of which are discussed in Chapter 3:

- Patient rights
- Identity verification
- Content of the practice's Notice of Privacy Practices
- Authorizations
- Requests from local, state, and federal public health or law enforcement officials

What to Do:

Develop an external communications plan.

How to Do It:

- Appoint or recruit an internal communications leadership team. In most cases, this includes the practice administrator, one or more physicians, the director of nursing, and the privacy and security officials. Some proactive practices also include a patient advocate on the communications team. Your risk management team will be an excellent addition to the communications team and can help think through possible scenarios that would require a quick response.
- Determine your communications strategy. You may wish to invite a communications professional to help define and deploy your communications plan. Local public relations societies or communications groups can be valuable resources should you need assistance. Input from patient advisory boards, and a written understanding of your target audiences, can be a preferred starting point.
- As you are building your communications plan, determine common communication goals to set the stage for your practice's culture. Decide on one or two common goals, such as the following:
  - ☐ Preparing everyone on staff to know what to do and say if there are patient inquiries, complaints, privacy breaches, or security incidents.
  - ☐ Creating an environment where everyone feels safe reporting a patient complaint, privacy breach, or security incident.
- A practice's communications plan should include:
  - ☐ The understanding of target audiences and what they want
  - ☐ A plan for outreach, such as via newsletters, Web sites, and/or social networking (discussed later in this chapter)
  - ☐ Patient advisory boards and how they will benefit your practice or clinic
  - ☐ Patient satisfaction surveys, and what you will do with the survey results
  - ☐ Disaster recovery and contingency plans (discussed in Chapter 4)
  - ☐ The Notice of Privacy Practices (discussed in Chapter 3)
  - ☐ Response to audits, credentialing boards, and public health on-site reviews
  - ☐ How the practice will manage internal messages (e-mails that do and do not contain PHI)
- Your communications team also should be aware that HIPAA violations may trigger a response from internal whistleblowers, patients, law enforcement officials, or business associates that casts the practice in an unfavorable light. Manage the conflict internally as best you can, and train workforce members to report possible problems to the privacy official. Provide your workforce members with tools to help conquer the fear of conflict with patients and coworkers.

TABLE 5.4

Sample Communications Template for HIPAA Messages

The first three messages are completed as an example.

Goal	Audience	Message	Threats, Issues	Outcomes
Acknowledge the patient's right to access the medical record.	Patients, their families, or personal representatives	We are happy to help. Please complete this form and let us know what part of your medical chart you would like to access.	Make sure the request is consistent with state law, for example with respect to minors. You also may deny access if you, in your professional opinion, believe access could harm the patient.	Patient understands how you will assist. Manage patient relationship.
Respond to a law enforcement or public health request to access medical chart data, and safeguard protected health information (PHI).	Law enforcement; local, state, or federal health and human services agent	May I see your credentials? Thank you. One moment, I will connect you with our privacy official.	Provide law enforcement with only the information requested.	Document the request and what you provided. Anticipate possible court order for additional information.
Patient wishes to correct PHI that the patient believes is incorrectly entered in the chart.	Patient or family member	The only person who can make that change is your physician. I'd be happy to connect you with our privacy official.	Adoption of electronic health records (EHRs) resulted in many records that needed updating or corrections. Ask medical assistants to check data such as medications during initial intake.	If you are participating in Centers for Medicare and Medicaid Services (CMS) quality incentives, you are providing patients with clinical summaries at each visit. Ask them to verify that the information is correct. Outcome is better patient engagement and communication.
Patient does not want to be contacted at home.				

Continued

TABLE 5.4 (continued)

Sample Communications Template for HIPAA Messages

Goal	Audience	Message	Threats, Issues	Outcomes
Patient believes privacy has been breached and wants to file a complaint with your privacy official.				
A personal representative or family member wishes to be in the exam room with a patient.				

You may choose to complete Table 5.4 for problematic HIPAA requests, and these talking points should be continually reinforced to all workforce members, especially during training and staff meetings. You may also consider developing a quick reference guide for the most common and most frequently misunderstood requests. The following list represents requests likely to create some confusion as a result of the HIPAA Omnibus Rule.

- Parents calling to request that immunization records be sent to a school. The practice must document the request, but parents no longer need to sign an authorization if the school requires immunization records.
- Patients requesting that medical information be withheld from a payer when paying in full and out of pocket for treatment.
- Patients requesting 60 days to complete an accounting of disclosures in an electronic environment. HIPAA Omnibus Rule did not change the timeline to respond to an accounting of disclosures request, which remains at 60 days from the date of request, with a one-time 30-day extension. [164.528 (c)(1)]
- Patients receiving an electronic clinical summary, providing an e-mail address, or signing on to secure patient portals.
- Responding to inquiries about the Genetic Information Nondiscrimination Act (GINA), a rule that applies to payers and not to health care professionals. As discussed in Chapter 3, GINA prevents health plans from requesting genomic information for underwriting purposes.

Electronic Communications and Health IT

Communications plays a vital role when a practice transitions into an electronic environment. An EHR software system is no substitute for people talking to each other, but privacy and security play a major role in workflow redesign.

Just as the business world turned e-mail, software, and mobile devices into tools, so now must physicians treat EHRs, e-mail, and mobile communication devices as tools that, when managed, will enhance the patient-physician relationship.

What to Do:

Establish rules on how you will manage e-mails, EHR messaging, texting, and other issues related to electronic communication and mobile devices.

How to Do It:

- Consistently use encryption. Unless your e-mails are encrypted, they are not secure.
- Create and implement policies and procedures for using e-mail. A practice should include in its policies and procedures how e-mail can and cannot be used. For example, e-mail using Microsoft Outlook may be used for practice-wide announcements or business-related messages. Workforce members must understand that unsecured internal e-mails may not contain any electronic PHI. Clinical information embedded in e-mails not only presents a privacy problem but also is not part of the medical chart; therefore, the physicians' clinical decision making is hampered when information is omitted from the medical chart.
- Use the EHR's messaging component for sending electronic PHI inside the practice. This EHR system feature or module allows the clinical care team involved in the patient's care to securely exchange information within the EHR software.
- Encrypted texting can be an effective way to securely communicate with patients, such as patient reminders. Unencrypted texting also presents a breach situation if the phone is stolen.
- Be aware of the risks of connecting to the Internet via smart phones. Most phones use public hotspots to access messages, exposing information on the phone, including user IDs and passwords, to potential attackers that intercept the information before it reaches the location the physician wanted to access.[7]
- Determine a policy for workforce members who want to bring their own devices to work. Organizations that allow physicians to use smart phones must require the physician to enable security features and also ensure that access to the server does not allow the physician to store information locally on the smart phone. The risk of losing or misplacing a phone is so common that this policy must be put in place.
    - Most smart phones provide a feature to help you establish passwords and patterns to make passwords invisible.
    - Establishing a password is not the same as encrypting the device. Encrypting a smart phone typically takes about an hour, but it is well worth the time and security. Consult any of several online resources for information technology (IT) professionals that provide reviews and discussion of encryption applications. These reviewers are likely to change their opinions of encryption

applications, but they offer insight into current encryption models. Resources include the following:

- TopTenReviews reviews encryption software.[8]
- eSecurityPlanet regularly reviews and posts comments on encryption applications for Android phones.[9] iPhones have a passcode locking feature that also encrypts email messages. The feature is located inside iTunes on your computer. To find a reviews of encryption for mobile devices, consult http://mobile-encryption-software-review.toptenreviews.com.

Physicians who use their phones for e-prescribing or accessing medical charts must ensure that the phone is encrypted. End-to-end encryption encrypts traffic from the physician's phone to the server.[10] Encryption allows the physician using a portable device while away from the practice to access the patient record in a secure manner prior to making a clinical decision.

Develop and Deploy an External Communication Plan

The policies and procedures that the internal communications team develops, approves, educates the workforce on, and delivers will impact how the external audience receives and responds to your message. Use these tips to be sure the message is delivered succinctly but kindly.

What to Do:

Ensure the internal training and communications infrastructure is in place.

How to Do It:

- Build on the internal communication plan by ensuring everyone in the practice knows what's inside the Notice of Privacy Practices.
- Regularly update your business associates list. Regularly communicate your policies and procedures with business associates to ensure theirs are not in conflict with yours. In particular, business associates who are involved in the daily management of PHI must be aware of your expectations and policies. Business associates are now under the direct jurisdiction of the OCR and must comply with the Security Rule and Breach Notification Rule, as well as some portions of the Privacy Rule. See Chapters 3 and 4 for additional guidance on business associates.
- Post signs that indicate you value the patient's safety and confidentiality.
- Decide who will be the spokesperson(s) for the practice. Depending on the situation, it may be the office manager in a business setting or a physician in a public or clinical setting.

Build a Breach Response Plan Before You Need It

If you know a physician who has been involved in a breach, you know that the physician's practice often feels as victimized as the patients whose charts may have been accessed. Stolen laptops, server attacks, or employee theft usually leaves the clinical staff numb from the unexpected assault. The sooner the practice takes the lead on managing the breach, the sooner the practice can get back to normal operations.

CRITICAL POINT

Planning for a breach before it happens is preventive medicine for a potentially hostile environment that could occur in the event of a breach.

What to Do:

Build a breach response plan.

How to Do It:

1. Expect difficulties, but manage internal behavior. Dealing with bad news is an art form. The practice is likely to experience a loss of productivity, face a period of organizational instability, and question workforce members' adherence to policies and documentation requirements. Leaders must immediately determine the extent of damage to customers, including patients and the physician community.
   a. Get as many details as possible on the first day you are informed of the breach. Information about what happened will be fresh and will enable you to begin to build a response plan. Specific details gathered should include:
      i. What happened
      ii. Date of the breach and date of discovery of the breach
      iii. A description of the types of unsecured PHI involved in the breach, such as name, Social Security numbers, address, account numbers, diagnosis, disability codes
   b. Write down the details and require the person reporting the breach to acknowledge your notes with a signature, but also allow the workforce member to add details as he or she remembers them.
   c. If the breach involves stolen property, you will likely need to report the incident to local law enforcement authorities.
2. Predetermine your core team of advisers. Include the following in your breach response plan, if they are not already part of your core team of advisers:
   a. Practice administrator
   b. Legal counsel
   c. Insurance agent
   d. Privacy and security officials
   e. Technology officer or system administrator
   f. Practice owners
3. Convene the team of advisers and ask them to help determine:
   a. Whether there was a breach; and
   b. Whether there is a "low probability" that PHI was compromised. The HIPAA Omnibus Rule clarified processes for determining damage resulting from a breach.[11] Consult Chapter 1 on breach notification or the HIPAA Omnibus Rule. The best course of action is to present the facts to the core team and ask them to collectively determine and document the events that occurred. The number of previous incidents will be a significant factor in determining regulatory activities, sanctions, and next steps. The OCR Web site[12] provides expanded guidance on the definition of a breach and instructions for covered entities to report a breach. Remember, covered entities and business associates have the burden of

proof to demonstrate that all required notifications have been provided or that a use or disclosure of unsecured PHI did not constitute a breach.[13] The physician office must provide notice to all persons affected by the breach within 60 calendar days after discovery of the breach.

4. After the core team of advisors determines whether PHI was compromised, consider the content of notification, as defined in the Breach Notification Rule,[14] as an outline for your next steps. Table 5.5 provides guidance on decisions you will make when developing this letter. Figure 5.1 provides a timeline for managing the breach.

TABLE 5.5

Decisions to Make When Developing Content for the Notification Letter

Content	Decisions to Make	Who Makes the Decisions?
Dear Patient	Which patients were affected?	System administrator
	Patient contact information	Practice administrator
	Patient or personal representative	Practice administrator
This is what happened	Date of discovery	Privacy official or practice administrator
	What was stolen (or hacked), and what protected health information (PHI) was involved?	Practice administrator System administrator
	How many records were affected?	System administrator
Safeguards already in place	What policies are currently in place?	Privacy or security official
	Did individual violate policy?	Lawyer, practice administrator
	Sanctions	Lawyer, practice administrator
	Document actions taken	Privacy official, lawyer, practice administrator
	Additional risk management (was this an unexpected risk?)	Privacy or security officials, practice administrator
How individuals should protect themselves	Research medical identity theft processes	Privacy or security official, insurance agent, lawyer
	How will we respond to unhappy patients?	Practice administrator
What we are doing	Identify all affected individuals	System administrator
	Arrange professional identity theft monitoring, including establishing an account	Practice administrator, lawyer, and/or insurance agent
	Manage any incidents that arise from stolen records	System administrator
	Establish hotline—who takes calls? Trained in what to say?	Practice administrator

FIGURE 5.1

Breach Notification Timeline

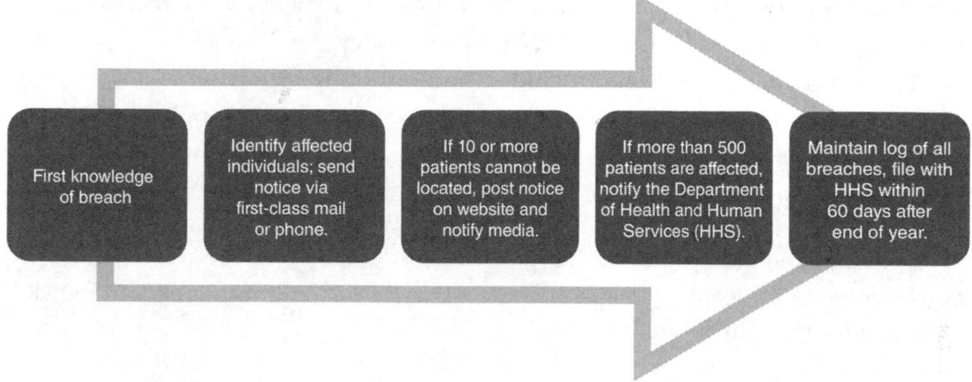
First knowledge of breach
Identify affected individuals; send notice via first-class mail or phone.
If 10 or more patients cannot be located, post notice on website and notify media.
If more than 500 patients are affected, notify the Department of Health and Human Services (HHS).
Maintain log of all breaches, file with HHS within 60 days after end of year.

Source: http://www.hhs.gov/ocr/privacy/hipaa/administrative/breachnotificationrule/index.html.

Managing an Audit from OCR

The Office for Civil Rights (OCR) enforces the Privacy Rule, Security Rule, and Breach Notification Rules in several ways:[15]

- As required by the HITECH Act, the Department of Health and Human Service (HHS) requires OCR to conduct periodic audits of covered entities and business associates to ensure compliance with the HIPAA Privacy Rule, Security Rule, and Breach Notification Rule.[16] The audit protocol is organized by privacy, security, and breach notification. At its discretion, the OCR may vary the combinations of these reviews. For example, OCR may ask to see the following:
  - ☐ The Notice of Privacy Practices
  - ☐ The practice's policy allowing patients to access their patient rights
  - ☐ Your training calendar and list of attendees
  - ☐ How you use and disclose PHI
  - ☐ Your encryption policy[17]
- One of the more common reasons for an audit is a patient complaint. In this case, a call from OCR is focused on the specifics embedded in the patient complaint. When OCR follows up on a patient request, a phone call and/or a letter will initiate the conversation. OCR does not send an e-mail to initiate the conversation, though it is likely the investigator will ask you to send documentation electronically (via e-mail) to the investigator.
- In the event of an audit following a patient complaint, OCR carefully reviews the complaint before determining whether to take action on the complaints. See Appendix C to learn more about the documentation an investigator will request. In most cases, the investigator will ask for the following:

- ☐ Your policy and procedure on managing PHI. For example, if a patient complains that he or she was denied access to the medical chart, the OCR investigator may request your policy on this patient right and the procedures your practice deploys to provide patients with access.
- ☐ Documentation that you followed your policy
- ☐ Documentation that you included training on this policy
- ☐ A list of attendees who participated in training on this topic
- ☐ What you have done (or are doing) to remediate this complaint
- ☐ What corrective action, if any, you implemented so that this complaint will not happen again. The corrective action should consistently follow your sanctions policy for all persons.

- If evidence indicates that the covered entity is not in compliance, the OCR will attempt to resolve the case.[18]

CRITICAL POINT

OCR does *not* want to see all of your policies and procedures, and you should not send all of them. Send only the policy referenced in the complaint.

Audit Prevention Strategies

One of the most effective messages you can convey to your workforce members is to listen when a patient says he or she believes the privacy of PHI has been violated. Both OCR and your practice's owners want you to manage the complaint internally using your own mitigation strategies and corrective action plan. Keep the following three quick responses on hand in the event an individual complains in person or by phone about a privacy issue.

- I am glad you brought this (event, situation, etc) to my attention. Please give me a moment to get our privacy official so that you can explain the situation to her (him).
- Do you mind if I take notes about this complaint? I'd like to be sure I get this down as accurately as possible. Our privacy official may want to follow up with you on this.
- This is a matter for our privacy official. Please wait a moment, and I will get him (her) for you.

When an individual believes his or her privacy has been violated, the first person to hear the complaint must also ensure the patient feels as though someone is listening. Often, we hear of patient complaints that could have been better managed if someone in the practice had not said the following:

- That's really not my problem.
- We are all busy right now. Please call our privacy official in the morning.
- That happens a lot around here. It's no big deal. Just let it go. This is a great practice.
- We don't have a privacy official. Privacy is managed by the hospital administrators.

What to Do:

Establish an initial response procedure for patient complaints.

How to Do It:

- Use the Patient Complaint form (see sample in Appendix A) or a blank piece of paper and write down the patient's comments. Or, ask the patient to tell you the reason for the complaint, and then ask the patient to complete the Patient Complaint form.
- Be sure to get the patient's signature and date on the bottom of the complaint.
- Follow up with the patient and let the individual know that you have taken steps to remediate the situation, and thank the patient for bringing the complaint to your attention.

Despite your practice's policy to listen to a complaint, the individual may still file a complaint with OCR. See Appendix C for information on what OCR considers during intake and review of a complaint.

PATIENT ENGAGEMENT

Physicians have always demonstrated patient engagement strategies by inviting patients into their offices, listening to their health needs, responding to on-call emergencies, and attempting to offer the highest clinical and ethical services to the patient and family.

Patient or consumer engagement is not at all a new concept, but combining it with health IT raises the bar on the definition. A definition of patient engagement by *Healthcare IT News* offers the following:

> Patient engagement refers to ongoing and constructive dialogue between patient and practitioner. Within the scope of healthcare IT, patient engagement is driven by technology ranging from patient portals, which enable patients to view test results and records online and communicate with doctors, to electronic data capturing platforms that result in more accurate and streamlined diagnostic information. A high emphasis has been placed on patient engagement in Stage 2 meaningful use.[19]

Patient engagement in health IT may include:

- Virtual computer-based video patient-physician office visits, or telemedicine
- Smart phone photos of wounds sent to a physician supporting patients with diabetes
- Patients requesting the medical chart be downloaded onto a handheld device
- A kiosk at the practice's entrance allowing patients to scan a card that identifies the patient, updates demographics, accepts co-pays, acknowledges payer information, and in some cases provides a quick reason for the visit
- Concierge services for patients desiring more focused attention from physicians and paying only with out-of-pocket funds
- Patients carrying an electronic copy of a CT scan to a specialist for consult and treatment

Patient engagement heightens the awareness patients have for the privacy and security of confidential health information. Since 2003, HIPAA has provided protections for individually identifiable health information, but mobile applications, or "apps," make it easier now for patients to be better informed about their health care.

In 2013, the Office of the National Coordinator for Health Information Technology launched two programs intended to motivate patients and consumers to become more actively engaged in their health care by creating health IT as another avenue for communicating with the patients. *Patient engagement* focuses on tools, key messages, and the use of physician-patient interaction both inside and outside the practice that further engages the patient in care management. *Consumer engagement policies and messaging* describes the benefits of health IT to consumers and presents a case for how health IT will reduce paperwork, get information accurately to physicians, coordinate care, and promote patient safety.[20]

To encourage patient engagement, health care professionals that participate in CMS incentive programs, such as the incentive program for meaningful use of certified EHR software,[21] must demonstrate how they extract information from the patient visit into a clinical summary.

Several HIPAA requirements overlap with the meaningful use incentives, the majority of which are discussed in the privacy and security risk management strategies provided in Chapters 3 and 4. For example:

- When providing patients with a clinical summary, normally completed before the patient leaves the practice, covered entities must match the summary with the correct patient.
- When uploading patient demographics into a patient portal, covered entities must ensure that the patient summary goes to the correct patient record.
- When building an interface between two entities, such as labs and the EHR, ample testing must ensure that the correct patient record is matched to the correct lab result.

One exciting, but cautionary, aspect of patient engagement is that consumers may begin to assume privacy and security are commonplace, especially as social networking sites, such as LinkedIn, Facebook, Twitter, YouTube, Google+, Meetup, Ning, Pinterest, and so forth, become part of the health care experience. The following section addresses privacy and security concerns related to social networking.

Social Networking

An online search for a definition of *social media*, also called social networking, generated more than 50 definitions, many of them captured in the Social Media Guide.[22] All definitions include words such as *content shared online*, *communication*, *promote engagement and response*, and *group thinking*, but the most powerful word is *instant*. When used in combination with health information, social media may be helpful or dangerous.

Physicians and their office staff are securely "texting health messages to patients, tracking disease trends on Twitter, identifying medical problems on Facebook pages and communicating with patients through email. . . . Many doctors still cling to pen and paper, and are most comfortable using e-technology to communicate with each other—not with patients."[23] While most doctors still prefer written communications managed by pen or computer and sent via the US postal service, some of the nation's top clinics realize patients want more interaction than the 15-minute appointment offers.

"Social media makes it easier than ever for patients and physicians to connect outside the exam room," writes Angela Haupt in a US News.com health article titled "How Doctors Are Using Social Media to Connect with Patients."[24] "And while most of the attention has centered on hospitals' efforts, which are often driven by marketing and have relatively large budgets, primary care and other private-practice doctors are building an online presence."[25] TwitterDoctors.net, for example, is a site where patients can learn whether their physician is on Twitter and can choose to follow, or subscribe to, their physician's "Tweets." (A Tweet is a very short message posted by a person with a Twitter account.)

Kevin Pho, a physician and popular medical blogger, engages his patients via Facebook and Twitter.[26] He cautions that patients should be skeptical of health information that is posted without linking the advice to a reputable physician. In his book, *Establishing, Managing, and Protecting Your Online Reputation: A Social Media Guide for Physicians and Medical Practices*, coauthored by Susan Gay,[27] Pho provides guidance on how to connect with the new generation of patients. Each week, his content development team, along with Pho supervising the content, subscribes to several online news feeds and accepts blog postings for his Web site from other physicians. They select 15 to 25 articles and post them with hyperlinks to the publication in subscriber e-mails and on Twitter and Facebook.

Glen Stream, a family physician and 2013 president of the American Academy of Family Physicians, uses Facebook to post reminders to patients about the Great American Smokeout and information about medical conferences and sessions he attends.[28]

Social media is not without its challenges, especially when it comes to patient engagement and protecting patient confidentiality. Once a message is posted online, it can remain unnoticed, or spread among closely linked communities and, within a day, become "viral" or so widely distributed that it becomes difficult to track.

For physicians, social media needs to be intentional, and much more strategic than opening a Facebook, Twitter, or LinkedIn account and beginning to post, though the creators of these sites have made it easy to do just that. Reputation management, confidentiality, and instant messaging can have long-range consequences for physicians giving medical advice over the Internet. Physician Adriana Tobar, in a blog post at KevinMD.com that is also available at the AMA Web site, recounts why medical students need to keep a clean profile: "Anything you say or do may end up on social media," she writes, recounting how one medical student's behavior at a party ended up on social media, and therefore discoverable during a future employer's background search.[29]

HIPAA and Social Media

"Social Media and HIPAA Are Not Enemies" is the topic of a webinar hosted by Mayo Clinic's Social Media Health Network.[30] The title sets the tone for how physicians should broadly approach social media, but HIPAA requirements, along with common sense, prevail when it comes to posting content that is freely accessed by the public.

Examples of unlawful posts include:

- Asking a patient for a date after seeing his or her profile on Facebook
- Posting a patient's photo on Facebook because it was "cute," without written authorization
- Posting frustrating details of a patient visit
- Posting videos of accident victims on YouTube
- Providing medical advice to a patient via Twitter

Examples of helpful posts include:

- Top news stories quoting trusted medical resources
- Tips on dealing with weight loss, strength training, or a medical condition such as depression, if the information is not targeted to a specific patient and is available to the public
- Links to disease-specific advocacy groups

What to Do:

Establish policies and procedures that govern how workforce members are allowed to post comments on networks such as YouTube, LinkedIn, Plaxo, Facebook, or Twitter.

How to Do It:

- Refer to your security risk analysis to determine potential exposures from social networking.
- Develop policies and procedures that govern how you and your workforce members using your practice's infrastructure will approach social networking. A sample list of considerations is shown in Table 5.6.

TABLE 5.6

Considerations Regarding Your Practice's Social Networking Policies

Issue	Our Practice's Position: *Yes, Yes with conditions,* or *No.*	Risk Managers: Who Is Assigned to Manage Social Networking and Suggested Policies?
Should the practice engage in social networking activities?	Yes, but only after we consider potential risks and benefits	Person hired to manage social networking should report directly to privacy and security officials.
Web site management	If possible, this is a great way to launch social networking, post educational materials, provide forms to patients, and in general engage patients.	Practice administrator, with help from privacy and security officials
Editorial control of content	Determine who may post, and who may not.	Privacy official will regularly monitor social media use.
Security of social networking sites	Include in risk assessment	Security official
Doctors may have a separate account outside of the practice	Yes, with conditions	Privacy official will regularly monitor social networking sites of employees.
Use of personal social networking sites	Determine whether and how the practice will have governance over these.	Practice administrator

If you plan to begin your social media efforts with a practice Web site, determine why you want customers to go to your site. Possible uses of the Web site include the following:

- Post updated Notice of Privacy Practices in English and Spanish.
- Allow patients to request an appointment.
- Post results from patient satisfaction surveys.
- Post referral forms so that patients and physicians can refer you.
- Provide patient educational materials. These often are offered by an outside source, such as the American Medical Association (AMA), medical specialty organizations, Krames StayWell, or WebMD.
- Provide forms to patients before they arrive for new patient interviews.
- Enable patients to connect to the patient portal.
- Allow patients to make payments online.
- Post an educational training video.
- Wish patients a happy holiday.
- Post informal or candid pictures of your workforce "being human"—but obtain permission if patients appear in any of the photos.
- Remind patients of an upcoming event, such as bringing on a new physician or opening a new office.

- Encourage health care professionals to submit an article or blog.
- Inform patients of Web sites for disease-specific advocacy groups.
- Inform patients about sudden cancellations resulting in an opening in the schedule.

Begin by building policies and procedures about how the Web site will be accessed and used.

WHAT'S NEXT?

In the appendices, you will find resources to help you comply with the HIPAA Omnibus Rule, train your audience, and search for clarification.

ENDNOTES

1. Alexandra Podrid, "HIPAA—Exceptions Providing Law Enforcement Officials and Social Service Providers Access to Protected Health Information," *Update* (National District Attorneys Association), v. 16, n. 4, 2003, http://www.ndaa.org/ncpca_update_v16_no4.html. Accessed April 12, 2013.
2. Department of Health and Human Services, Office of the Secretary, "45 CFR Parts 160 and 164: Modifications to the HIPAA Privacy, Security, Enforcement, and Breach Notification Rules Under the Health Information Technology for Economic and Clinical Health Act and the Genetic Information Nondiscrimination Act; Other Modifications to the HIPAA Rules; Final Rule," *Federal Register*, v. 78, n. 17, January 25, 2013, pp. 5566-5702. This document is available at http://www.gpo.gov/fdsys/pkg/FR-2013-01-25/pdf/2013-01073.pdf.
3. Office for Civil Rights, "Health Information Privacy: Enforcement Highlights," http://www.hhs.gov/ocr/privacy/hipaa/enforcement/highlights/index.html. Accessed May 7, 2013.
4. Office for Civil Rights, "Health Information Privacy: All Case Examples," http://www.hhs.gov/ocr/privacy/hipaa/enforcement/examples/allcases.html. Accessed May 7, 2013.
5. Institute of Medicine. *To Err Is Human: Building a Safer Health System*. Washington, DC: National Academy Press, 2000.
6. Robin Cohn. *The PR Crisis Bible: How to Take Charge of the Media When All Hell Breaks Loose*. New York: St. Martin's Press, 2000, p. 154.
7. "Security Issues With Smart Phones," Business Security Information, December 8, 2009, http://www.businesssecurityinformation.com/2009/12/security-issues-smartphones/. Accessed April 18, 2013.
8. TopTenReviews is available at http://encryption-software-review.toptenreviews.com/. Accessed April 20, 2013.
9. "Top 20 Android Security Apps," eSecurityPlanet, June 28, 2012, http://www.esecurityplanet.com/views/article.php/3901686/Top-20-Android-Security-Apps.htm. Accessed April 20, 2013.
10. "Security Issues With Smart Phones."
11. Ed Jones, "HIPAA Final Rule: Enforcement–Factors for Determining Civil Money Penalties for HIPAA Violations," HIPAA.com, February 25, 2013. http://www.hipaa.com/2013/02/hipaa-final-rule-enforcement-factors-for-determining-civil-money-penalties-for-hipaa-violations/. This article states:

    Today, we examine factors considered in determining the amount of a civil money penalty for a HIPAA violation that are modified in the Final Rule: *Modifications to the HIPAA Privacy, Security, Enforcement, and Breach Notification Rules Under the Health Information Technology for Economic and Clinical Health Act [HITECH Act] and the Genetic Information Nondiscrimination Act; Other Modifications of the HIPAA Rules*, which was published in the Federal Register on January 25, 2013. The effective date of the Final Rule is March 26, 2013, and covered entities and business associates must comply by September 23, 2013.

The Department of Health and Human Services (HHS) identified "five general factors" for modification of 45 CFR 160.408 in conformance with the HITECH Act:

- Nature and extent of the violation
- Nature and extent of the harm resulting from a violation
- History of prior compliance with the administrative simplification provision, including violations by the covered entity or business associate
- Financial condition of the covered entity or business associate
- Such other matters as justice may require.

Within each of the five general categories, HHS identified "specific factors" for consideration, the information relating to which would be collected and compiled during an investigation. As we pointed out in our enforcement posting last week, the modified 45 CFR 160.306, at 78 *Federal Register* 5690, provides for:

(c) *Investigation.*

(1) The Secretary will investigate any complaint filed under this section when a preliminary review of the facts indicates a possible violation due to willful neglect.

(2) The Secretary may investigate any other complaint filed under this section.

(3) An investigation under this section may include a review of the pertinent policies, procedures, or practices of the covered entity or business associate and of the circumstances regarding any alleged violation.

(4) At the time of the initial written communication with the covered entity or business associate about the complaint, the Secretary will describe the acts and/or omissions that are the basis of the complaint.

Here is the modified 45 CFR 160.408, at 78 *Federal Register* 5691, that outlines the five general factors and specific factors within each of the five:

Factors considered in determining the amount of a civil money penalty.

In determining the amount of any civil money penalty, the Secretary will consider the following factors, which may be mitigating or aggravating as appropriate:

(a) The nature and extent of the violation, consideration of which may include but is not limited to:

(1) The number of individuals affected; and

(2) The time period during which the violation occurred;

(b) The nature and extent of the harm resulting from the violation, consideration of which may include but is not limited to:

(1) Whether the violation caused physical harm;

(2) Whether the violation resulted in financial harm;

(3) Whether the violation resulted in harm to an individual's reputation; and

(4) Whether the violation hindered an individual's ability to obtain health care;

(c) The history of prior compliance with the administrative simplification provisions, including violations, by the covered entity or business associate, consideration of which may include but is not limited to:

(1) Whether the current violation is the same or similar to previous indications of noncompliance;

(2) Whether and to what extent the covered entity or business associate has attempted to correct previous indications of noncompliance;

(3) How the covered entity or business associate has responded to technical assistance from the Secretary provided in the context of a compliance effort; and

(4) How the covered entity or business associate has responded to prior complaints

(d) The financial condition of the covered entity or business associate, consideration of which may include but is not limited to:

(1) Whether the covered entity or business associate had financial difficulties that affected its ability to comply;

(2) Whether the imposition of a civil money penalty would jeopardize the ability of the covered entity or business associate to continue to provide, or to pay for, health care; and

(3) The size of the covered entity or business associate

(e) Such other matters as justice may require.

We recommend that you visit three of the sites that the Office for Civil Rights (OCR) maintains regarding enforcement: *Enforcement Process* [http://www.hhs.gov/ocr/privacy/hipaa/enforcement/process/index.html], *Case Examples and Resolution Agreements* [http://www.hhs.gov/ocr/privacy/hipaa/enforcement/examples/index.html], and *HIPAA Privacy & Security Audit Program* [http://www.hhs.gov/ocr/privacy/hipaa/enforcement/audit/index.html]. OCR is HHS' enforcement arm for HIPAA Privacy and Security Rules and the HITECH Act Breach Notification Rule. Each of these sites provides information on the enforcement process and examples of the type of information OCR seeks during an investigation to address the general and specific factors identified in 45 CFR 160.408 above, as modified and effective March 26, 2013.

12. Information on the Breach Notification Rule with guidance from the OCR is available at http://www.hhs.gov/ocr/privacy/hipaa/administrative/breachnotificationrule/index.html. Accessed April 23, 2013.

13. Ibid.

14. Breach Notification Rule, 45 CFR 164.404(c) and 164.530(j).

15. 45 CFR 160 and 164, Subparts A, C, and E.

16. As a result of pilot audit programs, OCR established a protocol for completing audits. The protocol is available at http://www.hhs.gov/ocr/privacy/hipaa/enforcement/audit/protocol.html.

17. These are a sampling of requests and do not represent any pattern of requests.

18. OCR, "Health Information Privacy: How OCR Enforces the HIPAA Privacy Rule," http://www.hhs.gov/ocr/privacy/hipaa/enforcement/process/howocrenforces.html. Accessed April 23, 2013.

19. "Healthcare IT News Index: Patient Engagement," Healthcare IT News, http://www.healthcareitnews.com/directory/patient-engagement. Updated March 28, 2013. Accessed May 30, 2013.

20. "Information Technology in Health Care: The Next Consumer Revolution," http://www.healthit.gov/policy-researchers-implementers/consumerpatient-engagement-power-team. Accessed May 7, 2013.

21. See Centers for Medicare and Medicaid Services (CMS), "EHR Incentive Programs," at http://www.kevinmd.com/blog/2013/01/online-reputation-doctors-comprehensive-social-media-guide.html.

22. http://thesocialmediaguide.com/social_media/50-definitions-of-social-media.

23. Lindsey Tanner, "Doctors Use Facebook, Twitter, Email to Connect With Patients," Associated Press and *Columbia Missourian*, June 10, 2012.

24. Angela Haupt, "How Doctors Are Using Social Media to Connect With Patients," *U.S. News and World Report*, November 11, 2011, http://health.usnews.com/health-news/most-connected-hospitals/articles/2011/11/21/how-doctors-are-using-social-media-to-connect-with-patients. Accessed May 14, 2013.

25. Ibid.

26. Ibid.

27. Pho, Kevin, and Susan Gay. *Establishing, Managing, and Protecting Your Online Reputation: A Social Media Guide for Physicians and Medical Practices*. Phoenix, MD: Greenbranch Publishing, 2013.

28. Haupt, "How Doctors Are Using Social Media."

29. "Medical Residents: Tips to Keep a Clean Social Media Profile," http://www.kevinmd.com/blog/2012/11/medical-residents-tips-clean-social-media-profile.html. Accessed June 20, 2013.

30. Mayo Clinic Social Media Health Network, "Webinar—Social Media and HIPAA Are NOT Enemies," May 25, 2011, http://network.socialmedia.mayoclinic.org/2011/05/25/webinar-social-media-and-hipaa-are-not-enemies-2/. Accessed May 31, 2013.

appendix A

HIPAA Forms

Table of Contents

Business Associate Agreements Tracking Form

Business Associate	**Contact Info**	**Signed Prior BA Agreement**	**Needs New BA Agreement**	**Status**
Company	Contact name, address, e-mail, phone number	Yes/No	Yes/No	**C**=completed **R**=in review **NB**=no longer in business

Privacy Official Job Responsibilities

General duties: Be the advocate that maintains the privacy of patients' protected health information (PHI) and oversee activities that keep our practice in compliance with rules that govern the privacy of protected health information in oral, written, and electronic form.

Specific duties: The privacy official has the following specific duties:

Management Advisor

Work with the medical practice's management team and lawyers to comply with federal and state laws governing the privacy of individually-identifiable health information. Stay current on privacy laws and updates in privacy technology. Immediately notify medical management of requested investigations and reviews by HHS or other governing agency.

Human Resources and Training

Develop, or serve as team leader in the development of, the practice's privacy policies and procedures. Integrate those policies into the practice's day-to-day activities and provide training, either as on-the-spot refresher courses or planned courses. Oversee sanctions according to our policies and procedures and bring them to the attention of the practice's leadership committee.

Risk Management

Collaborate with the security official to ensure privacy and security risks are analyzed and policies and procedures are developed, updated, and enforced to prevent unauthorized disclosures of PHI.

Business Associates

Lead the practice in updating business associate contracts and, with our lawyers, developing and executing business associate agreements in accordance with the HITECH, HIPAA, and Breach Notification Rules.

Patient Rights

Oversee patient requests to the practice and help the practice's employees understand how to address patient questions about the practice's privacy initiatives. Develop an effective internal and external communications effort to help patients and workforce understand how the practice protects patient rights.

Complaint Management

Implement and manage complaints regarding the practice's standards and protocols, including documenting and investigating and, if necessary, mitigating those complaints. Educate workforce on the practice's policies and procedures on complaints and prohibited retaliatory actions against individuals who exercise their patient rights.

Qualifications

Be familiar with medical and administrative functions of the practice. Have excellent communication, problem solving, and research skills. Have an interest in privacy laws and regulations; be recognized as having high integrity and detail oriented. Have strong organizational skills and work well with management and staff.

Workforce Training Session Attendee List

Name of Trainer: ______________________________

Trainer's Company Affiliation: ______________________________

Date of Training: ______________ Hours in Training: ______________

Topics Included in Training (or attach outline): ______________________________

____

____

Attendee List

Print Name	Signature	Date

Notice of Privacy Practices Receipt

Our Notice of Privacy Practices (NPP) provides information on how our practice may use and/or disclose protected health information about you for treatment, payment, and health care operations. A copy of our NPP can be found at http:///www.______________________________ and at the check-in desk.

I acknowledge that I have received a copy of

____ Notice of Privacy Practices.
(NAME OF PRACTICE)

Patient's Name: ____
(PRINT)

Patient's Signature: ____
(SIGNATURE)

Today's Date: ____

Patient's Date of Birth: ____

If signed by a personal representative:

Name of Personal Representative: ____
(PRINT)

Signature of Personal Representative: ____
(SIGNATURE)

Relationship to Patient: ____

Driver's License Number: ____________________________________ State: ________________

Today's Date: ____

\- -

For practice use only:

Patient's ID/Chart Number: ____

Signature of Employee: __________________________________ **Date:** ________________

Sample Authorization Form

Patient's Name: ______________________________

Patient's Date of Birth: ____________ Patient's ID/Chart No: ____________

I hereby authorize the use and disclosure of individually-identifiable health information relating to me as described below:

Specific Description of Information to be Used or Disclosed

Purpose for Disclosure

____

____

____

I authorize the following person(s) to use or disclose the above health information.

____

____

Person(s) receiving my authorized information include:

____

____

____

Check all that apply:

☐ I understand that I may revoke this authorization at any time by notifying ____________ ______________________ (Name of Practice) in writing. If I choose to do so, my revocation will not affect any actions taken by ____________ (Name of Practice) before receiving my revocation.

☐ I understand that I may refuse to sign this authorization; and that my refusal to sign in no way affects my treatment, payment, enrollment in a health plan, or eligibility for benefits.

This authorization expires on ______________________________.

Signature of Patient or Patient's Personal Representative

____

Date: ______________________________

If personal representative, print:

Name: ______________________________

Signature: ______________________________

Relationship to Patient: ______________________________

Driver's License Number: ______________________ State: ____________

For internal use only

Patient Chart/ID Number: ______________

Date: ______________ Physician: ________________________

Sample Verification Form/Patient Certification

Please provide us with the following information.

General Information

Name: ____

Address: ____

City: ______________________ State: __________ Zip: __________

Date of Birth: ____________________ SS#: ____________________

Driver's License Number: ______________________ State: __________

Insurance Information

Name of Subscriber: ____________________________________

Relationship to Subscriber: ______________________________

Group No: ________________ Individual No: ________________

Responsible Party

Who is responsible for your charges today?

Name: ____

Address: ____

City: ______________________ State: __________ Zip: __________

I certify that the above information is correct.

Signature of Patient: ______________________ Date: __________

Personal Representative

Name of Personal Representative: __________________________

Relationship to Patient: __________________________________

Driver's License Number: ______________________ State: __________

Sample Consent to Disclose PHI for Treatment, Payment, and Health Care Operations

This form must be completed by the individual whose protected health information is to be disclosed, or by a parent or guardian if the person is a minor under state law.

Name: ____

Date of Birth: ______________________ (for identification purposes)

I hereby authorize <physician practice> to release the following personal health information for (check all that apply):

☐ Medical services claims information

☐ Prescription, diagnostic, treatment, and/or care management services

☐ Reviews required by HHS or HIPAA-compliant health care operations

The above information may be released by:

☐ Phone ☐ Fax ☐ Mail ☐ Friend or Relative ______________

My Consent:

Effective: Today's Date: ______________________________

I want this consent to:

☐ Continue indefinitely ☐ Effective only until __________ (date).

I understand that consent may be revoked by me at any time. I understand why I have been asked to disclose this information and am aware that my patient rights are identified in the practice's Notice of Privacy Practices.

Signature of Patient: ______________________ Date: __________

Or Personal Representative: ______________________ Date: __________

Sample Marketing Authorization Form

Dear <Patient>

<Insert description of marketing activity>

The immediate benefit to our practice is that we will receive a financial incentive of up to <$XX.00> for each individual within our practice who signs up for this program. The immediate benefit to you is <xxxxx>.

Our goal is to safeguard your protected health information, and we will NOT provide information about you to this company without your authority.

If you have an interest in a representative from <company> contacting you about this marketing endeavor, please respond below with your authorization. You are under no obligation to respond, and we will continue to provide the highest quality of care regardless of your decision.

<Name, address, phone number>

Authorization to Market

I hereby authorize <physician practice> to provide only my name, address, and phone number to <company> for the purposes of reviewing a discount on my medical fees.

Print Patient Name: ______________________________

Date of Birth: ______________________ (for identification purposes, not to be disclosed to <company>.)

Patient's Signature: ______________________ Date: ____________

Personal Representative

Name of Personal Representative: ______________________________

Relationship to Patient: ______________________ Date: ____________

Driver's License Number: ______________________ State: ____________

Personal Representative Signature: ______________________________

Request to Access Records

Submitted to <Privacy Official, Contact Information>

Patient's Name: ______________________________
(PRINT)

Describe records requested and approximate dates of records you wish to review.

____

____

What would you like for us to do for you?

☐ I wish to inspect the requested records.

☐ I wish to obtain a copy of the requested records.

☐ I wish to inspect and copy the requested records.

Fees:

Our practice charges a reasonable fee to copy the records and also for postage to mail your requested records.

Questions?

Please contact our privacy official listed at the top of this page if you have any questions about your request to inspect or copy records.

Patient information

Patient Signature: ______________________________ Date: ______________

Date of Birth: ______________________________ (for identification purposes)

For the personal representatives of the patient:

Print the name of the personal representative: ______________________________

Relationship to Patient: ______________________________ Date: ______________

Driver's License Number: ______________________________ State: ______________

I certify that I have the legal authority under federal and state laws to make this request on behalf of the patient identified above.

Signature of Personal Representative: ______________________________

Response to Request to Access Records

Patient Name: ____

Address: ____

Access Request Date:

Dear _______________ (Patient):

In response to your request to access records, please see our response below.

Access is:

☐ Granted

Our practice grants you access to medical records specified below. Please contact _________________________, our privacy official, to arrange a convenient time for you to inspect and copy your requested records. You also may request that we send this information to you via US Postal Service. Our practice may charge a reasonable fee to cover the cost of copying and postage.

☐ Denied

Our practice denies your request to access records in whole or in part for the following reasons:

☐ Partially granted, partially denied

Review of Denial

You may request that our practice have the denial reviewed by a licensed health care professional who did not participate in the original decision to deny access.
To request a review, please contact our practice's privacy official.

Access Denial Log

<Name of Practice>

Patient Name	Chart ID Number	Date of Review	Reason for Denial	Date Patient Notified

Request to Amend Records

Directions: Please use this form to make a request that our practice amend or make corrections to information maintained about you. If mailing, please return this form to the privacy official listed on the bottom of this form.

Patient information

Name of Patient: ______________________________
(PRINT)

Signature of Patient: ______________________________

Date: ______________ Patient's Date of Birth: ______________

For Personal Representatives of the Patient

Your Name: ______________________________

Relationship to Patient: ______________________________

Your Driver's License Number: ______________ State: ______________

I hereby certify that I have legal authority under applicable law to make this request on behalf of the patient identified above.

Signature of Personal Representative: ______________________________

Date: ______________________________

Requested Amendment

Please describe in detail how you want your records amended.

Reason for Requested Amendment

Contact Person

Name: ______________________________

Phone number: ______________________________

Address: ______________________________

Please contact our practice's privacy official if you have any questions relating to your request to amend records.

Signature

Patient: ______________________________

Date: ______________________________

Response to Request to Amend Records

Patient Name: ______________________________

Patient Chart/ID Number: ______________________________

Date of Amendment Request: ______________________________

Dear <Patient>:

On <date>, you requested our practice amend certain information stored in our records about you. Your request has been:

☐ Granted

☐ Denied

☐ Partially Granted

If granted, our practice has made the following amendment to your records:

____

____

____

If denied, our practice denies your amendment request for the following specific reasons:

_____ The protected health information was not created by our practice.

_____ The PHI is not part of the designated record set maintained by our practice.

_____ The PHI is not available for inspection under the HIPAA Privacy Rule.

_____ The PHI is accurate and complete.

You have a right to submit a written statement disagreeing with our denial to the practice's privacy official. You also have a right to submit a complaint concerning the denial of this request to our privacy official and/or to the Secretary of the US Department of Health and Human Services at www.hhs.gov/ocr within 180 days of any alleged violation. Your complaint must describe the acts or omissions that you believe are in violation of the HIPAA Privacy Rule.

Please contact me if you have any questions regarding your amendment request.

Sincerely

<Name>

Privacy Official

Signature: ______________________________ Date: ________________

Request for Accounting of Disclosures

To our patient: You have requested an accounting of disclosures of protected health information that our practice has made during a specified time period. Use this form to complete your request.

Patient Name: ______________________________
(PRINT)

Date of Birth: ______________________________ (for identification purposes)

Specified Time Frame for Accounting

Start Date: ______________________ End Date: ______________________

Please specify if you wish to limit our accounting to:

_____ Certain types of disclosures _____ Disclosures to a specific entity[1]

Please provide details of the scope of disclosures for this request:

____

____

____

Patient Signature: ______________________ Today's Date: __________

For Personal Representative of the Patient

Print Name: ______________________________

Relationship to Patient: ______________________________

Driver's License: ______________________ State: __________

[1] Our practice is not required to keep disclosures for the following: to the patient, incidental disclosures; pursuant to a HIPAA-compliant authorization, for a facility directory, to persons involved in the patient's care, for national security or intelligence, to correctional institutions or law enforcement officials having custody of patient, in compliant limited data set disclosures, prior to April 14, 2003.

Response to Request for Accounting of Disclosures

Patient Name: ____________________

Address: ____________________

____

Chart/ID Number: ____________________

Request Date: ____________________

To our patient:

In response to your request for an accounting of disclosures of protected health information about you during the timeframe you requested, the following includes all disclosures we are required to make to you, according to the HIPAA Privacy Rule and our policies.

Time Period:

From: ____________________ To: ____________________

Date of Disclosure	Name and Address of Entity Receiving Disclosure	Description of PHI Disclosed	Purpose of Disclosure

Please contact me if you have any questions regarding your accounting of disclosures.

Privacy Official: ____________________

Phone number: ____________________

E-mail address: ____________________

Signature: ____________________

Date: ____________________

Request to Restrict Disclosure

In the presence of my physician, ______________________________, I am requesting that the medical practice withhold submitting health information to the health plan ______________________________ for purposes of payment or health care operations relating to the following items or services:

____

____

____

In return, I have paid in full out-of-pocket for the items and services itemized above.

______________________________ ______________________

Patient Signature Date

Patient's Date of Birth: ____________________

______________________________ ______________________

Physician or Administrator's Signature Date

Request to Terminate Restrictions

Patient Name: ____

Patient Date of Birth: ______________________________ (for identification purposes)

Today's Date: ____

I hereby consent to terminate additional restrictions on the use and disclosure of protected health information that were previously agreed to by the practice's privacy official on the date identified below. I understand the practice will continue to protect my PHI according to the HIPAA Privacy Rule, Breach Notification Rule, and the HITECH Rule.

Date of Agreed Restriction: ______________________________________

(Attach previously agreed restriction)

Patient Agreement to Terminate Restriction:

____

____

Patient Signature: ____

Date: ____

For Personal Representative of Patient

Name: ____

Relationship to Patient: ____

Driver's License Number: ____________________________ State: ____________

Signature of Personal Representative: ___________________________

Date: ____

Disclosure Log[1]

Patient Name	Chart/ID Number	Date of Disclosure	Name/ Entity Receiving Disclosure	Description of PHI Disclosed	Purpose of Disclosure

[1] You are not required to keep disclosures for the following: to the patient, incidental disclosures; pursuant to a HIPAA-compliant authorization, for a facility directory, to persons involved in the patient's care, for national security or intelligence, to correctional institutions or law enforcement officials having custody of patient, in compliant limited data set disclosures, prior to April 14, 2003.

Request for Alternative Communications

Note to patient: Use this form to request that our practice communicate with you other than at your primary phone number. Fill out this request in its entirety.

Patient Name: ____
(PRINT)

Alternative communication request (Please describe your request to be contacted at an alternative location or by alternative means.)

____

____

____

Payment Information

Your request to be contacted at an alternative location may affect our normal billing and payment procedure. Please specify your alternative method for handling payment.

____

____

____

Alternative Address or Alternative Means of Contact:

____

____

Our Contact Person

If you have any questions about this request, you may contact our privacy official:

Privacy Official: ____

Phone number: ____

E-mail address: ____

Patient Information

Signature of Patient: ______________________________ Date: __________

Date of Birth: ____

For personal representatives of the patient:

Print name of Personal Representative: ______________________________

Relationship to Patient: ____

Driver's License Number: ______________________________ Date: __________

Sample Complaint Form

Note to patient: We will follow up on your complaints, whether they are submitted to us in oral or written form. You are not required to complete a written report, but your comments are helpful to us as we continue to provide excellent service to our patients.

Date: ______________________________

Name of Complainant: ______________________________

Address: ______________________________

____

Phone: ______________________________

Description of Complaint:

Signature of Complainant: ______________________________

What would you like to happen?

_____ I want someone from the office to contact me by ____ phone ____ mail.

_____ I don't want to be contacted.

Other: ______________________________

____

For Internal Use Only

Date Reviewed: ______________________________

Reviewer: ______________________________

Details and Findings: ______________________________

____

____

Follow up:

_______ Phone _______ Mail _______ Both Phone and Mail

Sample Privacy Complaint Log

Note to Practice: Use this log to track patient privacy complaints and how they were mitigated. The first line has been completed as a reference. This document should be maintained by the privacy official.

Privacy Complaint	Individual's Name	Complaint Presented to:	Privacy Official's Action	Follow Up and Date
Patient presented evidence that an authorized workforce member accessed her account.	Betty Jo	Practice Administrator	Investigated complaint, conducted audit review of patient files. Noted that an employee accessed the record. Sanctions applied in accordance with our policies & procedures against the employee.	Letter to patient sent on 11/21/2013.

Minimum Necessary Checklist

Our practice has assigned access to the following PHI.

Name	Billing	Medical/ Clinical	Administrative Access	Scheduling
(Physician)				
(Physician)				
(Physician)				
(Nurse Practitioner)				
(Physician Assistant)				
(Medical Assistant)				
(Medical Assistant)				
(Receptionist)				

De-identification Checklist

To meet the requirements of a limited data set, our privacy official will eliminate the following identifiers from the record.

(a) Names

(b) Postal address information, other than town or city, state and zip code

(c) Telephone numbers

(d) Fax numbers

(e) Electronic mail addresses

(f) Social security numbers

(g) Medical record numbers

(h) Health plan beneficiary numbers

(i) Account numbers

(j) Certificate/license numbers

(k) Vehicle identifiers and serial numbers, including license plate numbers

(l) Device identifiers and serial numbers

(m) Web Universal Resource Locators (URLs)

(n) Internet protocol (IP) address numbers

(o) Biometric identifiers, including finger and voice prints

(p) Full face photographic images and any comparable images

Security-related Repair Form

Use this form to maintain a log of repairs that are made to ensure your physical location is secure.

Name of Practice: ______________________________

Facility Address: ______________________________

City: ____________________ State: __________ Zip: __________

Description of Repair	Date Scheduled	Date Repaired	Contractor		Cost	Approval[1]
			Name, Address	Phone		

[1] Security official or appointed representative should initial when the repair has been completed.

Emergency Access Log

Use this form to maintain a log of emergency access activities. Identify when emergency access involved emergency responders, such as the fire department, law enforcement, or emergency rescue. Also, log events that were the result of a workforce member's abusive activity and the sanctions imposed.

Name of Practice: ______________________________

Facility Address: ______________________________

City: ______________________ State: __________ Zip: __________

Describe Incident		**Who Initiated Access?**[1]	**Emergency Involved**		**Abusive Activity**		**Official**[2]
Description	**Date**	**Name**	**Yes/ No**	**Dept.**[3]	**Describe**	**Sanctions**	

[1] Identify the person who initiated emergency access procedures.

[2] Security official or delegated representative acting on the security official's behalf.

[3] Indicate the emergency responder.

Electronic Media and Hardware Movement Log

Use this form to check out and track the location of electronic media such as portable computers, laptops, and backup disks.

Name of Practice: ______________________________

Facility Address: ______________________________

City: ______________________ State: __________ Zip: __________

Workstation	Static IP Address	Assigned User		Check Out		Initials
		Name	Location	Out	In	

Acknowledgement of Responsibilities Regarding Access to Practice's Electronic Systems Containing Electronic Protected Health Information

Use this form for workforce to acknowledge their responsibilities when accessing the practice's electronic systems that contain protected health information.

Name of Practice: ______________________________

Facility Address: ______________________________

City: ______________________ State: __________ Zip: __________

Acknowledgement

I, ______________________________ (PRINT WORKFORCE MEMBER'S NAME), have read and understand that my job assignment grants me clearance to access protected health information (PHI) about individuals and/or their personal representatives. I also have read and understand our practice's policies and procedures on safeguarding PHI, including sanctions that may be imposed against me, regarding the electronic use and disclosure of protected health information.

I further understand that any questions about the security and privacy of protected health information should be addressed to our privacy and/or security official for guidance.

____

Signature of Employee

____

Signature of Security Official

Date: ______________________________

Consequences of Unauthorized Access to the Practice's Electronic Protected Health Information

Use this form to acknowledge that the workforce member has been informed of the consequences for abusing privileges to access electronic protected health information.

Name of Practice: ______________________________

Facility Address: ______________________________

City: ____________________ State: __________ Zip: __________

Acknowledgement

I, ______________________________ (PRINT WORKFORCE MEMBER'S NAME), have read and understand our policies and procedures and sanctions may be applied to me if I abuse the clearance assigned to me.

I also understand that my job responsibilities may change, eliminating my access to protected health information, and if I abuse my privileges and access PHI, even though access has changed, that the practice has the authority to terminate immediately my employment.

I also understand that if I lose or misplace electronic devices, or if I disable the encryption software safeguarding PHI, and thereby enable an unauthorized user to access protected health information, that I may be subject to legal action taken against me as an individual.

____

Signature of Employee

____

Signature of Security Official

Date: ______________________________

Workforce Member Exit Interview Checklist

Use this checklist to close out a workforce member's access to protected health information upon exiting the practice. Use this checklist irrespective of whether the workforce member left voluntarily or involuntarily.

Name of Practice: ______________________________

Facility Address: ______________________________

City: ____________________ State: __________ Zip: __________

Employee: ____________________ Employee ID: __________

Departure Effective Date: ______________________________

_____ Disable immediately user ID and passwords to practice management system

_____ Disable immediately user ID and password access to electronic health records

_____ Disable access to practice-hosted e-mail and e-mail server

_____ Credit cards returned; cancel online purchasing authority

_____ Retrieve any portable electronic devices

_____ Cancel telephone voice mail

_____ Retrieve keys, cancel card-key or biometric access privileges to facility

_____ Handbooks, including policies and procedures returned

Human Resources List

_____ Letter of resignation received; or notice of termination delivered

_____ Final timesheet and/or activity report delivered

_____ Final check sent to address provided by workforce member

_____ Forwarding address on file

_____ Benefits (health, retirement contributions, sick leave/vacation leave) discussed

Workforce Member Acknowledgement of Awareness and Understanding of Practice's Exit Interview

Use this form in an exit interview for the workforce member to acknowledge termination of a workforce member, irrespective of whether the workforce member is terminated voluntarily or involuntarily.

Name of Practice: ______________________________

Facility Address: ______________________________

City: ______________________ State: __________ Zip: __________

I, ______________________________, understand that in terminating my
(PRINT WORKFORCE MEMBER'S NAME)

employment, whether voluntarily or involuntarily, that the practice will take the following actions: (Workforce member initials each of the following.)

_____ My access to electronic protected health information is terminated and all authentication and authorization credentials for access are invalidated and, as appropriate, are removed.

_____ Keys, card-keys, and/or biometric access will be retrieved or canceled.

_____ The practice will refer any unauthorized attempts at access to the practice's electronic protected health information to appropriate authorities.

_____ A representative of the practice has completed an exit interview and I have provided a forwarding address.

____

Signature of Terminated Employee

____

Signature of Security Official

Date: ______________________________

Otherwise Permitted Uses and Disclosures (45 CFR 164.512)

Expanded from Step 2F, Chapter 3.

1. **Public Health Activities.**[1] Our practice may disclose protected health information without the individual's authorization for public health activities and purposes as follows:
   a. **Public Health Reporting.** Our practice may disclose protected health information without the individual's authorization to a public health authority that is authorized by law to collect or receive such information for the purposes of preventing or controlling disease, injury, or disability, including but not limited to the reporting of disease, injury, vital events such as birth or death, and the conduct of public health surveillance, public health investigations, and public health interventions; or, at the direction of a public health authority, to an official of a foreign government agency that is acting in collaboration with a public health authority.
   b. **Child Abuse or Neglect.** Our practice may disclose protected health information without the individual's authorization to a public health authority or other appropriate government authority authorized by law to receive reports of child abuse or neglect.
   c. **Food and Drug Administration (FDA).** Our practice may disclose protected health information without the individual's authorization about a person subject to the jurisdiction of the FDA with respect to an FDA-regulated product or activity for which that person has responsibility, for the purpose of activities related to the quality, safety, or effectiveness of such FDA-regulated product or activity.
   d. **Communicable Disease.** Our practice may disclose protected health information without the individual's authorization to a person who may have been exposed to a communicable disease or may otherwise be at risk of contracting or spreading a disease or condition, if the covered entity or public health authority is authorized by law to notify such person as necessary in the conduct of a public health intervention or investigation.
2. **Abuse, Neglect, or Domestic Violence**[2]
   a. **If disclosure is required by law.** In cases that do not involve reports of child abuse or neglect (see above), our practice shall not require an individual's authorization to disclose protected health information about an individual whom we reasonably believe to be a victim of abuse, neglect, or domestic violence to a government authority, including a social service or protective services agency, authorized by law to receive reports of such abuse, neglect, or domestic violence to the extent the disclosure is required by law and the disclosure complies with and is limited to the relevant requirements of such law.

---

[1] 45 C.F.R. § 164.512(b).

[2] 45 C.F.R. § 164.512(c).

b. **If disclosure is not required by law.** If disclosure is not required by law, and in our professional judgement we believe the disclosure is necessary to prevent serious harm to the individual or other potential victim, we will consult legal counsel to determine whether the disclosure is expressly authorized by statute or regulation and to determine if any other legal requirements have been met.

c. **Informing the individual.** If our practice makes such a permitted disclosure of abuse, neglect, or domestic violence, whether or not the individual agreed to the disclosure, we shall promptly inform the individual that such a report has been or will be made, except if:

   i. In the exercise of professional judgement, we believe informing the individual would place the individual at risk of serious harm, or

   ii. We would be informing a personal representative, and we reasonably believe the personal representative is responsible for the abuse, neglect, or other injury, and that informing such person would not be in the best interests of the individual as we determine in the exercise of professional judgement.

3. **Government Health Oversight Activities.**[3] If our practice receives a request for disclosure from a health oversight agency in connection with an activity such as an audit, investigation, inspection, licensure or disciplinary action, civil, administrative, or criminal proceeding or action, we shall contact legal counsel to determine how to respond and whether we must obtain authorization from the appropriate individual(s) prior to disclosing any requested protected health information. Examples of such activities include:

   a. Oversight of the health care system
   b. Government benefit programs such as Medicare and Medicaid
   c. Government regulatory programs
   d. Determining compliance with civil rights laws
   e. Investigation of an individual related to the receipt of health care, a claim for public benefits related to health, or qualification for public benefits or services when a patient's health is integral to his or her claim for public benefits or services.

4. **Judicial and administrative proceedings.**[4] If our practice receives an order of a court or administrative tribunal or a subpoena, discovery request, or other lawful process, we shall contact our legal counsel to determine:

   a. How to respond
   b. Whether we must obtain authorization from the appropriate individual(s) prior to disclosing any requested protected health information

[3] 45 C.F.R. § 164.512(d).

[4] 45 C.F.R. § 164.512(e).

c. Whether we must receive "satisfactory assurances" from the party seeking the information
d. Whether a "qualified protective order" is required
e. Whether we must give the individual notice of the request or obtain the individual's authorization prior to disclosing protected health information.

5. **Law Enforcement Official**[5]
   a. **Request.** Our practice shall promptly contact legal counsel if we receive a request for information for law enforcement purposes from a law enforcement official, including any of the following:
      i. A court order or court-ordered warrant, or a subpoena or summons issued by a judicial officer
      ii. A grand jury subpoena
      iii. An administrative request, including an administrative subpoena or summons, or a civil or an authorized investigative demand, or similar process authorized under law
      iv. A request for information about an individual who is or is suspected to be a victim of a crime
   b. **Response.** Before our practice responds to a request for a law enforcement purpose to a law enforcement official, we shall determine in consultation with our legal counsel how to respond, what information must be disclosed, whether any additional items (such as samples of body fluids or tissue must be disclosed), and whether we require authorization from the individual prior to disclosure.
   c. **Decedent.** If an individual has died and we suspect that the death may have resulted from criminal conduct, our practice may disclose protected health information to a law enforcement official about the individual for the purpose of alerting law enforcement of the death.
   d. **Crime on premises.** We may disclose to a law enforcement official protected health information that we believe in good faith constitutes evidence of criminal conduct that occurred on our premises.
   e. **Reporting crime in emergency.** If we provide emergency health care in response to a medical emergency (other than a medical emergency on our premises), we may disclose protected health information to a law enforcement official if the disclosure appears necessary to alert law enforcement to:
      i. The commission and nature of a crime
      ii. The location of the crime or the victim(s) of the crime, and
      iii. The identity, description, and location of the perpetrator of the crime.

   However, if we believe the medical emergency is the result of abuse, neglect, or domestic violence of the individual who needed emergency

[5] 45 C.F.R. § 164.512(f).

health care, our practice must follow the procedure in item 2, "Abuse, Neglect, and Domestic Violence."

6. **Coroners, Medical Examiners, and Funeral Directors.**[6] We may disclose protected health information to a coroner or medical examiner for the purpose of identifying a deceased person, determining a cause of death, or other duties as authorized by law. We may disclose protected health information to funeral directors, consistent with applicable law, as necessary to carry out their duties with respect to the decedent. If necessary for funeral directors to carry out their duties, we may disclose the protected health information prior to, and in reasonable anticipation, of the individual's death.
7. **Organ and Tissue Donation.**[7] We may use or disclose protected health information to organ procurement organizations or other entities engaged in the procurement, banking, or transplantation of cadaveric organs, eyes, or tissue for donation or transplantation.
8. **Research.**[8] Our dental practice shall not use or disclose protected health information for research purposes without consulting legal counsel to make sure all necessary requirements have been met. Examples of such requirements include approval by an Institutional Review Board or privacy board, reviews preparatory to research, review and approval procedures, and required signatures.
9. **Averting a Serious Threat to Health or Safety.**[9] Our practice will consult our legal counsel to determine whether HIPAA and other applicable law permit us to disclose protected health information if we believe in good faith that such disclosure is necessary:
   - **a.** To prevent or lessen a serious and imminent threat to the health or safety of a person or the public
   - **b.** For law enforcement authorities to identify or apprehend an individual where it appears from all the circumstances that the individual has escaped from a correctional institution or from lawful custody
   - **c.** For law enforcement authorities to identify or apprehend an individual because of a statement by an individual admitting participation in a violent crime that we reasonably believe may have caused serious physical harm to the victim.
10. **Specialized Government Functions.**[10] Our practice shall consult legal counsel to determine whether HIPAA and other applicable law permit us to disclose protected health information involving:
    - **a.** Military and veterans activities
    - **b.** National security and intelligence activities

---

[6] 45 C.F.R. § 164.512(g).
[7] 45 C.F.R. § 164.512(h).
[8] 45 C.F.R. § 164.512(i).
[9] 45 C.F.R. § 164.512(j).
[10] 45 C.F.R. § 164.512(k).

c. Protective services for the President and others
d. Correctional institutions and other law enforcement custodial situations

11. **Workers' Compensation.**[11] Our practice may disclose protected health information as authorized by and to the extent necessary to comply with laws relating to workers' compensation or other similar programs, established by law, that provide benefits for work-related injuries or illness without regard to fault.

Since 2003 when HIPAA Privacy Rules became enforceable, health care providers have exercised great caution not to disclose PHI. However, significant disasters, including earthquakes, hurricanes, and terrorist activities, have caused confusion as to what to disclose and what not to disclose. As a result, the HHS Office for Civil Rights (OCR) issued, and continues to issue, guidance such as Communicating with Friends and Family, FAQs for Family Members, and the Emergency and Disaster Disclosure Decision Tree, which are included in this appendix.

[11] 45 C.F.R. § 164.512(l).

Communicating with a Patient's Family, Friends, or Others Involved in the Patient's Care

US Department of Health and Human Services • Office for Civil Rights

This guide explains when a health care provider is allowed to share a patient's health information with the patient's family members, friends, or others identified by the patient as involved in the patient's care under the Health Insurance Portability and Accountability Act of 1996 (HIPAA) Privacy Rule. HIPAA is a federal law that sets national standards for how health plans, health care clearinghouses, and most health care providers are to protect the privacy of a patient's health information.[1]

Even though HIPAA requires health care providers to protect patient privacy, providers are permitted, in most circumstances, to communicate with the patient's family, friends, or others involved in their care or payment for care. This guide is intended to clarify these HIPAA requirements so that health care providers do not unnecessarily withhold a patient's health information from these persons. This guide includes common questions and a table that summarizes the relevant requirements.[2]

---

[1] The HIPAA Privacy Rule applies to those health care providers that transmit any health information in electronic form in connection with certain standard transactions, such as health care claims. See the definitions of "covered entity," "health care provider," and "transaction" at 45 C.F.R. §160.103.

[2] The full text of these requirements can be found at 45 C.F.R. § 164.510(b). Note that this guide does not apply to a health care provider's disclosure of psychotherapy notes, which generally requires a patient's written authorization. See 45 C.F.R. §164.508(a)(2).

Common Questions About HIPAA

1. If the patient is present and has the capacity to make health care decisions, when does HIPAA allow a health care provider to discuss the patient's health information with the patient's family, friends, or others involved in the patient's care or payment for care?

If the patient is present and has the capacity to make health care decisions, a health care provider may discuss the patient's health information with a family member, friend, or other person if the patient agrees or, when given the opportunity, does not object. A health care provider also may share information with these persons if, using professional judgement, he or she decides that the patient does not object. In either case, the health care provider may share or discuss only the information that the person involved needs to know about the patient's care or payment for care.

Here are some examples:

- An emergency room doctor may discuss a patient's treatment in front of the patient's friend if the patient asks that her friend come into the treatment room.
- A doctor's office may discuss a patient's bill with the patient's adult daughter who is with the patient at the patient's medical appointment and has questions about the charges.
- A doctor may discuss the drugs a patient needs to take with the patient's health aide who has accompanied the patient to a medical appointment.
- A doctor may give information about a patient's mobility limitations to the patient's sister who is driving the patient home from the hospital.
- A nurse may discuss a patient's health status with the patient's brother if she informs the patient she is going to do so and the patient does not object.

BUT:

- A nurse may *not* discuss a patient's condition with the patient's brother after the patient has stated she does not want her family to know about her condition.

2. If the patient is not present or is incapacitated, may a health care provider still share the patient's health information with family, friends, or others involved in the patient's care or payment for care?

Yes. If the patient is not present or is incapacitated, a health care provider may share the patient's information with family, friends, or others as long as the health care provider determines, based on professional judgement, that it is in the best interest of the patient. When someone other than a friend or family member is involved, the health care provider must be reasonably sure that the patient asked the person to be involved in his or her care or payment for care. The health care provider may discuss only the information that the person involved needs to know about the patient's care or payment.

Here are some examples:

- A surgeon who did emergency surgery on a patient may tell the patient's spouse about the patient's condition while the patient is unconscious.
- A pharmacist may give a prescription to a patient's friend who the patient has sent to pick up the prescription.
- A hospital may discuss a patient's bill with her adult son who calls the hospital with questions about charges to his mother's account.
- A health care provider may give information regarding a patient's drug dosage to the patient's health aide who calls the provider with questions about that particular prescription.

BUT:

- A nurse may *not* tell a patient's friend about a past medical problem that is unrelated to the patient's current condition.
- A health care provider is *not* required by HIPAA to share a patient's information when the patient is not present or is incapacitated, and can choose to wait until the patient has an opportunity to agree to the disclosure.

3. Does HIPAA require that a health care provider document a patient's decision to allow the provider to share his or her health information with a family member, friend, or other person involved in the patient's care or payment for care?

No. HIPAA does not require that a health care provider document the patient's agreement or lack of objection. However, a health care provider is free to obtain or document the patient's agreement, or lack of objection, in writing, if he or she prefers. For example, a provider may choose to document a patient's agreement to share information with a family member with a note in the patient's medical file.

4. May a health care provider discuss a patient's health information over the phone with the patient's family, friends, or others involved in the patient's care or payment for care?

Yes. Where a health care provider is allowed to share a patient's health information with a person, information may be shared face-to-face, over the phone, or in writing.

5. **If a patient's family member, friend, or other person involved in the patient's care or payment for care calls a health care provider to ask about the patient's condition, does HIPAA require the health care provider to obtain proof of who the person is before speaking with them?**

   No. If the caller states that he or she is a family member or friend of the patient, or is involved in the patient's care or payment for care, then HIPAA doesn't require proof of identity in this case. However, a health care provider may establish his or her own rules for verifying who is on the phone. In addition, when someone other than a friend or family member is involved, the health care provider must be reasonably sure that the patient asked the person to be involved in his or her care or payment for care.

6. **Can a patient have a family member, friend, or other person pick up a filled prescription, medical supplies, X-rays, or other similar forms of patient information, for the patient?**

   Yes. HIPAA allows health care providers to use professional judgement and experience to decide if it is in the patient's best interest to allow another person to pick up a prescription, medical supplies, X-rays, or other similar forms of information for the patient.

   For example, the fact that a relative or friend arrives at a pharmacy and asks to pick up a specific prescription for a patient effectively verifies that he or she is involved in the patient's care. HIPAA allows the pharmacist to give the filled prescription to the relative or friend. The patient does not need to provide the pharmacist with their names in advance.

7. **May a health care provider share a patient's health information with an interpreter to communicate with the patient or with the patient's family, friends, or others involved in the patient's care or payment for care?**

   Yes. HIPAA allows covered health care providers to share a patient's health information with an interpreter without the patient's written authorization under the following circumstances:

   - A health care provider may share information with an interpreter who works for the provider (eg, a bilingual employee, a contract interpreter on staff, or a volunteer).

   For example, an emergency room doctor may share information about an incapacitated patient's condition with an interpreter on staff who relays the information to the patient's family.

- A health care provider may share information with an interpreter who is acting on its behalf (but is not a member of the provider's workforce) if the health care provider has a written contract or other agreement with the interpreter that meets HIPAA's business associate contract requirements.

For example, many providers are required under Title VI of the Civil Rights Act of 1964 to take reasonable steps to provide meaningful access to persons with limited English proficiency. These providers often have contracts with private companies, community-based organizations, or telephone interpreter service lines to provide language interpreter services. These arrangements must comply with the HIPAA business associate agreement requirements at 45 C.F.R. 164.504(e).

- A health care provider may share information with an interpreter who is the patient's family member, friend, or other person identified by the patient as his or her interpreter, if the patient agrees, or does not object, or the health care provider determines, using his or her professional judgement, that the patient does not object.

For example, health care providers sometimes see patients who speak a certain language and the provider has no employee, volunteer, or contractor who can competently interpret that language. If the provider is aware of a telephone interpreter service that can help, the provider may have that interpreter tell the patient that the service is available. If the provider decides, based on professional judgement, that the patient has chosen to continue using the interpreter, the provider may talk to the patient using the interpreter.

8. Where can I find additional information about HIPAA?

The Office for Civil Rights, part of the Department of Health and Human Services, has more information about HIPAA on its Web site. Visit www.hhs.gov/ocr/hipaa for a wide range of helpful information, including the full text of the Privacy Rule, a HIPAA Privacy Rule Summary, fact sheets, over 200 frequently asked questions, as well as many other resources to help health care providers and others understand the law.

HIPAA Privacy Rule Disclosures to a Patient's Family, Friends, or Others Involved in the Patient's Care or Payment for Care

	Family Member or Friend	Other Persons
Patient is present and has the capacity to make health care decisions	Provider may disclose relevant information if the provider does one of the following: (1) obtains the patient's agreement (2) gives the patient an opportunity to object and the patient does not object (3) decides from the circumstances, based on professional judgement, that the patient does not object Disclosure may be made in person, over the phone, or in writing.	Provider may disclose relevant information if the provider does one of the following: (1) obtains the patient's agreement (2) gives the patient the opportunity to object and the patient does not object (3) decides from the circumstances, based on professional judgement, that the patient does not object Disclosure may be made in person, over the phone, or in writing.
Patient is not present or is incapacitated	Provider may disclose relevant information if, based on professional judgement, the disclosure is in the patient's best interest. Disclosure may be made in person, over the phone, or in writing. Provider may use professional judgement and experience to decide if it is in the patient's best interest to allow someone to pick up filled prescriptions, medical supplies, X-rays, or other similar forms of health information for the patient.	Provider may disclose relevant information if the provider is reasonably sure that the patient has involved the person in the patient's care and in his or her professional judgement, the provider believes the disclosure to be in the patient's best interest. Disclosure may be made in person, over the phone, or in writing. Provider may use professional judgement and experience to decide if it is in the patient's best interest to allow someone to pick up filled prescriptions, medical supplies, X-rays, or other similar forms of health information for the patient.

Emergency and Disaster Disclosure Decision Tree

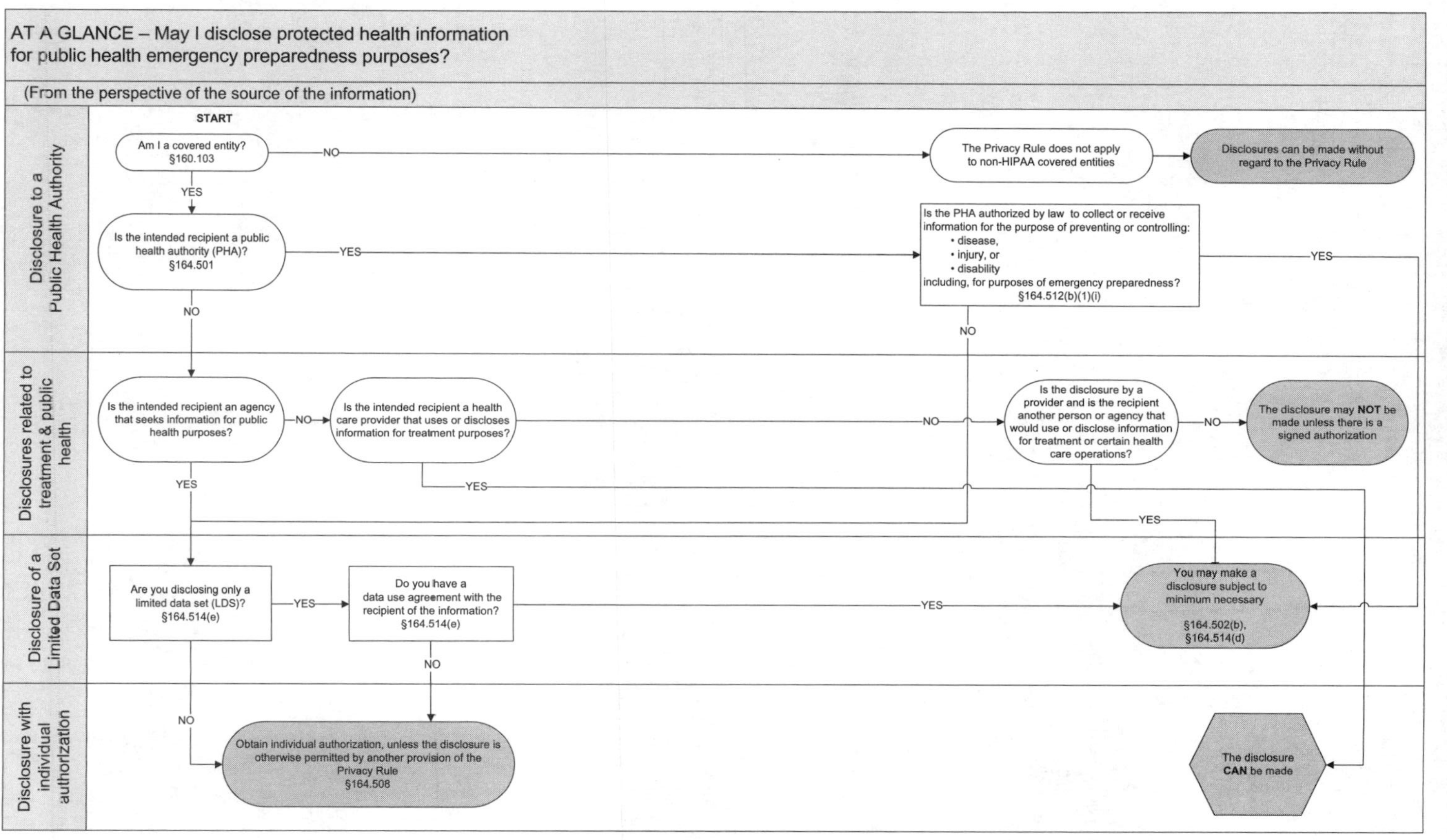

HIPAA for Behavioral Health in an Electronic Environment

Carolyn P. Hartley, MLA

ABSTRACT

Security and privacy issues play a large part in behavioral health care as practitioners measure and manage risks for patients needing integrated care. Behavioral healthcare was largely excluded from Stage 1 Meaningful Use measures, but HR 6043 promises to correct the oversight, setting the stage for the behavioral health (BH) community[1] to participate in incentives for electronic health record adoption. As few practitioners outside the behavioral health community realize the extent of integrated care required in treating BH patients, this white paper serves as a platform to increase awareness across the clinical spectrum and also refresh BH communities on their obligations to safeguard protected health information (PHI). This white paper is provided for educational purposes only. Consult a health law attorney for concerns related to privacy and security requirements.

OPERATIONALIZING HIPAA PRIVACY AND SECURITY

Of the five HIPAA[2] patient rights defined in the Privacy Rule,[3] the two that create the most headaches for behavioral health organizations are (1) Request to access and copy PHI and (2) Request an accounting of disclosures (Figure 1). This was the experience reported by nearly 475 attendees of a May 2012 Webinar titled "HIPAA for Behavioral Health in an Electronic Environment." (To receive an electronic copy of the Webinar, please visit http://sigmund software.com/contact_us.aspx and type "HIPAA Webinar Request" in the comments section.)

FIGURE 1

HIPAA Patient Rights Reported as Biggest Headaches by Behavioral Health Organizations

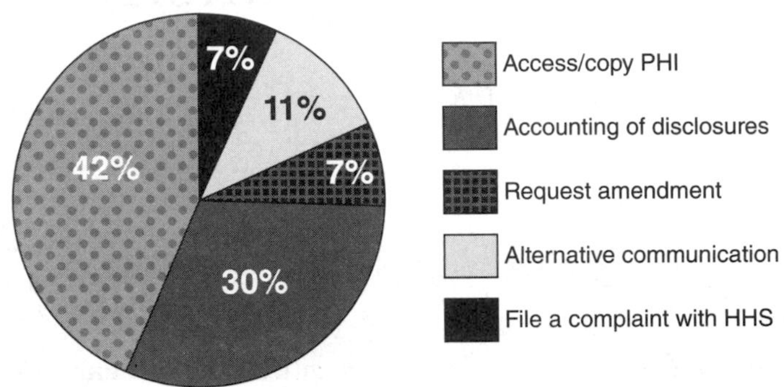

The audience also reported that their staff often confused the safeguards embedded in HIPAA's Privacy Rule with requirements for HIPAA's Security Rule. This is not at all uncommon, since both Privacy safeguards and the Security Rule implementation specifications are divided into three categories: administrative, physical, and technical safeguards.

The framers of both rules intentionally designed the overlap. Privacy Rule safeguards, effective April 14, 2003, served as a stopgap measure until Security Rule specifications became effective two years later, on April 20, 2005. The Privacy Rule[4] gained widespread recognition when thousands of health law attorneys, consulting groups, medical societies, and publishers helped spread the word of the rule's compliance standards. The Security Rule, designed to put good security business practices in place, really came of age when Congress approved the HITECH Act's[5] investment of $20+ billion to build a health information technology infrastructure. The HITECH Act also required HHS to significantly beef up enforcement penalties and corrective action plans for covered entities' privacy breaches and willful neglect of security and privacy safeguards.

As one of three agencies within HHS[6] assigned to regulate privacy and security, the Office of the National Coordinator for Health Information Technology (ONC) included a requirement that eligible professionals (EPs) and eligible hospitals (EHs) demonstrate how they safeguard PHI in Core Measure #15 for EPs and Core Measure #14 for EHs. The measures are met by attesting that the EP or EH has completed a risk analysis and *also* put in place measures to mitigate those risks.

A *risk analysis* is a series of queries with responses determining where risks have been, where they might be, and how to mitigate them. The National Institute for Standards and Technology (NIST.gov) poses 492 questions you should include in a risk analysis in its Toolkit[7] available online. While the questions are directed at larger organizations, some of the administrative requirements applicable to BH providers include:

- Did you appoint a security official?
- Did you conduct a risk assessment and build your policies and procedures based on risks you identified in that assessment?
- Have you trained your workforce on those policies and procedures?
- Do you monitor reports of persons who access systems and patient files?
- Do you have a disaster recovery plan in place? Have you tested it?
- Do you also comply with other state and federal privacy requirements?

BEHAVIORAL HEALTH PRIVACY AND SECURITY RISK MANAGEMENT

Predating HIPAA by more than two decades[8] are federal privacy provisions protecting the confidentiality of alcohol and drug abuse treatment records in 42 Code of Federal Regulations (CFR), Part 2. The stigma associated with substance abuse and fear of prosecution deterred people from entering treatment. If misused, information could lead to the loss of a patient's job or occupational licensing.[9]

In the adoption of electronic health records (EHRs), the importance of best practices in managing confidentiality becomes even more heightened in behavioral health clinics, especially as staff migrates charts from paper into the EHR. (See Risk #4 below.) Protected health information (PHI) turns into ePHI, requiring user and password protection, time out monitoring, audit controls to monitor who has had access and what the user changed, deleted, or modified during access, encryption software, protections from malicious software, and network protection. Of the 40+ implementation specifications defined in HIPAA's Security Rule, confidentiality is often most compromised when PHI/ePHI hovers between paper and electronic records during chart abstraction and migration into an EHR.

To meet Core Measure #15, and also comply with HIPAA, you must not only identify the organization's vulnerabilities and threats, but mitigate those risks with policies and procedures and train staff on those processes.

The seven risks presented here may not apply to all situations, but they do reflect the state of privacy in behavioral health as the community transitions into EHRs. Risks also apply in an integrated care delivery system that includes behavioral health services.

Risk #1: Health Information Exchange with Hospitals, Accountable Care Organizations, and Super Groups

The framers of HIPAA leveraged mental health privacy laws by providing a higher degree of protection on the use of behavioral health notes, requiring additional patient consent before releasing any mental health notes. To that end, behavioral health clinics can only partially rely on authorization forms developed for most medical environments. A hospital, for example, that diagnoses, refers, or provides treatment to a substance abuse patient must meet additional consent requirements identified in this "Behavioral Health Consent" list:

- Name or general designation of the program or person permitted to make the disclosure
- Name or title of the individual or name of the organization to which disclosure is to be made
- Name of the patient
- Purpose of the disclosure
- How much and what kind of information is to be disclosed
- Signature of patient (and, in some states, a parent or guardian)
- Date on which consent is signed
- Statement that the consent is subject to revocation at any time except to the extent that the program has already acted on it
- Date, event, or condition upon which consent will expire if not previously revoked
- Privacy Rule Add-ons:
  - ☐ Organization will not withhold treatment if patient doesn't sign consent form (45 CFR 164.508)
  - ☐ Organization provides patient with copy of signed form (45 CFR 164.508 (c)(4))
  - ☐ Keep a copy for six years (45 CFR 164.508(b)(6))

Policies and procedures must be put in place to ensure PHI will be used and disclosed with utmost confidentiality in behavioral health referrals and treatment facilities.

As hospitals acquire ambulatory medical practices, establish accountable care organizations that include BH services, or take leadership roles in state and local health information exchanges (HIEs), privacy policies may need to be reviewed and updated, especially if BH patients transition between primary care and BH providers.

Risk Prevention Strategies

- Participate in HIE governance structures. Part of their governance is intended to determine privacy and security policies between members as well as sanctions if an organization fails to protect privacy.
- Ask for assurance that HIE interoperability standards will meet 42 CFR, Part 2.
- If part of a hospital system, read the consent forms to ensure PHI safeguards meet behavioral health requirements.
- As this is a legal issue, consult a health law attorney for additional guidance.

Risk #2: Privacy Risks in the Integrated Care Setting

Physicians and BH providers need little convincing that the patient's outcome is best served if mental health issues and physical problems are co-managed. According to California's Integrated Behavioral Health Project,[10] the best integrated outcomes have occurred when combining treatment for depression and chronic medical conditions.

One frustration in an electronic health record environment is that the medical practice sets permissions on the EHR administration panel that, in accordance with HIPAA, add protected access to patients diagnosed with a behavioral health disorder. As much as the EHR vendors claim you need them for physician referrals, referrals still initiate with a phone call between colleagues. But the actual exchange of information is handled in many ways. Therein lies the risk.

If the referral is made within the organization, the BH provider may, or may not, have access due to protected settings and the selected system. As a work-around, a nurse creates a password-protected PDF file. But since either most physicians are not yet using secure e-mail, or the firewalls are too secure and won't allow the PDF out of the network, the nurse uses an unsecured email account, such as Yahoo!, Gmail, or AOL, to send the password-protected file to a referring BH clinic. Outside the secure network, the file is subject to any number of free unlocking software programs unless the PDF is embedded in document security software.

Risk Prevention Strategies

- Seek an encrypted and secure patient portal for internal PHI exchange.
- For external exchanges between credentialed health care professionals, consider using services such as mdEmail.md or a similar application such as DIRECT Project. DIRECT Project is a public-private collaborative that allows physicians to securely send messages containing PHI to another health care provider.
- Use the EHR's messaging components for internal communication.
- Encrypt systems that contain PHI, such as scanned images, claims payment appeals, and copies of remittance advices.
- Develop or update policies and procedures that govern access processes, as well as use and disclosure rights.

Key Terms and How Adoption of Health IT Complicates Them

While Privacy and Security Rules contain relevant definitions, five terms stand out as being more complex in the electronic environment.[11]

Key Term	Abbreviated Definition	Complication
Protected Health Information, or Individually-identifiable Information	The individual's past, present, or future* physical or mental health or condition in oral, written, or electronic format Provision of health care to individual, or past, present, or future payment for the provision of health care to the individual	In migrating to an electronic health record (EHR), the paper chart becomes a hybrid chart until the paper chart has been retired to storage. A chart migration plan must include a strategy for protecting paper, not only for privacy, but also for patient safety. Results of genetic testing can no longer be used to determine insurance eligibility.
Use	Create, retrieve, revise, or delete PHI	Access now means setting access controls, identifying who has access and how, reviewing audit trails to identify who had access, when, and what they accessed or changed.
Disclose	Release, transfer, divulge, or allow access to PHI outside the holding entity	PHI is stored in multiple systems such as imaging, voice records, and hybrid (part paper, part EHR) records. This inhibits the ability to pull together a complete record or know where PHI is located.
Data at rest	Stored in paper and electronic charts, networks, or devices	PHI is stored now on portable notebooks, servers, handheld devices.
Data in motion	During transmission	Transmission carriers that do not require access to PHI are not regarded as business associates in the HIPAA Omnibus Rule. (Section 13408) ePrescribing gateways, for example are business associates.[12]

* Future refers to genomic information that payers may not use for underwriting purposes.

Risk #3: Access Control and Audit Controls

Access Control in HIPAA's Security Rule is a companion to the Minimum Necessary requirement in the Privacy Rule. In both rules, the covered entity is required to determine the minimum amount of access to PHI necessary to effectively perform a job. For example, a psychologist, psychiatrist, psychiatric nurse practitioner, and in most cases a social worker may need access to clinical information while a registration clerk or scheduler most likely will not require the same access privileges.

Audit controls, a required specification in the Security Rule, allows administrators to see who has had access to ePHI, when they had access, and what they created, viewed, modified, or deleted. Risks associated with access control and audit controls come with several issues.

Access control = who can have access according to their role?

Audit controls = who had access, and what did they create, change, modify, delete, or download, and when?

- Some EHR vendors don't train administrators how to run the audit control feature.
- Audit controls take up space on the server and can slow the system.
- Some EHR vendors embed administrative functions, such as scanning driver's licenses and payer cards into the clinical screens. So when a front office admits a patient, they may immediately compromise role-based policies and procedures to gain access to the patient's insurance information or authenticate the patient by looking at the driver's license.
- The clinic may need to develop a script to run an audit control report.
- Employees may not access another patient's chart if they are not directly involved in the patient's care.

If you have not yet implemented the audit control feature of your EHR system, talk to the system's technical support team as this feature will be invaluable in the event of a breach in which, for example, you need to know what patient information was downloaded onto a tablet.

Risk #4: Managing the Hybrid Record is the Solution; the Risk is the Hybrid Record

During the chart abstraction process, a medical assistant (MA)[13] opens the paper chart and selects information that the clinic has determined may be scanned and data that must be directly entered into the EHR, such as medications, dosages, allergies and adverse events, progress notes, and vitals as discrete data in the system. The MA then marks pages that have been scanned or entered as discrete data. In most cases, the scanning strategy then is to shred pages that have been scanned, and keep pages with discrete data to ensure quality control of data entry. The internal policy then is to shred all paper by the end of the day. All too frequently, the paper is shredded when the MA remembers to shred it, such as at the end of the week. Over several days, the pile of paper builds to overflow. The MA picks up a piece of paper from the trash, scribbles a grocery list, and accidentally leaves the grocery list in the cart. On the flip side of the list are a patient's progress notes. The employee could have simply tossed the records into a dumpster, which likely would have set off greater risks for a large-scale breach notification process. Until the clinic establishes, trains, and enforces policies and procedures for how they will manage the hybrid record, the chart will remain a combination of paper and EHR, creating both patient safety and privacy issues as well as a missing one of the most significant benefits of an EHR—having the patient's record in one place. Hybrid records also can present unmanageable privacy exposures.

Risk Prevention Strategies

- Put in place policies that require paper to be shredded at the end of each workday. Enforce this policy.
- Build a strategy for managing hybrid medical charts. This is part of your go-live strategy and should be part of your strategic implementation plan.
- Ask your EHR vendor how they plan to help you comply with access and audit controls.

Risk #5: Lack of Clarity Concerning Data Ownership

Consider this scenario: A group of primary care physicians recently achieved Patient-Centered Medical Home certification status. They are committed to work with the state and local HIE and would like for the behavioral health providers not only to join the HIE, but also to share clinical and medication findings within the HIE. The hospital supporting the HIE believes sharing of information will improve delivery of care, particularly on weekends when episodes are more likely to occur. You know that BH patients rarely sign consent forms to participate in the HIE, but the physicians involved in the patients' integrated care do not see an immediate problem since the HIE has stringent privacy policies. Social workers, however, have learned that some of their patients report being discriminated against in the emergency department.

Until recently, BH has not been a stakeholder at local and state HIE governance meetings. Complex privacy issues, along with widespread misinformation about integrated care for BH patients, kept BH providers from weighing in on protocols, privacy and interoperability standards, and data exchange. To some extent, BH also has been late to the table and has some serious catching up to do.

Spokespersons from the Substance Abuse and Mental Health Services Administration (SAMHSA), including administrator H. Westley Clark, MD, JD, MPH, CAS, FASAM, and Elaine Perry, MS, Director, Office of Management, Technology, and Operations, have initiated an awareness campaign to include BH as participants in HIEs.[14]

Risk Prevention Strategies

If you are asked to participate in an HIE, ask these questions.

- What PHI can a BH provider put into the HIE and expect that it will be protected with 42 CFR, Part 2 standards?
- If erroneous information is provided by another caregiver, how will it be corrected?
- Who owns the record and is responsible for its upkeep?

Risk #6: Privacy, Mobility, and Breach Notification

The question about mobility is not whether your organization will embrace handheld devices but rather how, when, and what secure solutions, including encryption, you will put in place to protect patient confidentiality. Considerable debate has emerged regarding bring your own device (BYOD) policies, and how an organization will protect ePHI when it resides on a device owned by a provider, not the organization. Organizations may put policies in effect, but the real measure of this policy is how BYOD is enforced with sanctions applied consistently across the organization.

As BH providers join the ranks of iPad and smart phone users, the BH organization must begin to assess and mitigate risks in the rapidly expanding mobile environment. In patient care, providers can access the patient record from home in the event of an episode, hospitalization, or setback to quickly identify medication and behavioral histories.

One of the most intimidating HIPAA questions for an office manager comes from a patient asking, "I'd like to know where my protected health information has been used and disclosed."

In an informal gathering of New York[15] primary care providers, they collectively said they received from one to three requests for an accounting of disclosures each month. Participants in the May 2012 Webinar on privacy and behavioral health in an electronic environment reported they received approximately 30 requests a month.

Lost, stolen, or missing mobile devices also are the leading cause of breaches that must be reported to the Office for Civil Rights, either once yearly (less than 500 records affected) or within 60 days of the breach (500 or more records). Fines have dramatically escalated, rebuffing the notion that OCR was a sleeper agency. The Alaska Department of Health and Human Services recently paid $1.7 million to OCR for a breach in which a USB hard drive possibly containing ePHI was stolen from the vehicle of a DHHS employee.

> Over the course of the investigation, OCR found that Alaska DHHS did not have adequate policies and procedures in place to safeguard ePHI. Further, DHHS had not completed a risk analysis, implemented sufficient risk management measures, completed security training for its workforce members, implemented device and media controls, or addressed device and media encryption as required by the HIPAA Security Rule.[16]

In a recent "war game" with 23 EHR consultants enrolled in Breach Communication and Issues Management,[17] the task they struggled through the most was how to identify the location of patient records.

Risk Prevention Strategies

- Conduct a PHI gap analysis and identify the location of PHI within your facility.
- Encrypt mobile devices.
- Prevent download of patient information onto mobile devices, including USB hard drives, by locking PHI onto the server. Clinicians can still access patient information but through a secure Virtual Private Network (VPN).
- As your organization transitions into electronic health records, be sure the EHR you select not only meets the clinical and functional elements for behavioral health[18] but also has the technical capacity to electronically provide you with these disclosures.
- Put in place a strategy that will help you identify patient records *before* a breach occurs.

Risk #7: Consumer Complaints

Every organization should put in place a process that encourages patients to file complaints to someone inside the clinic. These complaints are easier to manage than having to work through an OCR audit. An audit from any organization is time consuming, but OCR audits are much more investigative in nature. They may begin with a phone and email investigation, but could quickly ramp up to onsite visits, deeper investigations into multiple policies, fines, and penalties, as well as additional investigation into potential fraud and abuse activities.

If a patient does file a complaint with the Office for Civil Rights (www.hhs.gov/ocr), the four consistently asked questions are these:

1. What is your policy for this complaint? For example, a patient says your clinic disclosed information to another clinic without consent. In response, you would provide your written policy for use and disclosure for treatment, payment, and health care operations.
2. What is your training policy and when did you last train on this policy? You would provide a list of attendees at a HIPAA training session, the topic, and the date of training.
3. What is your sanction policy, and did you follow it? Sanctions often are applied inconsistently. You would provide a log of instances of applied sanctions.
4. What is your plan to remediate this complaint? Document steps you are taking to repair damage, if any, to the patient.

On its Web site, the Office for Civil Rights says it has processed 71,849 HIPAA complaints since April 2003. Figure 2 shows the volume of cases and outcomes.

FIGURE 2

HIPAA Complaints Managed by OCR

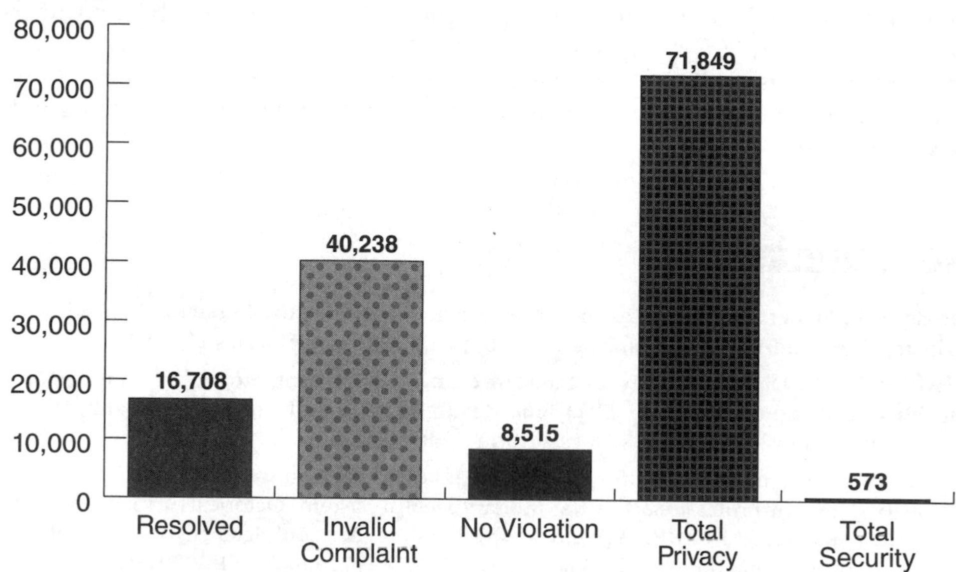

The most common types of covered entities that have been required to take corrective action to achieve voluntary compliance are, in order of frequency:[19]

1. Private practices
2. General hospitals
3. Outpatient facilities
4. Health plans (group health plans and health insurance issuers)
5. Pharmacies

Risk Prevention Strategies

- Train staff on privacy and security policies and procedures on a regular basis.
- Ensure staff knows what is included in your Notice of Privacy Policies.
- Privacy officials should participate in organizational workgroups, such as those aligned with the Workgroup for Electronic Data Interchange (WEDI.org), to keep up to date on privacy and security situations and best practices.
- Consult a health law attorney if you receive a call from the Office for Civil Rights.
- Train staff on how to respond to a complaint and refer complainants to the privacy official.

SUMMARY

Timing is of the essence as BH professionals become eligible professionals and eligible hospitals[20] attesting to meeting Meaningful Use measures. Take advantage of the availability of Meaningful Use funds, including one of the core (required) measures that calls for an annual risk analysis. Put privacy and security measures in place not only because it's the law, but also because it is good business sense.

RESOURCES

Druss, BG., Mauer, Barbara, "Health Care Reform and Care at the Behavioral Health–Primary Care Interface," *Psychiatr Serv*, 2010, doi: 10.1176/appi.ps.61.11.1087.

Clark, HW. MD, Director, Center for Substance Abuse Treatment, Strategic Initiative #6: Health Information Technology, Electronic Health Records and Behavioral Health. http://www.samhsa.gov/about/siDocs/healthIT.pdf.

A Quality Management System for Licensed Mental Health Counselors and Other Behavioral Health Professionals in the Military Health System, October 13-15 Workshop Transcript sponsored by TRICARE and the National Academy of Sciences Institute of Medicine. http://iom.edu/~/media/Files/Activity%20Files/MentalHealth/TRICARE MentalHealth/TRICARE-Transcripts.pdf.

A Delicate Balance: Behavioral Health, Patient Privacy, and the Need to Know, George Washington University School of Public Health and Health Services, published by California Health Care Foundation, March 2008.

ENDNOTES

1. For this white paper, the term "behavioral health" includes services provided for mental health, substance abuse, and addiction therapies.
2. Health Insurance Portability and Accountability Act (HIPAA). To learn more, go to www.hhs.gov/ocr.
3. To view all patient rights, go to Office for Civil Rights Web site, www.hhs.gov/ocr/privacy.
4. HIPAA's Privacy Rule went into effect on April 14, 2003. Consult www.hhs.gov/ocr/privacy for details on the Privacy Rule. Select the Health Information Privacy tab.
5. Health Information Technology for Economic and Clinical Health Act (HITECH Act) was embedded in the American Recovery and Reinvestment Act (ARRA, www.recovery.gov).
6. The Office for Civil Rights (OCR) is the enforcement agency for both HIPAA's Privacy Rule and Security Rule. The Office of the National Coordinator for Health Information Technology (ONC) requires eligible professionals and eligible hospitals demonstrate they are managing protected health information in a secure environment, and the Centers for Medicare and Medicaid Services (CMS) regulate and enforce use of HIPAA standard transactions.

7. NIST has posted a free risk HIPAA Security Rule Toolkit (HSR) available at www.scap.nist.gov/hipaa.
8. Wattenberg, Sarah A., MSW, Project Officer, Substance Abuse and Mental Health Services Administration (SAMSHA), http://www.samhsa.gov/healthprivacy/docs/ehr-faqs.pdf, 42 CFR, Part 2 codified in "Applying the Substance Abuse Confidentiality Regulations to Health Information Exchange."
9. "A Delicate Balance: Behavioral Health, Patient Privacy, and the Need to Know," March 2008, California Healthcare Foundation, 1-2.
10. California's Integrated Behavioral Health Project is a joint project of the Tides Center, www.tides.org, and The California Endowment, www.calendow.org.
11. Reprinted with permission from Physicians EHR, Inc. Copyright 2012.
12. HIPAA Omnibus Final Rule, Federal Register. Vol. 78, p. 5572.
13. Or other health care professional, based on state law regarding who can access PHI.
14. Substance Abuse and Mental Health Services Administration, www.samhsa.gov, provides a wealth of details, tool kits, and resources for behavioral health providers.
15. Medical society meeting in 2009 where the author was a speaker and polled the audience.
16. Headline news at hhs.gov/ocr/privacy and also in multiple television markets.
17. Breach Communication and Issues Management is a course offered by Physicians EHR, www.physiciansehr.com.
18. Clinical and Functional Elements of Behavioral Health can be downloaded at www.physiciansehr.com, Resource Library.
19. www.hhs.gov/ocr/privacy. Select Enforcement Activities on the left menu.
20. www.cms.gov/EHRIncentivePrograms.

appendix B

Additions to HIPAA Training Program

Training on HIPAA privacy and security is an ongoing process. A 12-month training program that includes content from the HIPAA Omnibus Rule is provided for you here. Following the month-by-month calendar of training topics is a sample training presentation for you to customize and present to all workforce members.

If you already have a robust training program in place, the elements in this table should be added to your curriculum.

New HIPAA Omnibus Rule Additions to Training Program

New in HIPAA Omnibus Rule	Our Policy and Procedure	Training Schedule
Business associates must directly comply with HIPAA Security, some portions of HIPAA Privacy, and Breach Notification Rule—also applies to business associate subcontractors	Update your business associate agreements	Inform workforce members on new business associate requirements and timelines. BA subcontractors also must comply with new requirements.
Marketing and fundraising	Covered entities required to seek written authorization for all subsidized treatment and health care operations communications when the covered entity receives financial remuneration from the third party whose products and services are being marketed. State rules may apply; some states are opt-out only and/or have other requirements Requires a covered entity to include a clear and conspicuous opportunity to opt out of fundraising communications and permits a covered entity to provide an individual who has opted out of receiving fundraising communications with a method to opt back in	Train marketing team on marketing, fundraising, and any opt-out requirements before sending anything to patients
Updated notice of privacy practices	All workforce members must know what is included in our NPP	Train on updated NPP
Individual rights	Right to withhold information from payer if paid out of pocket and in full Right to request accounting of disclosures including those sent from the EHR	Train on updated individual rights.
Immunization records to schools that require records	Individuals do not have to sign authorization form to submit immunization records to schools. Phone and e-mail requests okay, but document request in patient chart.	Front office likely to need additional training on this request.
E-mails through patient portals	Include in patient registration form. Ask patient to approve providing e-mail address to access patient portal. No PHI may be submitted to an e-mail address outside the secure EHR network. A patient portal must be securely networked to the EHR.	
Encrypt data at rest	Any device or server storing PHI must be encrypted. This also applies to all mobile devices.	Training, including sanctions critical for this new requirement
Genomic Information Non-discriminatory Act	Health plans cannot utilize genomic information for underwriting purposes	Train all workforce members; this question is likely to arise in many departments

Month-by-Month Suggested HIPAA Training Calendar

First Month (45 Minutes)	Second Month (20 Minutes)	Third Month (10-15 minutes)
Topic: What's New with HIPAA Omnibus Rule Resources: Chapter 1; PowerPoint; updated Notice of Privacy Practices Customize the PowerPoint file provided with this book to explain updated HIPAA Omnibus Rule requirements and those requirements that did not change. Also discuss your updated Notice of Privacy Practices and when to present to patients.	Topic: Security Risk Management Resources: Chapter 4 Leveraging findings from your security risk assessment, explain the risks identified and focus on how your practice, in general, focuses on security measures. If possible, assign risk managers to be department resources, available to manage higher-frequency and/or costlier risks.	Topic: Access and Audit Controls, Minimum Necessary Resources: Chapters 3, 4 Explain to all workforce members access requirements and how an EHR system tracks activities through access controls (user ID/password), and how audit controls help track who has accessed the system and what that user did while on the system. Provide guidance on the importance of data integrity and confidentiality in the event of a breach or complaint.
Fourth Month (10 minutes)	**Fifth Month** (10 minutes)	**Sixth Month** (15 minutes)
Topic: Managing Patient Complaints Resources: Chapter 3; OCR Web site for filing patient complaints; How OCR Enforces the HIPAA Privacy Rule (see Appendix B) Workforce members should know your internal process for managing patients who believe the privacy of their PHI has been compromised. Talking points and training will help mitigate complaints.	Topic: Encryption Resources: Chapter 4; OCR guidance* HIPAA Omnibus Rule provides additional rules for when PHI must be encrypted; for example, on devices where data is stored. Overlap your encryption policies with impacts of breach notification.	Topic: Workplace Devices Resources: Chapters 3, 4; CyberSecure games available at www.healthIT.gov** Resources: Chapters 3, 4 Mobile devices present a new risk that must be managed. Also present your policies on workstation use, automatic log-offs, how workstations are accessed by business associates, workforce members or volunteers, offline access, and tracking the placement of workplace stations.
Seventh Month (10 minutes)	**Eighth Month** (10–15 minutes)	**Ninth Month** (15 minutes)
Topic: HIPAA, Friends and Family Resources: Chapters 3, 4; Friends and Family Guidance (see Appendix A) Present policies and procedures on how to discuss PHI in the presence of a friend or family; also policies on authorizations for when friends or family members can be granted PHI to the benefit of the patient, and under what circumstances PHI cannot be disclosed.	Topic: Disaster Recovery Resource: Chapter 4; your contingency plan Provide instruction on how the practice would recover from an emergency or disaster. Your plan should be documented and stored with important papers (scanned documents). Introduce workforce members to your emergency decision tree, call plan, and resources management in the event of a disaster.	Topic: Managing Business Associates Resource: Chapters 3, 4 Many practices now require business associates, vendors, and sales representatives to sign a log and also be escorted through the physical location. If this is your policy, provide instruction on who this applies to and how it will be enforced.

Continued

Month-by-Month Suggested HIPAA Training Calendar (continued)

Tenth Month (10-15 Minutes)	**Eleventh Month** (10 Minutes)	**Twelfth Month** (30 Minutes)
Topic: Patient Engagement and Patient Portals Resources: Chapters 3, 4, 5 If you are on a meaningful use Stage 1, 2, or 3 track, you are familiar with providing patients with clinical summaries, patient portals, and HHS's plan to get patients engaged in managing their health. This presents new workflow processes, bringing together business associates (patient portal or personal health record companies, your EHR), and PHI to ensure patients have information needed to participate in clinical decisions and care management.	Topic: Disclosures to Law Enforcement, Public Health Officials, HHS Resources: Chapters 3, 5 Ensure all members of the workforce know how to respond to requests from law enforcement, public health, attorneys, or HHS from state, local and federal agencies. Consider talking points presented in Chapters 3 and 5.	Topic: Year-end Evaluation Resources: Chapters 1, 3, 4 As your practice expands or purchases new hardware, adds new physicians or plans a merger, your practice also will identify new risks. Evaluate those new risks and build policies and processes to manage those expanded risks. Train workforce members on expanded risks and how you plan to manage them.

* Guidance to render unsecured protected health information unreadable or indecipherable to unauthorized individuals: http://www.hhs.gov/ocr/privacy/hipaa/administrative/breachnotificationrule/brguidance.html.

** Privacy and security training games: www.healthit.gov/providers-professionals/privacy-security-training-games.

How OCR Enforces the HIPAA Privacy Rule*

The Office for Civil Rights (OCR) is responsible for enforcing the HIPAA Privacy and Security Rules (45 C.F.R. Parts 160 and 164, Subparts A, C, and E). One of the ways that OCR carries out this responsibility is to investigate complaints filed with it. OCR may also conduct compliance reviews to determine if covered entities are in compliance, and OCR performs education and outreach to foster compliance with requirements of the Privacy and Security Rules.

OCR may only take action on certain complaints. See "What OCR Considers During Intake and Review of a Complaint" below for a description of the types of cases in which OCR cannot take an enforcement action.

If OCR accepts a complaint for investigation, OCR will notify the person who filed the complaint and the covered entity named in it. Then the complainant and the covered entity are asked to present information about the incident or problem described in the complaint. OCR may request specific information from each to get an understanding of the facts. Covered entities are required by law to cooperate with complaint investigations.

If a complaint describes an action that could be a violation of the criminal provision of HIPAA (42 U.S.C. 1320d-6), OCR may refer the complaint to the Department of Justice for investigation.

OCR reviews the information, or evidence, that it gathers in each case. In some cases, it may determine that the covered entity did not violate the requirements of the Privacy or Security Rule. If the evidence indicates that the covered entity was not in compliance, OCR will attempt to resolve the case with the covered entity by obtaining:

- Voluntary compliance;
- Corrective action; and/or
- Resolution agreement.

Most Privacy and Security Rule investigations are concluded to the satisfaction of OCR through these types of resolutions. OCR notifies the person who filed the complaint and the covered entity in writing of the resolution result.

If the covered entity does not take action to resolve the matter in a way that is satisfactory, OCR may decide to impose civil money penalties (CMPs) on the covered entity. If CMPs are imposed, the covered entity may request a hearing in which an HHS administrative law judge decides if the penalties are supported by the evidence in the case. Complainants do not receive a portion of CMPs collected from covered entities; the penalties are deposited in the US Treasury.

* Excerpted from the Office for Civil Rights Web site: www.hhs.gov/ocr/privacy/hipaa/enforcement/process/howocrenforces.html.

What OCR Considers During Intake and Review of a Privacy Complaint*

The Office for Civil Rights (OCR) is the agency within the US Department of Health and Human Services that investigates complaints about failures to protect the privacy of health information. It does so under its authority to enforce the Privacy and Security Rules.

OCR carefully reviews all complaints that it receives. Under the law, OCR only may take action on complaints that meet the following conditions:

- The alleged action must have taken place after the dates the Rules took effect. Compliance with the Privacy Rule was not required until April 14, 2003. Compliance with the Security Rule was not required until April 20, 2005. Therefore, OCR cannot investigate complaints about actions that took place before these dates.
- The complaint must be filed against an entity that is required by law to comply with the Privacy and Security Rules. Not all organizations are covered by the Privacy and Security Rules. Entities subject to the Privacy and Security Rules are considered "covered entities." Briefly, a covered entity is:
  - A health plan, including but not limited to health insurance companies, company health plans; or
  - A health care provider that electronically transmits any health information in connection with certain financial and administrative transactions (such as electronically billing insurance carriers for services), including but not limited to:
    - Doctors
    - Clinics
    - Hospitals
    - Psychologists
    - Chiropractors
    - Nursing homes
    - Pharmacies
    - Dentists
    - Health care clearinghouses

* Excerpted from the Office for Civil Rights Web site: www.hhs.gov/ocr/privacy/hipaa/enforcement/process/whatocrconsiders.html.

- Examples of organizations that are not required to comply with the Privacy and Security Rules include:
  - ☐ Life insurers
  - ☐ Employers
  - ☐ Workers compensation carriers
  - ☐ Many schools and school districts
  - ☐ Many state agencies like child protective service agencies
  - ☐ Many law enforcement agencies
  - ☐ Many municipal offices
- A complaint must allege an activity that, if proven true, would violate the Privacy or Security Rule. For example, OCR generally could not investigate a complaint that alleged that a physician sent a person's demographic information to an insurance company to obtain payment, because the Privacy Rule generally permits doctors to use and disclose such information to bill for their services.
- Complaints must be filed within 180 days of when the person submitting the complaint knew or should have known about the alleged violation of the Privacy or Security Rule. OCR may waive this time limit if it determines that the person submitting the complaint shows good cause for not submitting the complaint within the 180 day time frame (eg, such as circumstances that made submitting the complaint within 180 days impossible).

appendix C

Because resources and guidance are continually posted and updated, the authors have compiled a list of resources that they regularly check for guidance on topics, such as

- Encryption
- De-identification standards workshop
- Consumer education on HIPAA Privacy
- Enforcement activities
- Breach management and reasons for breaches

Please reference these additional sites discussed throughout *HIPAA Plain & Simple,* third edition.

Topic	Description	Link to Content
Guidance Material for Consumers	Available in multiple languages, these materials provide guidance to consumers on patient rights	http://www.hhs.gov/ocr/privacy/hipaa/understanding/consumers/index.html
Guidance Materials for Covered Entities	Provides a summary of the Privacy Rule, Guidance on Significant Aspects of the Privacy Rule, and Summary of the Security Rule	http://www.hhs.gov/ocr/privacy/hipaa/understanding/cover edentities/index.html
Peer-to-Peer (P2P) Security Issues	Designed for businesses that collect and store sensitive information	http://business.ftc.gov/documents/bus46-peer-peer-file-sharing-guide-business
De-identification	Workshop on HIPAA Privacy Rule's De-identification Standard	http://www.hhs.gov/ocr/privacy/hipaa/understanding/cover edentities/De-identification/deidentificationworkshop2010.html
Enforcement Activities and Results	Learn how OCR enforces HIPAA and about corrective action plans obtained by OCR from covered entities	http://www.hhs.gov/ocr/privacy/hipaa/enforcement/index.html
Enforcement Data	Enforcements by state and annual number of cases resolved	http://www.hhs.gov/ocr/privacy/hipaa/enforcement/data/index.html
Breach Notification Rule	Breach Notification details, including how to submit a breach to the HHS secretary	http://www.hhs.gov/ocr/privacy/hipaa/administrative/breach notificationrule/index.html
List of Breaches	As required by the HITECH Act, these breaches must be posted if a breach affects 500 or more individuals	http://www.hhs.gov/ocr/privacy/hipaa/administrative/breach notificationrule/breachtool.html
What Is Encryption?	Encryption quiz to test your knowledge	http://myappsecurity.com/encryption-quiz/

Continued

Topic	Description	Link to Content
Guidance for Selecting Encryption	Provides guidance that secures PHI, rendering it unreadable, unusable or indecipherable	http://www.hhs.gov/ocr/privacy/hipaa/administrative/breachnotificationrule/brguidance.html
Encryption Details	Guidance for this addressable standard	http://www.hhs.gov/ocr/privacy/hipaa/faq/securityrule/2001.html
Genetic Information Nondescrimination Act (GINA)	HIPAA Omnibus Rule includes genetic information as protected health information, prohibiting health plans from using or disclosing genetic information for underwriting purposes	http://www.hhs.gov/ocr/privacy/hipaa/understanding/special/genetic/
Business Associates Preparedness	Presentation by David Holtzman, OCR, "HITECH & The Cloud: Control and Accessibility of Data Downstream"	http://csrc.nist.gov/news_events/hipaa-2013/presentations/day1/holtzman_david_koenig_james_lesueur_ted_day1_115_cloud_computing_vendor_assurance.pdf

glossary

Except as otherwise provided, the following definitions apply to subpart sections as noted:*

Access means the ability or the means necessary to read, write, modify, or communicate data/information or otherwise use any system resource. (This definition applies to "access" as used in this subpart, not as used in subparts D or E of this part.) **§164.304**

Act means the Social Security Act. **§160.103**

Addressable refers to the determination a covered entity makes regarding "whether each implementation specification is a reasonable and appropriate safeguard in its environment, when analyzed with reference to the likely contribution to protecting the entity's or business associate's electronic protected health information." 68 Federal Register 8377.

Administrative safeguards are administrative actions, and policies and procedures, to manage the selection, development, implementation, and maintenance of security measures to protect electronic protected health information and to manage the conduct of the covered entity's or business associate's workforce in relation to the protection of that information. **§164.304**

Administrative simplification provision means any requirement or prohibition established by:

(1) 42 U.S.C. 1320d—1320d–4, 1320d–7, 1320d–8, and 1320d-9

(2) Section 264 of Public Law 104–191

(3) Sections 13400-13424 of Public Law 111-5

(4) This subchapter. **§160.103**

---

* The HIPAA Administrative Simplification definitions in this section are from the *Electronic Code of Federal Regulations* (eCFR), which is available at http://www.ecfr.gov, and from the Department of Health and Human Services, Office of the Secretary, 45 CFR Parts 160 and 164: Modifications to the HIPAA Privacy, Security, Enforcement, and Breach Notification Rules Under the Health Information Technology for Economic and Clinical Health Act and the Genetic Information Nondiscrimination Act; Other Modifications to the HIPAA Rules: Final Rule, *Federal Register*, v.78, n.17, January 25, 2013, pp. 5566-5702. The Final Rule is effective March 26, 2013, and covered entities and business associates must comply by September 23, 2013.

They are also from Title 45 (Public Welfare), Subtitle A (Department of Health and Human Services), Subchapter C (Administrative Data Standards and Related Requirements), Parts 160 (General Administrative Requirements), 162 (Administrative Requirements), and 164 (Security and Privacy). At the end of each definition, in bold, is the location designator of the part and subpart section where the definition is located. For example, the definition, *Administrative safeguards*, is located in **§164.304.**

ALJ means Administrative Law Judge. **§160.103**

ANSI stands for the American National Standards Institute. **§160.103**

Authentication means the corroboration that a person is the one claimed. **§164.304**

Availability means the property that data or information is accessible and useable upon demand by an authorized person. **§164.304**

Board means the members of the HHS Departmental Appeals Board, in the Office of the Secretary, who issue decisions in panels of three. **§160.502**

Breach means the acquisition, access, use, or disclosure of protected health information in a manner not permitted under subpart E of this part which compromises the security or privacy of the protected health information.

(1) Breach excludes:

(i) Any unintentional acquisition, access, or use of protected health information by a workforce member or person acting under the authority of a covered entity or a business associate, if such acquisition, access, or use was made in good faith and within the scope of authority and does not result in further use or disclosure in a manner not permitted under subpart E of this part.

(ii) Any inadvertent disclosure by a person who is authorized to access protected health information at a covered entity or business associate to another person authorized to access protected health information at the same covered entity or business associate, or organized health care arrangement in which the covered entity participates, and the information received as a result of such disclosure is not further used or disclosed in a manner not permitted under subpart E of this part.

(iii) A disclosure of protected health information where a covered entity or business associate has a good faith belief that an unauthorized person to whom the disclosure was made would not reasonably have been able to retain such information.

(2) Except as provided in paragraph (1) of this definition, an acquisition, access, use, or disclosure of protected health information in a manner not permitted under subpart E is presumed to be a breach unless the covered entity or business associate, as applicable, demonstrates that there is a low probability that the protected health information has been compromised based on a risk assessment of at least the following factors: **§164.402**

(i) The nature and extent of the protected health information involved, including the types of identifiers and the likelihood of re-identification;

(ii) The unauthorized person who used the protected health information or to whom the disclosure was made;

(iii) Whether the protected health information was actually acquired or viewed; and

(iv) The extent to which the risk to the protected health information has been mitigated.

Business associate:

(1) Except as provided in paragraph (4) of this definition, business associate means, with respect to a covered entity, a person who:

(i) On behalf of such covered entity or of an organized health care arrangement (as defined in this section) in which the covered entity participates, but other than in the capacity of a member of the workforce of such covered entity or arrangement, creates, receives, maintains, or transmits protected health information for a function or activity regulated by this subchapter, including claims processing or administration, data analysis, processing or administration, utilization review, quality assurance, patient safety activities listed at 42 CFR 3.20, billing, benefit management, practice management, and repricing; or

(ii) Provides, other than in the capacity of a member of the workforce of such covered entity, legal, actuarial, accounting, consulting, data aggregation (as defined in §164.501 of this subchapter), management, administrative, accreditation, or financial services to or for such covered entity, or to or for an organized health care arrangement in which the covered entity participates, where the provision of the service involves the disclosure of protected health information from such covered entity or arrangement, or from another business associate of such covered entity or arrangement, to the person.

(2) A covered entity may be a business associate of another covered entity.

(3) *Business associate* includes:

(i) A Health Information Organization, E-prescribing Gateway, or other person that provides data transmission services with respect to protected health information to a covered entity and that requires access on a routine basis to such protected health information.

(ii) A person that offers a personal health record to one or more individuals on behalf of a covered entity.

(iii) A subcontractor that creates, receives, maintains, or transmits protected health information on behalf of the business associate.

(4) *Business associate* does not include:

(i) A health care provider, with respect to disclosures by a covered entity to the health care provider concerning the treatment of the individual.

(ii) A plan sponsor, with respect to disclosures by a group health plan (or by a health insurance issuer or HMO with respect to a group health plan) to the plan sponsor, to the extent that the requirements of §164.504(f) of this subchapter apply and are met.

(iii) A government agency, with respect to determining eligibility for, or enrollment in, a government health plan that provides public benefits and is administered by another government agency, or collecting protected health information for such purposes, to the extent such activities are authorized by law.

(iv) A covered entity participating in an organized health care arrangement that performs a function or activity as described by paragraph (1)(i) of this definition for or on behalf of such organized health care arrangement, or that provides a service as described in paragraph (1)(ii) of this definition to or for such organized health care arrangement by virtue of such activities or services.

Contrary, when used to compare a provision of State law to a standard, requirement, or implementation specification adopted under this subchapter, means:

(1) A covered entity or business associate would find it impossible to comply with both the State and Federal requirements; or

(2) The provision of State law stands as an obstacle to the accomplishment and execution of the full purposes and objectives of part C of title XI of the Act, section 264 of Public Law 104–191, or sections 13400–13424 of Public Law 111–5, as applicable. **§160.103**

Civil money penalty or **penalty** means the amount determined under §160.404 of this part and includes the plural of these terms. **§160.103**

CMS stands for Centers for Medicare & Medicaid Services within the Department of Health and Human Services. **§160.103**

Code set means any set of codes used to encode data elements, such as tables of terms, medical concepts, medical diagnostic codes, or medical procedure codes. A code set includes the codes and the descriptors of the codes. **§162.103**

Code set maintaining organization means an organization that creates and maintains the code sets adopted by the Secretary for use in the transactions for which standards are adopted in this part. **§162.103**

Common control exists if an entity has the power, directly or indirectly, significantly to influence or direct the actions or policies of another entity. **§164.103**

Common ownership exists if an entity or entities possess an ownership or equity interest of 5 percent or more in another entity. **§164.103**

Compliance date means the date by which a covered entity or business associate must comply with a standard, implementation specification, requirement, or modification adopted under this subchapter. **§160.103**

Confidentiality means the property that data or information is not made available or disclosed to unauthorized persons or processes. **§164.304**

Contrary, when used to compare a provision of state law to a standard, requirement, or implementation specification adopted under this subchapter, means:

(1) A covered entity or business associate would find it impossible to comply with both the state and federal requirements; or

(2) The provision of state law stands as an obstacle to the accomplishment and execution of the full purposes and objectives of part C of title XI of the Act, section 264 of Public Law 104–191, or sections 13400-13424 of Public Law 111–5, as applicable. **§160.202**

Controlling health plan (CHP) means a health plan that—

(1) Controls its own business activities, actions, or policies; or (2)(i) is controlled by an entity that is not a health plan; and (ii) if it has a subhealth plan(s) (as defined in this section), exercises sufficient control over the subhealth plan(s) to direct its/their business activities, actions, or policies. **§162.103**

Correctional institution means any penal or correctional facility, jail, reformatory, detention center, work farm, halfway house, or residential community program center operated by, or under contract to, the United States, a state, a territory, a political subdivision of a state or territory, or an Indian tribe, for the confinement or rehabilitation of persons charged with or convicted of a criminal offense or other persons held in lawful custody. *Other persons* held in lawful custody includes juvenile offenders adjudicated delinquent, aliens detained awaiting deportation, persons committed to mental institutions through the criminal justice system, witnesses, or others awaiting charges or trial. **§164.501**

Covered entity means:

(1) A health plan.

(2) A health care clearinghouse.

(3) A health care provider who transmits any health information in electronic form in connection with a transaction covered by this subchapter. **§160.103**

Covered functions means those functions of a covered entity the performance of which makes the entity a health plan, health care provider, or health care clearinghouse. **§164.103**

Covered health care provider means a health care provider that meets the definition at paragraph (3) of the definition of "covered entity" at §160.103. **§162.103**

Data aggregation means, with respect to protected health information created or received by a business associate in its capacity as the business associate of a covered entity, the combining of such protected health information by the business associate with the protected health information received by the business associate in its capacity as a business associate of another covered entity, to permit data analyses that relate to the health care operations of the respective covered entities. **§164.501**

Data condition means the rule that describes the circumstances under which a covered entity must use a particular data element or segment. **§162.103**

Data content means all the data elements and code sets inherent to a transaction, and not related to the format of the transaction. Data elements that are related to the format are not data content. **§162.103**

Data element means the smallest named unit of information in a transaction. **§162.103**

Data set means a semantically meaningful unit of information exchanged between two parties to a transaction. **§162.103**

Descriptor means the text defining a code. **§162.103**

Designated record set means:

(1) A group of records maintained by or for a covered entity that is:

  (i) The medical records and billing records about individuals maintained by or for a covered health care provider;

  (ii) The enrollment, payment, claims adjudication, and case or medical management record systems maintained by or for a health plan; or

  (iii) Used, in whole or in part, by or for the covered entity to make decisions about individuals.

(2) For purposes of this paragraph, the term *record* means any item, collection, or grouping of information that includes protected health information and is maintained, collected, used, or disseminated by or for a covered entity. **§164.501**

Designated standard maintenance organization (DSMO) means an organization designated by the Secretary under §162.910(a). **§162.103**

Direct treatment relationship means a treatment relationship between an individual and a health care provider that is not an indirect treatment relationship. **§164.501**

Direct data entry means the direct entry of data (for example, using dumb terminals or Web browsers) that is immediately transmitted into a health plan's computer. **§162.103**

Disclosure means the release, transfer, provision of access to, or divulging in any manner of information outside the entity holding the information. **§160.103**

EIN stands for the employer identification number assigned by the Internal Revenue Service, U.S. Department of the Treasury. The EIN is the taxpayer identifying number of an individual or other entity (whether or not an employer) assigned under one of the following:

(1) 26 U.S.C. 6011(b), which is the portion of the Internal Revenue Code dealing with identifying the taxpayer in tax returns and statements, or corresponding provisions of prior law.

(2) 26 U.S.C. 6109, which is the portion of the Internal Revenue Code dealing with identifying numbers in tax returns, statements, and other required documents. **§160.103**

Electronic media means:

(1) Electronic storage material on which data is or may be recorded electronically, including, for example, devices in computers (hard drives) and any removable/transportable digital memory medium, such as magnetic tape or disk, optical disk, or digital memory card;

(2) Transmission media used to exchange information already in electronic storage media. Transmission media include, for example, the Internet, extranet or intranet, leased lines, dial-up lines, private networks, and the physical movement of removable/transportable electronic storage media. Certain transmissions, including of paper, via facsimile, and of voice, via telephone, are not considered to be transmissions via electronic media if the information being exchanged did not exist in electronic form immediately before the transmission. **§160.103**

Electronic protected health information means information that comes within paragraphs (1)(i) or (1)(ii) of the definition of *protected health information* as specified in this section. **§160.103**

Employer is defined as it is in 26 U.S.C. 3401(d). **§160.103**

Encryption means the use of an algorithmic process to transform data into a form in which there is a low probability of assigning meaning without use of a confidential process or key. **§164.304**

Facility means the physical premises and the interior and exterior of a building(s). **§164.304**

Family member means, with respect to an individual:

(1) A dependent (as such term is defined in 45 CFR 144.103), of the individual; or

(2) Any other person who is a first- degree, second-degree, third-degree, or fourth-degree relative of the individual or of a dependent of the individual. Relatives by affinity (such as by marriage or adoption) are treated the same as relatives by consanguinity (that is, relatives who share a common biological ancestor). In determining the degree of the relationship, relatives by less than full consanguinity (such as half-siblings, who share only one parent) are treated the same as relatives by full consanguinity (such as siblings who share both parents).

   (i) First-degree relatives include parents, spouses, siblings, and children.

   (ii) Second-degree relatives include grandparents, grandchildren, aunts, uncles, nephews, and nieces.

(iii) Third-degree relatives include great-grandparents, great-grandchildren, great aunts, great uncles, and first cousins.

(iv) Fourth-degree relatives include great-great grandparents, great-great grandchildren, and children of first cousins. **§160.103**

Format refers to those data elements that provide or control the enveloping or hierarchical structure, or assist in identifying data content of, a transaction. **§162.103**

Genetic information means:

(1) Subject to paragraphs (2) and (3) of this definition, with respect to an individual, information about:

(i) The individual's genetic tests;

(ii) The genetic tests of family members of the individual;

(iii) The manifestation of a disease or disorder in family members of such individual; or

(iv) Any request for, or receipt of, genetic services, or participation in clinical research which includes genetic services, by the individual or any family member of the individual.

(2) Any reference in this subchapter to genetic information concerning an individual or family member of an individual shall include the genetic information of:

(i) A fetus carried by the individual or family member who is a pregnant woman; and

(ii) Any embryo legally held by an individual or family member utilizing an assisted reproductive technology.

(3) Genetic information excludes information about the sex or age of any individual. **§160.103**

Genetic services means:

(1) A genetic test;

(2) Genetic counseling (including obtaining, interpreting, or assessing genetic information); or

(3) Genetic education. **§160.103**

Genetic tests the analysis detects genotypes, mutations, or chromosomal changes. Genetic test does not include an analysis of proteins or metabolites that is directly related to a manifested disease, disorder, or pathological condition. **§160.103**

Group health plan (also see definition of *health plan* in this section) means an employee welfare benefit plan (as defined in section 3(1) of the Employee Retirement Income and Security Act of 1974 (ERISA), 29 U.S.C. 1002(1)), including insured and self-insured plans, to the extent that the plan provides medical care (as defined in section 2791(a)(2) of the Public Health Service Act (PHS Act), 42 U.S.C. 300gg–91(a)(2)), including items and services paid for as medical care, to employees or their dependents directly or through insurance, reimbursement, or otherwise, that:

(1) Has 50 or more participants (as defined in section 3(7) of ERISA, 29 U.S.C. 1002(7)); or

(2) Is administered by an entity other than the employer that established and maintains the plan. **§160.103**

Guidance refers to opinions and explanations offered by a Federal Agency that has oversight over a federal rule. Guidance is issued after the publication of a final rule that generates questions that require an explanation. Guidance material for privacy and security can be found at http://www.hhs.gov/ocr/privacy/hipaa/understanding/coveredentities/index.html.

HCPCS stands for the Health [Care Financing Administration] Common Procedure Coding System. **§162.103**

HHS stands for the Department of Health and Human Services. **§160.103**

Health care means care, services, or supplies related to the health of an individual. *Health care* includes, but is not limited to, the following:

(1) Preventive, diagnostic, therapeutic, rehabilitative, maintenance, or palliative care, and counseling, service, assessment, or procedure with respect to the physical or mental condition, or functional status, of an individual or that affects the structure or function of the body; and

(2) Sale or dispensing of a drug, device, equipment, or other item in accordance with a prescription. **§160.103**

Health care clearinghouse means a public or private entity, including a billing service, repricing company, community health management information system or community health information system, and "value-added" networks and switches, that does either of the following functions:

(1) Processes or facilitates the processing of health information received from another entity in a nonstandard format or containing nonstandard data content into standard data elements or a standard transaction.

(2) Receives a standard transaction from another entity and processes or facilitates the processing of health information into nonstandard format or nonstandard data content for the receiving entity. **§160.103**

Health care component means a component or combination of components of a hybrid entity designated by the hybrid entity in accordance with §164.105(a)(2)(iii)(C). **§164.103**

Health care operations means any of the following activities of the covered entity to the extent that the activities are related to covered functions:

(1) Conducting quality assessment and improvement activities, including outcomes evaluation and development of clinical guidelines, provided that the obtaining of generalizable knowledge is not the primary purpose of any studies resulting from such activities; patient safety activities (as defined in 42 CFR 3.20); population-based activities relating to improving health or reducing health care costs, protocol development, case management and

care coordination, contacting of health care providers and patients with information about treatment alternatives; and related functions that do not include treatment;

(2) Reviewing the competence or qualifications of health care professionals, evaluating practitioner and provider performance, health plan performance, conducting training programs in which students, trainees, or practitioners in areas of health care learn under supervision to practice or improve their skills as health care providers, training of non-health care professionals, accreditation, certification, licensing, or credentialing activities;

(3) Except as prohibited under §164.502(a)(5)(i),underwriting, premium rating, and other activities relating to the creation, renewal, or replacement of a contract of health insurance or health benefits, and ceding, securing, or placing a contract for reinsurance of risk relating to claims for health care (including stop-loss insurance and excess of loss insurance), provided that the requirements of §164.514(g) are met, if applicable;

(4) Conducting or arranging for medical review, legal services, and auditing functions, including fraud and abuse detection and compliance programs;

(5) Business planning and development, such as conducting cost-management and planning-related analyses related to managing and operating the entity, including formulary development and administration, development or improvement of methods of payment or coverage policies; and

(6) Business management and general administrative activities of the entity, including, but not limited to:

(i) Management activities relating to implementation of and compliance with the requirements of this subchapter;

(ii) Customer service, including the provision of data analyses for policy holders, plan sponsors, or other customers, provided that protected health information is not disclosed to such policy holder, plan sponsor, or customer.

(iii) Resolution of internal grievances;

(iv) The sale, transfer, merger, or consolidation of all or part of the covered entity with another covered entity, or an entity that following such activity will become a covered entity and due diligence related to such activity; and

(v) Consistent with the applicable requirements of §164.514, creating de-identified health information or a limited data set, and fundraising for the benefit of the covered entity. **§164.501**

Health care provider means a provider of services (as defined in section 1861(u) of the Act, 42 U.S.C. 1395x(u)), a provider of medical or health services (as defined in section 1861(s) of the Act, 42 U.S.C. 1395x(s)), and any other person or organization who furnishes, bills, or is paid for health care in the normal course of business. **§160.103**

Health information means any information, including genetic information, whether oral or recorded in any form or medium, that:

(1) Is created or received by a health care provider, health plan, public health authority, employer, life insurer, school or university, or health care clearinghouse; and

(2) Relates to the past, present, or future physical or mental health or condition of an individual; the provision of health care to an individual; or the past, present, or future payment for the provision of health care to an individual. **§160.103**

Health insurance issuer (as defined in section 2791(b)(2) of the PHS Act, 42 U.S.C. 300gg–91(b)(2) and used in the definition of *health plan* in this section) means an insurance company, insurance service, or insurance organization (including an HMO) that is licensed to engage in the business of insurance in a state and is subject to state law that regulates insurance. Such term does not include a group health plan. **§160.103**

Health maintenance organization (HMO) (as defined in section 2791(b)(3) of the PHS Act, 42 U.S.C. 300gg–91(b)(3) and used in the definition of *health plan* in this section) means a federally qualified HMO, an organization recognized as an HMO under state law, or a similar organization regulated for solvency under state law in the same manner and to the same extent as such an HMO. **§160.103**

Health oversight agency means an agency or authority of the United States, a state, a territory, a political subdivision of a state or territory, or an Indian tribe, or a person or entity acting under a grant of authority from or contract with such public agency, including the employees or agents of such public agency or its contractors or persons or entities to whom it has granted authority, that is authorized by law to oversee the health care system (whether public or private) or government programs in which health information is necessary to determine eligibility or compliance, or to enforce civil rights laws for which health information is relevant. **§164.501**

Health plan means an individual or group plan that provides, or pays the cost of, medical care (as defined in section 2791(a)(2) of the PHS Act, 42 U.S.C. 300gg–91(a)(2)).

(1) **Health plan** includes the following, singly or in combination:

(i) A group health plan, as defined in this section.

(ii) A health insurance issuer, as defined in this section.

(iii) An HMO, as defined in this section.

(iv) Part A or Part B of the Medicare program under title XVIII of the Act.

(v) The Medicaid program under title XIX of the Act, 42 U.S.C. 1396, *et seq.*

(vi) The Voluntary Prescription Drug Benefit Program under Part D of title XVIII of the Act, 42 U.S.C. 1395w–101 through 1395w–152.

(vii) An issuer of a Medicare supplemental policy (as defined in section 1882(g)(1) of the Act, 42 U.S.C. 1395ss(g)(1)).

(viii) An issuer of a long-term care policy, excluding a nursing home fixed indemnity policy.

(ix) An employee welfare benefit plan or any other arrangement that is established or maintained for the purpose of offering or providing health benefits to the employees of two or more employers.

(x) The health care program for uniformed services under title 10 of the United States Code.

(xi) The veterans' health care program under 38 U.S.C. chapter 17

(xii) The Indian Health Service program under the Indian Health Care Improvement Act, 25 U.S.C. 1601, *et seq.*

(xiii) The Federal Employees Health Benefits Program under 5 U.S.C. 8902, *et seq.*

(xiv) An approved state child health plan under title XXI of the Act, providing benefits for child health assistance that meet the requirements of section 2103 of the Act, 42 U.S.C. 1397, *et seq.*

(xv) The Medicare Advantage program under Part C of title XVIII of the Act, 42 U.S.C. 1395w–21 through 1395w–28.

(xvi) A high risk pool that is a mechanism established under state law to provide health insurance coverage or comparable coverage to eligible individuals.

(xvii) Any other individual or group plan, or combination of individual or group plans, that provides or pays for the cost of medical care (as defined in section 2791(a)(2) of the PHS Act, 42 U.S.C. 300gg–91(a)(2)).

(2) **Health plan** excludes:

(i) Any policy, plan, or program to the extent that it provides, or pays for the cost of, excepted benefits that are listed in section 2791(c)(1) of the PHS Act, 42 U.S.C. 300gg–91(c)(1); and

(ii) A government-funded program (other than one listed in paragraph (1)(i)–(xvi) of this definition):

(A) Whose principal purpose is other than providing, or paying the cost of, health care; or

(B) Whose principal activity is:

(1) The direct provision of health care to persons; or

(2) The making of grants to fund the direct provision of health care to persons. **§160.103**

Hybrid entity means a single legal entity:

(1) That is a covered entity;

(2) Whose business activities include both covered and non-covered functions; and

(3) That designates health care components in accordance with paragraph §164.105(a)(2)(iii)(C). **§164.103**

Implementation specification means specific requirements or instructions for implementing a standard. **§160.103**

Incidental Use and Disclosure refers to administrative, technical, and physical safeguards that protect against uses and disclosures not permitted by the Privacy Rule. An incidental use, for example, may be inadvertent access to multiple electronic medical charts when searching for one patient's chart in particular. Incidental uses cannot be a by-product of an underlying use or disclosure that violates reasonable Privacy Rule safeguards. **45 CFR 164.502(a)(1)(iii)**

Indirect treatment relationship means a relationship between an individual and a health care provider in which:

(1) The health care provider delivers health care to the individual based on the orders of another health care provider; and

(2) The health care provider typically provides services or products, or reports the diagnosis or results associated with the health care, directly to another health care provider, who provides the services or products or reports to the individual. **§164.501**

Individual means the person who is the subject of protected health information. **§160.103**

Individually identifiable health information is information that is a subset of health information, including demographic information collected from an individual, and:

(1) Is created or received by a health care provider, health plan, employer, or health care clearinghouse; and

(2) Relates to the past, present, or future physical or mental health or condition of an individual; the provision of health care to an individual; or the past, present, or future payment for the provision of health care to an individual; and

(i) That identifies the individual; or

(ii) With respect to which there is a reasonable basis to believe the information can be used to identify the individual. **§160.103**

Information system means an interconnected set of information resources under the same direct management control that shares common functionality. A system normally includes hardware, software, information, data, applications, communications, and people. **§164.304**

Inmate means a person incarcerated in or otherwise confined to a correctional institution. **§164.501**

Integrity means the property that data or information have not been altered or destroyed in an unauthorized manner. **§164.304**

Law enforcement official means an officer or employee of any agency or authority of the United States, a state, a territory, a political subdivision of a state or territory, or an Indian tribe, who is empowered by law to:

(1) Investigate or conduct an official inquiry into a potential violation of law; or

(2) Prosecute or otherwise conduct a criminal, civil, or administrative proceeding arising from an alleged violation of law. **§164.103 & §164.501**

Maintain or **maintenance** refers to activities necessary to support the use of a standard adopted by the Secretary, including technical corrections to an implementation specification, and enhancements or expansion of a code set. This term excludes the activities related to the adoption of a new standard or implementation specification, or modification to an adopted standard or implementation specification. **§162.103**

Malicious software means software, for example, a virus, designed to damage or disrupt a system. **§164.304**

Manifestation or manifested means, with respect to a disease, disorder, or pathological condition, that an individual has been or could reasonably be diagnosed with the disease, disorder, or pathological condition by a health care professional with appropriate training and expertise in the field of medicine involved. For purposes of this subchapter, a disease, disorder, or pathological condition is not manifested if the diagnosis is based principally on genetic information. **§160.103**

Marketing means:

(1) Except as provided in paragraph (2) of this definition, marketing means to make a communication about a product or service that encourages recipients of the communication to purchase or use the product or service.

(2) Marketing does not include a communication made:

(i) To provide refill reminders or otherwise communicate about a drug or biologic that is currently being prescribed for the individual, only if any financial remuneration received by the covered entity in exchange for making the communication is reasonably related to the covered entity's cost of making the communication.

(ii) For the following treatment and health care operations purposes, except where the covered entity receives financial remuneration in exchange for making the communication:

(A) For treatment of an individual by a health care provider, including case management or care coordination for the individual, or to direct or recommend alternative treatments, therapies, health care providers, or settings of care to the individual;

(B) To describe a health-related product or service (or payment for such product or service) that is provided by, or included in a plan of benefits of, the covered entity making the communication, including communications about: the entities participating in a health care provider network or health plan network; replacement of, or enhancements to, a health plan; and health-related products or services available only to a health plan enrollee that add value to, but are not part of, a plan of benefits; or

(C) For case management or care coordination, contacting of individuals with information about treatment alternatives, and related functions to the extent these activities do not fall within the definition of treatment.

(3) *Financial remuneration* means direct or indirect payment from or on behalf of a third party whose product or service is being described. Direct or indirect payment does not include any payment for treatment of an individual. **§164.501**

Maximum defined data set means all of the required data elements for a particular standard based on a specific implementation specification. **§162.103**

Minimum Necessary: refers to the minimum amount of information that can be accessed, used, and disclosed to complete a task. Applying the minimum necessary standard is a condition of the permissibility of many uses and disclosures of protected health information. Thus, a business associate is not making a permitted use or disclosure under the Privacy Rule if it does not apply the minimum necessary standard, where appropriate. Additionally, the HITECH Act at section 13405(b) addresses the application of minimum necessary and, in accordance with 13404(a), also applies such requirements to business associates. **§164.502(b**

Modify or **modification** refers to a change adopted by the Secretary, through regulation, to a standard or an implementation specification. **§160.103**

More stringent means, in the context of a comparison of a provision of state law and a standard, requirement, or implementation specification adopted under subpart E of part 164 of this subchapter, a state law that meets one or more of the following criteria:

(1) With respect to a use or disclosure, the law prohibits or restricts a use or disclosure in circumstances under which such use or disclosure otherwise would be permitted under this subchapter, except if the disclosure is:

  (i) Required by the Secretary in connection with determining whether a covered entity or business associate is in compliance with this subchapter; or

  (ii) To the individual who is the subject of the individually identifiable health information.

(2) With respect to the rights of an individual, who is the subject of the individually identifiable health information, regarding access to or amendment of individually identifiable health information, permits greater rights of access or amendment, as applicable.

(3) With respect to information to be provided to an individual who is the subject of the individually identifiable health information about a use, a disclosure, rights, and remedies, provides the greater amount of information.

(4) With respect to the form, substance, or the need for express legal permission from an individual, who is the subject of the individually identifiable health information, for use or disclosure of individually identifiable health information, provides requirements that narrow the scope or duration, increase the privacy protections afforded (such as by expanding the criteria for), or reduce the coercive effect of the circumstances surrounding the express legal permission, as applicable.

(5) With respect to recordkeeping or requirements relating to accounting of disclosures, provides for the retention or reporting of more detailed information or for a longer duration.

(6) With respect to any other matter, provides greater privacy protection for the individual who is the subject of the individually identifiable health information. **§160.202**

Office for Civil Rights is the Agency within the Department of Health and Human Services that oversees the HIPAA Privacy, Security, Enforcement and Breach Notification Rules under the HITECH Act and the Genetic Information Nondiscrimination Act (GINA). www.hhs.gov/ocr/privacy/index.html.

Operating rules means the necessary business rules and guidelines for the electronic exchange of information that are not defined by a standard or its implementation specifications as adopted for purposes of this part. **§162.103**

Organized health care arrangement means:

(1) A clinically integrated care setting in which individuals typically receive health care from more than one health care provider;

(2) An organized system of health care in which more than one covered entity participates and in which the participating covered entities:

  (i) Hold themselves out to the public as participating in a joint arrangement; and

  (ii) Participate in joint activities that include at least one of the following:

    (A) Utilization review, in which health care decisions by participating covered entities are reviewed by other participating covered entities or by a third party on their behalf;

    (B) Quality assessment and improvement activities, in which treatment provided by participating covered entities is assessed by other participating covered entities or by a third party on their behalf; or

    (C) Payment activities, if the financial risk for delivering health care is shared, in part or in whole, by participating covered entities through the joint arrangement and if protected health information created or received by a covered entity is reviewed by other participating covered entities or by a third party on their behalf for the purpose of administering the sharing of financial risk.

(3) A group health plan and a health insurance issuer or HMO with respect to such group health plan, but only with respect to protected health information created or received by such health insurance issuer or HMO that relates to individuals who are or who have been participants or beneficiaries in such group health plan;

(4) A group health plan and one or more other group health plans each of which are maintained by the same plan sponsor; or

(5) The group health plans described in paragraph (4) of this definition and health insurance issuers or HMOs with respect to such group health plans, but only with respect to protected health information created or received by such health insurance issuers or HMOs that relates to individuals who are or have been participants or beneficiaries in any of such group health plans. **§160.103**

Password means confidential authentication information composed of a string of characters. **§164.304**

Patient Safety Organization provides functions and activities undertaken on behalf of a covered entity to gives rise to a business associate relationship. PSOs must be treated as business associates when they receive reports of patient safety events or concerns from providers and provide analyses of events to reporting providers. **42 CFR 3.10**

Payment means:

(1) The activities undertaken by:

  (i) Except as prohibited under §164.502(a)(5)(i), a health plan to obtain premiums or to determine or fulfill its responsibility for coverage and provision of benefits under the health plan; or

  (ii) A health care provider or health plan to obtain or provide reimbursement for the provision of health care; and

(2) The activities in paragraph (1) of this definition relate to the individual to whom health care is provided and include, but are not limited to:

  (i) Determinations of eligibility or coverage (including coordination of benefits or the determination of cost sharing amounts), and adjudication or subrogation of health benefit claims;

  (ii) Risk adjusting amounts due based on enrollee health status and demographic characteristics;

  (iii) Billing, claims management, collection activities, obtaining payment under a contract for reinsurance (including stop-loss insurance and excess of loss insurance), and related health care data processing;

(iv)Review of health care services with respect to medical necessity, coverage under a health plan, appropriateness of care, or justification of charges;

(v)Utilization review activities, including precertification and preauthorization of services, concurrent and retrospective review of services; and

(vi)Disclosure to consumer reporting agencies of any of the following protected health information relating to collection of premiums or reimbursement:

(A) Name and address;

(B) Date of birth;

(C) Social Security number;

(D) Payment history;

(E) Account number; and

(F) Name and address of the health care provider and/or health plan. **§164.501**

Person means a natural person, trust or estate, partnership, corporation, professional association or corporation, or other entity, public or private. **§160.103**

Personal Representative refers to a person, guardian or entity legally authorized by the patient or the courts to participate in health care decisions on behalf of the patient. A personal representative must provide authentication documentation that says they are who they say they are; for example, a legal durable power of attorney or court order. The personal representative for a decedent is the executor, administrator, or other person who has authority under applicable law to act on behalf of the decedent or the decedent's estate. **§164.502(f)**

Physical safeguards are physical measures, policies, and procedures to protect a covered entity's or business associate's electronic information systems and related buildings and equipment, from natural and environmental hazards, and unauthorized intrusion. **§164.304**

Plan sponsor is defined as at section 3(16)(B) of ERISA, 29 U.S.C. 1002(16)(B). **§164.103**

Protected health information means individually identifiable health information:

(1) Except as provided in paragraph (2) of this definition, that is:

(i) Transmitted by electronic media;

(ii) Maintained in electronic media; or

(iii) Transmitted or maintained in any other form or medium.

(2) Protected health information excludes individually identifiable health information:

(i) In education records covered by the Family Educational Rights and Privacy Act, as amended, 20 U.S.C. 1232g;

(ii) In records described at 20 U.S.C. 1232g(a)(4)(B)(iv);

(iii) In employment records held by a covered entity in its role as employer; and

(iv) Regarding a person who has been deceased for more than 50 years. **§160.103**

Psychotherapy notes means notes recorded (in any medium) by a health care provider who is a mental health professional documenting or analyzing the contents of conversation during a private counseling session or a group, joint, or family counseling session and that are separated from the rest of the individual's medical record. *Psychotherapy notes* excludes medication prescription and monitoring, counseling session start and stop times, the modalities and frequencies of treatment furnished, results of clinical tests, and any summary of the following items: Diagnosis, functional status, the treatment plan, symptoms, prognosis, and progress to date. **§164.501**

Public health authority means an agency or authority of the United States, a state, a territory, a political subdivision of a state or territory, or an Indian tribe, or a person or entity acting under a grant of authority from or contract with such public agency, including the employees or agents of such public agency or its contractors or persons or entities to whom it has granted authority, that is responsible for public health matters as part of its official mandate. **§164.501**

Reasonable cause means an act or omission in which a covered entity or business associate knew, or by exercising reasonable diligence would have known, that the act or omission violated an administrative simplification provision, but in which the covered entity or business associate did not act with willful neglect. **§160.401**

Reasonable diligence means the business care and prudence expected from a person seeking to satisfy a legal requirement under similar circumstances. **§160.401**

Relates to the privacy of individually identifiable health information means, with respect to a state law, that the state law has the specific purpose of protecting the privacy of health information or affects the privacy of health information in a direct, clear, and substantial way. **§160.202**

Required by law means a mandate contained in law that compels an entity to make a use or disclosure of protected health information and that is enforceable in a court of law. *Required by law* includes, but is not limited to, court orders and court-ordered warrants; subpoenas or summons issued by a court, grand jury, a governmental or tribal inspector general, or an administrative body authorized to require the production of information; a civil or an authorized investigative demand; Medicare conditions of participation with respect to health care providers participating in the program; and statutes or regulations that require the production of information, including statutes or regulations that require such information if payment is sought under a government program providing public benefits. **§164.103**

Research means a systematic investigation, including research development, testing, and evaluation, designed to develop or contribute to generalizable knowledge. **§164.501**

Respondent means a covered entity or business associate upon which the Secretary has imposed, or proposes to impose, a civil money penalty. **§160.103**

Secretary means the Secretary of Health and Human Services or any other officer or employee of HHS to whom the authority involved has been delegated. **§160.103**

Security or **Security measures** encompass all of the administrative, physical, and technical safeguards in an information system. **§164.304**

Security incident means the attempted or successful unauthorized access, use, disclosure, modification, or destruction of information or interference with system operations in an information system. **§164.304**

Segment means a group of related data elements in a transaction. **§162.103**

Small health plan means a health plan with annual receipts of $5 million or less. **§160.103**

Social Networking is electronic and online-based communication between organizations, person to person, or person to groups. Social networking is often used by physician practices to announce a new physician, dates and hours of service, or other general information about the practice. As social networking activities occur in an open forum, a covered entity may not post protected health information about a specific person, but may post general medical educational information that apply to multiple audiences.

Stage 1 payment initiation means a health plan's order, instruction or authorization to its financial institution to make a health care claims payment using an electronic funds transfer (EFT) through the ACH Network. **§162.103**

Standard means a rule, condition, or requirement:

(1) Describing the following information for products, systems, services or practices:

(i) Classification of components.

(ii) Specification of materials, performance, or operations; or

(iii) Delineation of procedures; or

(2) With respect to the privacy of protected health information. **§160.103**

Standard setting organization (SSO) means an organization accredited by the American National Standards Institute that develops and maintains standards for information transactions or data elements, or any other standard that is necessary for, or will facilitate the implementation of, this part. **§160.103**

Standard transaction means a transaction that complies with an applicable standard and associated operating rules adopted under this part. **§162.103**

State refers to one of the following:

(1) For a health plan established or regulated by federal law, state has the meaning set forth in the applicable section of the United States Code for such health plan.

(2) For all other purposes, *state* means any of the several states, the District of Columbia, the Commonwealth of Puerto Rico, the Virgin Islands, and Guam, American Samoa, and the Commonwealth of the Northern Mariana Islands. **§160.103**

State law means a constitution, statute, regulation, rule, common law, or other state action having the force and effect of law. **§160.202**

Subcontractor means a person to whom a business associate delegates a function, activity, or service, other than in the capacity of a member of the workforce of such business associate. **§160.103**

Subhealth plan (SHP) means a health plan whose business activities, actions, or policies are directed by a controlling health plan. **§162.103**

Technical safeguards means the technology and the policy and procedures for its use that protect electronic protected health information and control access to it. **§164.304**

Trading partner agreement means an agreement related to the exchange of information in electronic transactions, whether the agreement is distinct or part of a larger agreement, between each party to the agreement. (For example, a trading partner agreement may specify, among other things, the duties and responsibilities of each party to the agreement in conducting a standard transaction.) **§160.103**

Transaction means the transmission of information between two parties to carry out financial or administrative activities related to health care. It includes the following types of information transmissions:

(1) Health care claims or equivalent encounter information.

(2) Health care payment and remittance advice.

(3) Coordination of benefits.

(4) Health care claim status.

(5) Enrollment and disenrollment in a health plan.

(6) Eligibility for a health plan.

(7) Health plan premium payments.

(8) Referral certification and authorization.

(9) First report of injury.

(10) Health claims attachments.

(11) Health care electronic funds transfers (EFT) and remittance advice.

(12) Other transactions that the Secretary may prescribe by regulation. **§160.103**

Treatment means the provision, coordination, or management of health care and related services by one or more health care providers, including the coordination or management of health care by a health care provider with a third party; consultation between health care providers relating to a patient; or the referral of a patient for health care from one health care provider to another. **§164.501**

Unsecured protected health information means protected health information that is not rendered unusable, unreadable, or indecipherable to unauthorized persons through the use of a technology or methodology specified by the Secretary in the guidance issued under section 13402(h)(2) of Public Law 111–5. **§164.402**

Use means, with respect to individually identifiable health information, the sharing, employment, application, utilization, examination, or analysis of such information within an entity that maintains such information. **§160.103**

User means a person or entity with authorized access. **§164.304**

Violation or **violate** means, as the context may require, failure to comply with an administrative simplification provision. **§160.103**

Willful neglect means conscious, intentional failure or reckless indifference to the obligation to comply with the administrative simplification provision violated. **§160.401**

Workforce means employees, volunteers, trainees, and other persons whose conduct, in the performance of work for a covered entity or business associate, is under the direct control of such covered entity or business associate, whether or not they are paid by the covered entity or business associate. **§160.103**

Workstation means an electronic computing device, for example, a laptop or desktop computer, or any other device that performs similar functions, and electronic media stored in its immediate environment. **§164.304**

index

Page numbers for tables and figures in this index are printed in italics.

I

R

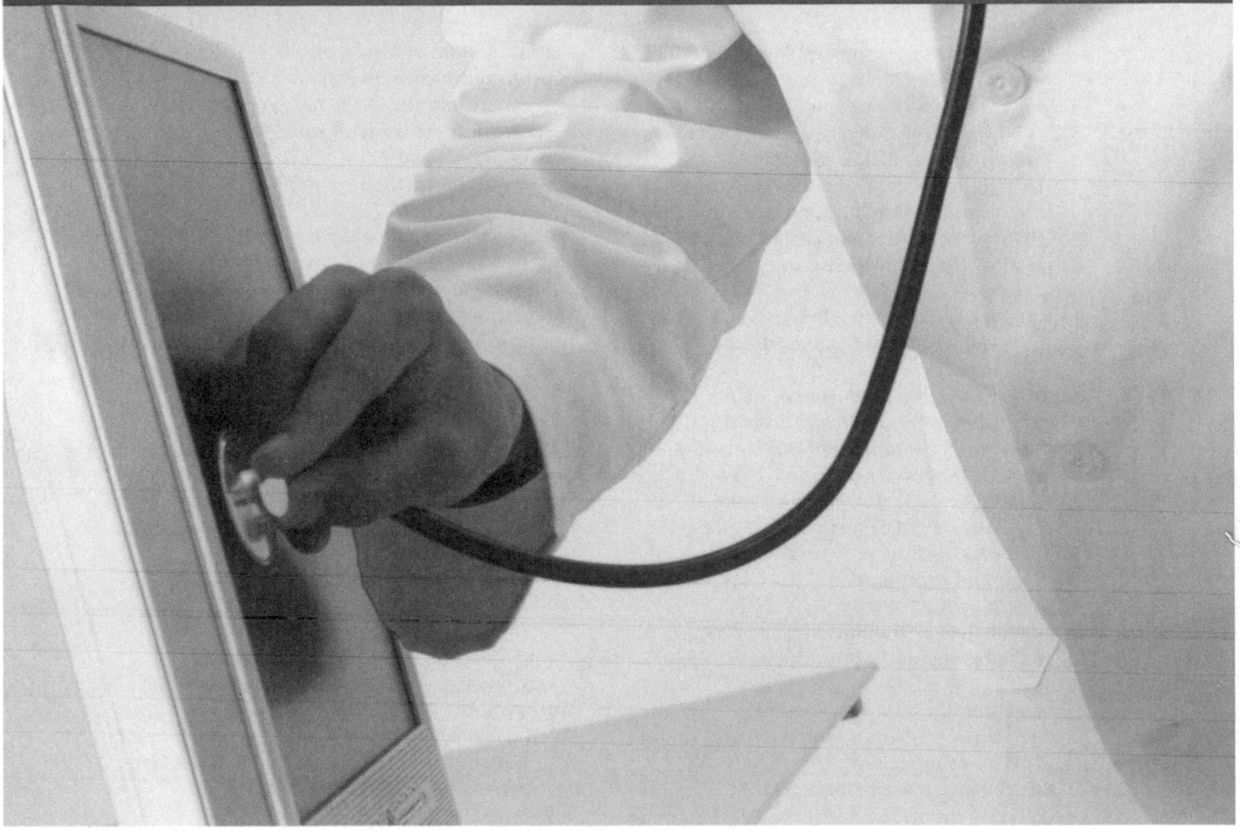

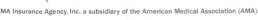

U

V

W

X

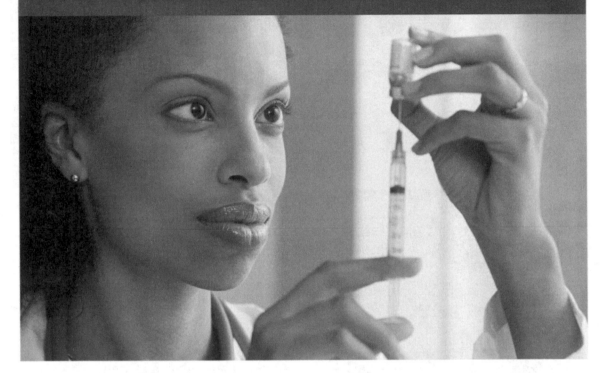

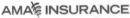